Skeletal Circulation in Clinical Practice

Skeletal Circulation in Clinical Practice

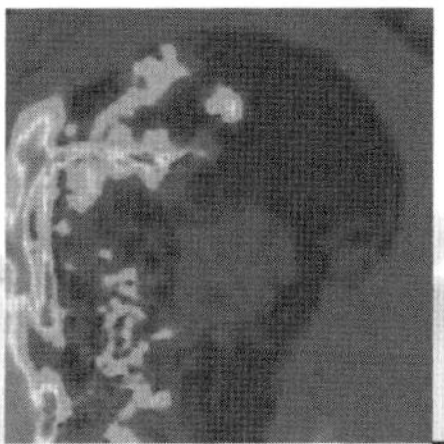

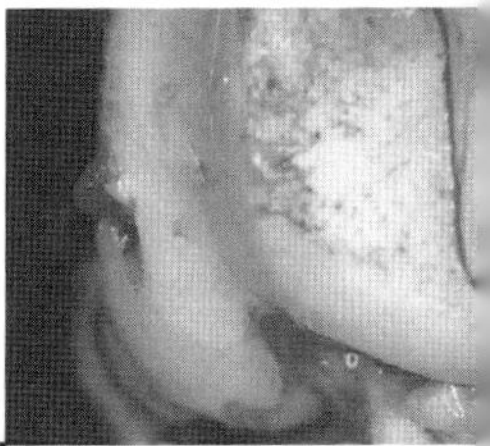

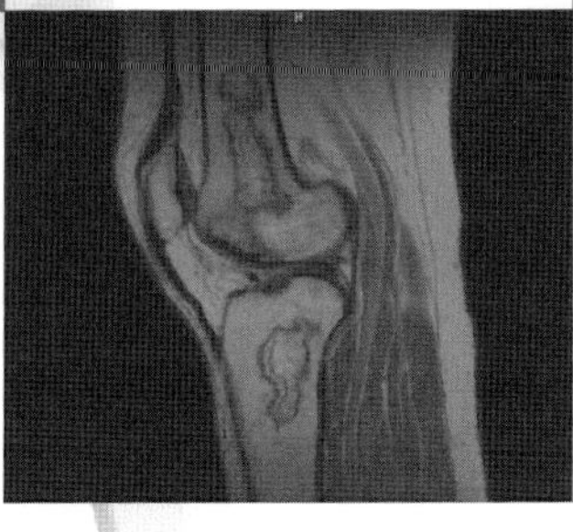

Editor

Roy K Aaron

Brown University, USA

World Scientific

EW JERSEY • LONDON • SINGAPORE • BEIJING • SHANGHAI • HONG KONG • TAIPEI • CHENNAI • TOKYO

Published by

World Scientific Publishing Co. Pte. Ltd.
5 Toh Tuck Link, Singapore 596224
USA office: 27 Warren Street, Suite 401-402, Hackensack, NJ 07601
UK office: 57 Shelton Street, Covent Garden, London WC2H 9HE

Library of Congress Cataloging-in-Publication Data
Names: Aaron, Roy K., editor.
Title: Skeletal circulation in clinical practice / editor, Roy K. Aaron.
Description: New Jersey : World Scientific, 2016. | Includes bibliographical references.
Identifiers: LCCN 2015042221 | ISBN 9789814713757 (hardcover : alk. paper)
Subjects: | MESH: Bone and Bones--blood supply. | Diagnostic Techniques, Cardiovascular. | Osteonecrosis--physiopathology. | Osteoporosis--physiopathology. | Regional Blood Flow--physiology.
Classification: LCC RC931.O8 | NLM WE 202 | DDC 616.7/1--dc23
LC record available at http://lccn.loc.gov/2015042221

British Library Cataloguing-in-Publication Data
A catalogue record for this book is available from the British Library.

Typeset by Stallion Press
Email: enquiries@stallionpress.com

Printed in Singapore

To Papa, Yudy, and everyone else who by example showed me the way.

PREFACE

Circulatory physiology, basic to all healthy organs and most diseases, has been difficult to study in the skeleton. The biological regulation of blood flow is complex and the tissues have been relatively inaccessible to measurement. In recent years, however, advances have been made in understanding circulatory physiology and fluid flow in bone, functional measurement of blood flow, and the roles of circulation in bone turnover and repair. These advances have enhanced our insights into bone homeostasis and the interrelationships of circulation and skeletal biology, including repair and osteonecrosis, osteoarthritis, and osteoporosis.

The first part of this book presents contemporary information on circulatory physiology of bone and fluid flow through bone matrix. The second part describes techniques of quantifying and imaging bone circulation with the expectation that functional imaging will yield further physiological information in the near future. The third part presents circulatory elements of diseases of the skeleton that may provide insight into pathophysiology and may serve as diagnostic biomarkers or therapeutic targets.

I have been extremely fortunate in having charismatic and influential mentors during formative stages in my education. As an undergraduate, Louis Stableford focused my nascent interest in experimental biology. In medical school, Philip Sawyer and Supramaniam Srinivasan developed my interest in vascular biology and taught me how to think scientifically about clinical problems. From my time at the National Institutes of Health (NIH), I owe a debt of gratitude to John Pisano, of the National Heart, Lung, and Blood Institute for encouraging me to apply experimental laboratory methods to clinical medicine, and to Vincent Hascall and Hari Reddi, then at the National Institute of Dental Research, for their guidance toward a musculoskeletal context.

I am indebted to these creative scientists and generous gifted teachers who understood how to lead and inspire by example. They have enabled me to interpret clinical problems in a biological context and to apply critical, translational approaches to clinical medicine. Any missteps and errors along the way have been mine alone.

Roy Kenneth Aaron
Providence, RI

ACKNOWLEDGEMENTS

Ms. Jennifer Racine has done essential and thoughtful work to bring this book to completion. The National Institute of Arthritis, Musculoskeletal, and Skin Diseases, NIH, provided the time to organize the book through a K24 award.

CONTENTS

Part 1

Physiology

CHAPTER 1

THE PHYSIOLOGY OF BONE CIRCULATION

IAN MCCARTHY

University College London Institute of Orthopaedics and Musculoskeletal Science

Royal National Orthopaedic Hospital, Brockley Hill, Stanmore, UK

INES REICHERT

Department of Orthopaedic Surgery

King's College Hospital, Denmark Hill, London, UK

1.1 Introduction

Maintenance, regular turnover, and repair of bone are critically dependent on a sufficient vascular supply and responsive hemodynamics. Bone circulation obviously acts as a conduit to provide nutrients for cell in bone, but in addition, it has an important role in mineral homeostasis, the control of bone turnover, and the response to injury. Any event such as a fracture or surgical intervention to bone poses a challenge due to disruption of the blood supply, and requires an intact vascular response for successful repair.

1.2 Organization of the Vascular System in Bone

The specific anatomical organization of the vascular system in the skeleton varies from bone to bone, and details have been described.[16,29] There are, however, common underlying principles for the vascular organization in all bones, and these are important for many of the physiological functions of the vascular system. This section, therefore, will provide an overview of the anatomic sources of blood flow to bone, and their hemodynamic interconnections.

Following historical accounts by Langer[72] and Lexer,[74] there is agreement that the blood supply of bone has three main sources of vessels supplying the cortex of long bones:[16,63] the epiphyseal-metaphyseal arteries, the nutrient artery, and the periosteum.

1.2.1 *Medullary circulation*

Bone marrow is perfused by blood vessels arising from the one or two nutrient arteries which have pierced the bone. In over 90% of the human tibiae examined by Menck *et al.* there was one nutrient foramen evident, but in a few cases there were two such foramina.[92] The nutrient vessels will not solely supply marrow, but cortical bone as well. In the diaphyseal marrow of tubular long bones, the nutrient artery divides into ascending and descending branches and, together with the medullary branches of the metaphyseal arteries, is responsible for the blood supply to the fatty and haemopoietic bone marrow.

1.2.1.1 *Parallel supply of marrow and cortex by the nutrient artery*

Lopez-Curto *et al.* used stereo light-microscopy for three-dimensional examination of the vasculature in the adult dog tibia and showed that the vasculature of the cortex and the medulla did not communicate at an arteriolar or capillary level.[80] They concluded that the nutrient artery supplied the marrow and cortex in parallel.

1.2.2 *Metaphyseal circulation*

The periosteal vascular plexus, the Hunter's vascular circle, around the metaphysis perforates the cortex in a pattern constant throughout the life of an individual. These arteries divide within the metaphyseal area and anastomose with branches of the nutrient artery.[142] Anecdotal evidence suggests that the metaphyseal arteries are capable of sufficiently supplying the diaphysis in long bones with congenitally absent nutrient foramina.[16] Following the closure of the epiphysis, intraosseous — in addition to the existing extra-osseous — anastomoses occur between the metaphyseal and epiphyseal arteries. The vascular network thus formed is referred to as the epiphysio-metaphyseal vascular system.[99,138,140]

1.2.3 *Venous system*

The arrangement of the venous system of the marrow is different from that of the arterial system. A central venous sinus with a diameter approximately four times that of the nutrient artery, but with a thinner wall, runs medullo-central the full length of the diaphysis.[16] The nutrient vein branches off the central venous sinus as well as other emissary vessels and traverses the cortex.[15,80]

1.2.4 *Periosteal circulation*

The periosteum forms a thin surrounding layer of soft tissue which envelopes bone. It is most distinct at the level of the diaphysis and particularly well established in the young organism. A fracture of the juvenile skeleton is often referred to as a "greenstick" fracture when the periosteal layer has stayed intact. The periosteum forms the interconnection of cortical bone with the musculature and connective tissue. The periosteum consists ultra-structurally of three layers of tissue: close to bone the cambium layer contains osteogenic cells, in the midzone a highly vascular layer contributes to the blood supply of the cortical bone, and in the periphery there is a dense layer of collagen bundles and fibers.[45] The periosteum is responsive to injury two-fold: its osteogenic layer forms the peripheral callus in fracture healing and its vascularity acts as reserve supply should the medullary system fail.

Menck *et al.* have given a detailed account of the anatomy of the arterial supply to the periosteum of the human tibia.[92] They dissected 30 legs after the injection of Berlin Blue Gelatine and found crucially that the distal diaphysis is supplied exclusively by semicircular branches of the anterior tibial artery. In contrast, the proximal diaphysis is supplied by periosteal branches of the anterior and posterior tibial artery. As clinically observed, it is in the distal tibia that fracture healing is often impaired.

1.2.5 *Structure and blood supply of the diaphyseal cortex*

The vasculature in cortical bone utilizes the spaces provided by the longitudinal Haversian system and the transverse Volkmann canals, although the causative relationship is probably the reverse. A description of the structure of compact bone will outline the arrangement of the angioarchitecture of bone.

Cortical bone is structured in a highly organized fashion and intracortical vessels play a central role. The osteon is a term often used interchangeably with the Haversian system and should be preferred if the structure is addressed. The osteon constitutes the basic morphological unit of most of the compact (cortical) bone, together with the circumferential and interstitial lamellae that are deposited at the periosteal and endosteal surfaces.[23] The vessels in the osteons were found to be continuous with vessels coursing in endosteal lamellae, most of which pierce the subendosteal lamellae. The network of osteons follows a spiral around the axis of the bone.

A Volkmann canal — a term for a vascular channel which is not surrounded by concentric lamellae of bone — forms a radial connecting canal passing through circumferential lamellae.[26]

1.2.5.1 *Ultrastructure of Haversian systems*

Cooper *et al.* performed electronmicroscopic studies on the Haversian system. Within each osteon they found one or two vessels with the ultrastructure of capillaries.[26] The vessels are lined by endothelial cells and often connected by a special single-layered membrane. Immediately adjacent, but not forming a complete ring, pericytes were seen. The basement membrane splits to include the pericytes.[34] Usually there were unmyelinated and sometimes myelinated nerve fibers 5–9 μm in diameter seen.[26]

Mature osteons gradually transform into resorption spaces and new osteons will be formed in such spaces. All osteons are demarcated from their neighbors by a jagged-edged cement line which may mark the limit of bone erosion prior to the formation of an osteon.[23] Similar basophilic lines also occur in the absence of erosion when bony growth is interrupted and then resumed (resting lines). Canaliculi may sometimes pass through the cement lines, thus providing a route for exchange between interstitial bone and osteons.[5] Most individual blocks of interstitial lamellae were structurally continuous with osteons, either distally or proximally, thus providing an axial pathway for diffusion of fluid through compact bone between the periosteal and endosteal surfaces.[23]

1.2.5.2 *Intracortical anastomoses*

Based on the anatomical basis of the cortical structure is the concept of a vascular connection between the different sources. Thus, a compensatory response between systems becomes possible if one system fails. There has been a considerable debate and opponents have denied intracortical anastomoses between the medullary and periosteal vascular systems.[16] However, a number of workers have described communications between the periosteal and medullary sources of cortical blood flow, as early as Drinker & Drinker.[40] Using the Spalteholz method of clearance and stereo-lightmicroscopy, Trias and Féry described the Haversian and

Volkmann canals and arrived at a network-like model of the vasculature of the canine femur.[137]

Lopez-Curto *et al.* observed transcortical periosteal-medullary arterioles, conduit vessels, which form anastomoses between branches of the nutrient artery and the periosteal vessels in the adult dog tibiae following perfusion with Microfil.[80] Skawina *et al.* support with their work using corrosion casting to investigate the human fetal long bone the existence of intracortical anastomoses.[128] Crock concurs showing illustrations of those in his atlas.[29]

The descriptive work of the vascular structure of cortical bone has been marred by methodological difficulties. Most injection studies use the nutrient artery as a route to inject the material to visualize the arterial system, thus demonstrating solely the centrifugal route of flow. Often the periosteum is removed from the illustrated specimens.

Of importance is the concept of sufficient intracortical vascular connections, anastomosing between the medullary, metaphyseal, and periosteal sources of blood flow. As suggested by Trias and Féry[137] the existence of intracortical anastomoses gives the anatomical basis for blood flow direction to change according to the prevailing physiological conditions.[139]

1.3 Distribution of Bone Blood Flow

Techniques for the measurement of blood flow to the skeleton are described in later chapters of this book. Bone poses specific problems for the measurement of blood flow: (1) there are 206 separate bones in the skeleton; (2) as discussed above, each bone has multiple arterial inputs and venous outflows; (3) each bone is heterogeneous, comprising varying proportions of cortical bone, cancellous bone, and marrow (both hematopoietic and fatty). Because of this heterogeneity of the tissue, it is important to specify precisely the region of bone that is being measured. These issues probably account for some of the variation in values of bone blood flow reported in the literature.

It is now generally accepted that approximately 5% of the cardiac output goes to the skeleton.[123] Within this overall figure, there is wide variation in absolute blood flow values between different bones[132] as well as between cortical bone, trabecular bone, bone marrow, and periosteum. Typical values of blood flow to these tissues are shown in Table 1.1. Trabecular bone has a higher rate of turnover than cortical bone, as well as containing marrow, and this is reflected in a higher blood flow in trabecular bone.

Table 1.1. Typical values of bone and periosteal blood flow.

	Blood Flow (ml/min/100g)
Cortical Bone	1
Trabecular Bone	5
Cortical Marrow	1
Periosteum	5

Source: Reichert ILH (2000).[118]

The periosteum also has significantly higher absolute blood flow than cortical bone,[118] reflecting its higher cellularity.

Although cortical bone appears relatively poorly perfused, the cellular volume in cortical bone is also low (see section 1.3.3). This has led to the suggestion that cortical bone perfusion is higher than that required to meet the metabolic needs of the tissue, and that the magnitude of bone blood flow is determined by requirements for bone to act as a buffer in mineral exchange for calcium homeostasis.[116] It is interesting to do some simple arithmetic, combining these fluid space data with blood flow data presented earlier. Although blood flow to cortical bone is relatively low in absolute terms, it is very high if expressed in terms of cellular mass of the tissue. This is also consistent with the observations of active control of mineral ion transport discussed later.

1.3.1 *Hemodynamics of flow direction in cortical bone*

Several means of examining blood flow to and in the diaphyseal cortex have been used to determine the normal blood flow direction. Brånemark used intravital microscopy to directly observe the blood flow in rabbit fibulae and found that the capillaries coming from the marrow arterioles enter the Haversian canals to supply the endosteal diaphysis only.[12] The capillaries then return to the marrow to empty into the sinusoids. Since only the endosteal diaphysis is centrifugally supplied, the remainder of the diaphyseal cortex must be supplied centripetally.

1.3.1.1 *Quantitative flow partition experiments*

Occluding a given source of blood flow by ligation or obliteration followed by blood flow measurement will give an estimate of the contribution of this source. Such experiments aiming for quantified flow partition have also indicated that blood flow is centrifugal. Kelly used the hydrogen washout technique to measure blood flow in the canine tibia and reported that 71% of nutrient artery flow supplies the cortex and 30% the marrow.[64] Cortical blood flow has been measured using the indicator fractionation technique with radio-labeled microspheres which is widely regarded as the gold standard method. Values of 2–5 ml/min/100g of blood flow have been measured in the diaphyseal cortex of canine long bone.[75] Tothill and McPherson used this technique and measured regional blood flow in cortical bone with radio-labeled microspheres pre- and post-ligation of the nutrient artery.[136] They reported that the nutrient artery contributes 70% of total diaphyseal cortical flow. Willans obtained lower figures of 62% contribution by the nutrient artery to total cortical flow in the canine tibial diaphysis.[153] Kowalski *et al.* performed a similar study measuring the contribution of the periosteum to cortical bone, in that they scraped the periosteum off the diaphysis, and found a reduction of cortical flux by 20% using laser Doppler flowmetry.[69]

1.3.2 *Intramedullary pressure*

Measurements of the intramedullary pressure (IMP) provide the most conclusive evidence for normal centrifugal flow. Fluid moves down the pressure gradient. Pressure in the marrow cavity has been measured in experimental animals and human subjects by a number of investigators and found to be higher than the surrounding soft tissues. The most meticulous measurement has been performed by Wilkes and Vischer,[152] who were able to remove the cortical bone to expose the endosteal membrane and to place the pressure transducer directly on this tissue layer. Thus they maintained the entity of the medullary cavity whilst performing the measurement. IMP is reported to be between 45 mmHg and 60 mmHg in the human.[16] The blood pressure in the nutrient artery must be correspondingly high for flow to access the medullary cavity. Tøndevold measured in dogs that arterial inflow into the medullary cavity stopped when the arterial blood pressure fell below 80 mmHg.[135] Extra-osseous capillaries in surrounding soft tissues measure a pressure in the range of 12 to 15 mmHg, which is lower than pressure in the medullary cavity.[16] Thus, the vascular driving pressure is centrifugal across the cortex from marrow to periosteum and blood flow direction is normally centrifugal.

1.3.3 *Compensatory vascular responses in cortical bone*

Based on the structural as well vascular connectivity between the vascular systems of cortical bone it is reasonable to suggest a compensatory response if that is required by the haemodynamic situation. Trueta, a surgeon as well as researcher, proposed the following suggestion, based on clinical observation: "... if one vascular system breaks down another takes over."[139]

The capacity of the cortical vasculature to respond to afferent breakdown has been studied by occluding one or two of the three afferent systems and examining the cortical viability using a variety of histological, angiographic, and quantitative methods. Clinically relevant is the investigation on cortical and periosteal blood flow following intramedullary reaming as a surgical procedure prior to intramedullary nailing, which occludes the nutrient artery and occludes the medullary system. The indicator fractionation technique has been extended to measure blood flow in the periosteum in a large animal model to establish the effect of reaming on blood flow in the tibia. The results show a six-fold increase in periosteal blood flow 30 minutes after intramedullary reaming and no change in net cortical blood flow.[117] This indicates an acute compensation for the occlusion of the medullary vascular system by the periosteum.

1.4 Bone Microcirculation

1.4.1 *Capillary ultrastructure*

Capillary structure is conventionally characterized as either continuous or fenestrated, or sinusoids. Capillaries in cortical bone are described as continuous, and microcirculatory vessels in bone marrow are commonly characterised as sinusoids.

1.4.1.1 *Capillary characterization by surface markers*

Beyond this gross classification of capillary morphology, it is now appreciated that vascular endothelial cells have tissue-specific characteristics dependent on cell surface markers. In bone, endothelial cells exhibit enhanced surface expression of the chemotractant SDF-1, and have characteristic heparin sulphate proteoglycan and adhesion molecule profiles.[59] However, not only does bone differ from other tissuesbut there is also important variation within bones. Recently, detailed characterisation of cell surface markers of capillaries has shown heterogeneity of surface markers even within the same bone. In mouse tibiae and femora, staining vessels for CD31 and endomucin (emcn) has indicated that there are two types of vessels — those staining strongly for CD31 and emcn ($CD31^{hi}Emcn^{hi}$ — type H) and those staining weakly for the same markers ($CD31^{lo}Emcn^{lo}$ — type L).[71]

Type H vessels were primarily observed near the metaphysis, and osteoprogenitor cells were selectively positioned around type H vessels, even though type H vessels only make up around 1.8% of the vessels. It was also shown that the proportion of type H vessels decreases with age, suggesting that these type H vessels may be implicated in bone changes observed in osteoporosis. The heterogeneity was not observed in most other tissues, and apart from bone, type H vessels were only found elsewhere in the liver.[71]

1.4.2 *Transcapillary exchange*

Transcapillary transport can be classified as flow-limited or diffusion-limited. In the former, transcapillary transport is very rapid, and the rate of delivery of solutes to tissue is limited by the flow to the tissue; in the latter, the rate limiting factor is transcapillary exchange rather than flow to the tissue. It has been shown that transcapillary transport is diffusion-limited, rather than flow-limited. Studies of capillary permeability in bone were developed by Patrick Kelly at the Mayo Clinic, who adapted the outflow dilution technique applied to other organs for use in bone Perfusing the tibial nutrient artery at a controlled rate, radioactive traces of a range of molecular weights and/or chemical properties would be injected as a bolus into the nutrient artery, and passage of the tracer through bone could be studied by collecting blood from the femoral vein. Such studies characterized the transcapillary exchange as being passive and diffusion-limited.[73] It was also possible to use this technique to investigate the kinetics of tracer movement beyond the capillary wall,[85] using, for example, calcium and potassium analogues to investigate extravascular transport rates.

1.4.3 *Bone fluid spaces*

Although "dry as a bone" is a common expression, bone has a significant fluid space. This fluid space is portioned between vascular, cellular, and extravascular extracellular. In mature cortical bone, the fluid space amounts to about 0.287 ml/ml bone by volume of the cortex.[97] The distribution of bone fluid between vascular, cellular, and interstitial (extravascular and extracellular) spaces is illustrated in Fig. 1.1. Vascular space comprises 6.3% of the total fluid space, and the cellular and interstitial spaces comprise 25.1% and 68.6%, respectively. These values are for mature cortical bone; fluid spaces are larger in immature bone.[108]

For a while, it was suggested that there was a discrete bone extracellular (BECF) fluid space, which was separated from the perivascular

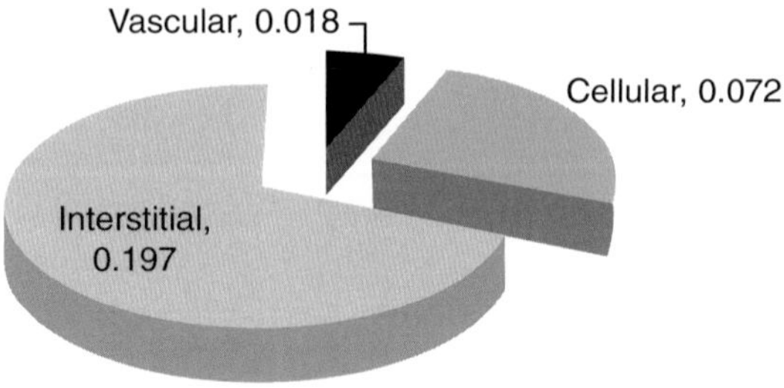

Fig. 1.1. Distribution of fluid spaces in cortical bone; values shown are in ml/ml bone.

fluid space in the Haversian canals.[17,101] It was originally proposed that there was a membrane delineating the bone fluid space, identified as a potassium-rich bone fluid space.[103] However, such a discrete potassium-rich space has not been found, and the potassium content of bone can probably be accounted for by the cellular space.[108] It is possible, though, that cells can regulate the composition of the pericellular extravascular fluid.

1.4.4 *Ion exchange in bone*

Although it has been difficult to investigate the composition of a specific BECF, other experiments indicate that an active transport system may contribute to short-term plasma calcium homeostasis without a contribution from bone remodeling. The rates of calcium exchange at the bone-plasma interface have been estimated to be about 50 to 100 mM Ca per day. This is about ten times higher than the daily flux due to bone remodeling, and three times than the daily flux in the kidney under PTH control.[115] Two experiments have aimed specifically at measuring any active component in mineral influx and efflux.[86,89] McCarthy and Hughes used the outflow dilution technique described above in the perfused tibia, and compared the effect of potassium cyanide in the perfusate on Sr^{86} (Ca analogue) and potassium (intracellular ion) outflow; Marenzana *et al.* measured real time Ca++ efflux from mouse weanling metatarsal bones, using the scanning ion-selective electrode technique (SIET).[91] Although very different in approach, both experiments showed passive influx of calcium into bone, but a small active component of efflux from bone. The exact mechanism of active control is uncertain, but the results are consistent with a pump-leak mechanism, probably under the control of an osteocyte-bone lining cell syncytium.

1.4.5 *Extravascular solute transport*

Another issue concerning extravascular transport in bone, irrespective of active control of calcium fluxes in ion exchange, is the nature of movement through the BECF, particularly for larger protein molecules.[18] Typically, an osteon within cortical bone is approximately 200 μm in diameter. This means that osteocytes within the bone matrix can be up to 100 μm from a capillary. Cortical bone has a very extensive network of channels allowing communication between plasma and bone matrix. Canaliculi, approximately 0.1 μm in diameter, radiate from the Haversian canal and form a complex network connecting osteocytes with the Haversian canal and other osteocytes. Radiating from the canaliculi are submicroscopic interfibrillar spaces of bone matrix. The extent of these networks is so great that it has been estimated that the surface area of the canalicular system is approximately 250 mm^2/mm^3, and the interfibrillar spaces represent an exchange area of the order of 35,000 mm^2/mm^3.

It has been speculated that, because distances between osteocytes and capillaries are relatively large in microvascular terms, diffusion may not be sufficient to supply these cells and that a more rapid turnover of interstitial fluid in bone aids the process of cell nutrition. The role of IMP in determining the direction of blood flow in cortical bone has been discussed above; similarly, IMP is thought to have a role in fluid movement through interstitial space. Experimental evidence suggesting that convective flow may contribute to the nutrient of osteocytes comes mainly from studies on the movement of labeled protein molecules (such as albumin, thorotrast, or ferritin) through both unloaded and loaded bone.[33,96,113] One problem with this type of experiment is to confirm that there is no movement of these tracers post-mortem during processing of the tissues; another problem is that bones are processed at specific times after injection of the tracer, providing isolated snapshots of tracer movement.

Using mathematical modeling, it was argued that mechanical loading would enhance perfusion and aid nutrition of osteocytes,[107] but Yang argued that the nutritional requirements of osteocytes were unknown, but presumably relatively low, and that mechanical load may not be required.[90] Enhancement of extravascular transport resulting from mechanical loading has been demonstrated.[134] Recently the technique of fluorescence bleaching after photobleaching (FRAP) has enabled dynamic measurement of solute movement in extravascular fluid in the murine tibia.[78,111,150] Using sodium fluorescein (376 Da) as a probe, no effect of vascular pressure on transport into bone was observed, and theoretical model for small (376 Da) and large (43,000 Da) molecules indicated that vascular pressure-driven convection was at least an order of magnitude smaller than diffusion in transport of solutes through bone interstitial fluid.[78] In contrast, mechanical loading inducing about 400–500 microstrain enhanced the transport of sodium fluorescein (+31%) and parvalbumin (+50%).[111,113,150]

In addition to contributing to solute movement through bone interstitial fluid space, mechanical loading also provides a mechano-transduction signal mediated by shear forces generated by load-induced transient fluid movement acting on osteocytes.[67] Details of the osteocyte response to load are beyond the scope of this chapter, but among factors released is vascular endothelial growth factor (VEGF), which not only stimulates blood vessel formation, but also stimulates osteoblastogenesis.[21]

1.4.6 *Fluid pressure and bone density*

Although the role of vascular intramedullary pressure on fluid movement through bone is equivocal, there are many instances in which there is an association between vascular pressure and bone density. The response of bone to load is site-specific, related to local interstitial fluid pressure.[141] In environments in which the distribution of cardiovascular pressures is changed (such as microgravity), bone density changes correlate with pressure changes, and there is apparent increase in bone density in regions with positive changes in cardiovascular pressures.[92] Rat tail suspension is an experimental approach to mimic the effects of microgravity, and bone density is decreased in the lower limb. Ligation of the femoral vein reduces the bone loss associated with tail suspension;[7] ligation also produced a significant increase in intramedullary pressure, and it was proposed that this increase in pressure resulted in enhanced interstitial fluid flow through bone, which mediated the bone response. Another experimental study ligating the popliteal artery in the caprine tibia caused intraosseous hypertension and resulted in significant increases in periosteal, endocortical, and trabecular bone formation.[151] However, theoretical studies suggested that the pressure changes were insufficient to have much effect of fluid flow, and that pressurization of the periosteum may be the causal link.[149]

Dynamic pressure application has been shown to be effective in modifying bone mass. In a rat tail suspension model, dynamic hydraulic stimulation at a frequency of 2 Hz for 20 minutes a day was able to induce peak-to-peak variations of IMP of either 10 or 15 mm Hg.[57] This intervention was found to eliminate the loss of bone volume fraction in the tibia caused by tail suspension. It was argued that the hydraulic stimulation produced direct muscle coupling, temporarily occluding vessels in bone, and generating an A-V pressure gradient driving fluid flow.[57]

There are also clinical examples of an association of vascular pressures and bone density. For example, Arnoldi *et al.* observed bone density changes in patients with intra-calcaneal hypertension.[4] It has also been shown that hypertension is associated with higher bone mineral density measurements for both women and men.[53] Atherosclerosis has been shown to be associated with reduced bone density.[100] Although these observations show an association between vascular pressures and bone density, it is not clear at the moment as to the nature of this association. An alternative explanation for this association could be that endothelin signaling could serve as a nexus for the convergence of vascular and skeletal modeling.[149]

1.5 Control of Bone Blood Flow

1.5.1 *Perivascular innervation*

Values of bone blood flow quoted above are typical values. However, as in most tissues, neural, humoral, and metabolic parameters all contribute to the regulation of blood flow and vascular resistance in bone. Bone and periosteum are innervated by both sympathetic and sensory nerves.[8,27,59,87,126] Several different staining techniques have been used to study the distribution of nerve fibers in bone. Most nerves are perivascular, and the periosteum, metaphysis, and epiphysis are more densely innervated than cortical bone. As well as noradrenergic sympathetic fibers, peptidergic nerves containing substance P (SP), calcitonin gene-related peptide (CGRP), vasoactive intestinal peptide (VIP), and neuropeptide Y have also been described.[9] Many SP- and CGRP-immunoreactive fibers were observed in association with blood vessels in both periosteum and cortical bone. During fracture repair, periosteal CGRP-containing nerve fibers are very actively proliferating elements, and it has been suggested that vascular control and stimulation of angiogenesis are major functions of CGRP during the fracture healing process.[59]

1.5.2 *Vascular reactivity*

The most precise physiological measurements of vascular reactivity of bone have been performed in experimental preparations that perfuse the nutrient supply of a long bone at a constant flow rate, and in which perfusion pressure is continuously monitored to investigate changes in vascular resistance in response to the injection of vasoactive agents into the perfusion circuit.[14,28,30,38,39,51,91] An alternative approach has been to study isolated resistance arteries from bone.[37,81]

In general, it has been shown that the vasculature in bone responds to most vasoconstrictor and vasodilator substances. However, comparing the vasoreactive responses in bone with those in other tissues, it has been proposed that bone is relatively hypersensitive to vasoconstrictors, and relatively hyposensitive to vasodilators.[14] Responsiveness to α- and β-adrenergic agonists has been observed, as well as the presence of prostaglandin H_2/thromboxane A_2 receptors. Table 1.2 summarizes some of the major observations of vascular reactivity in bone.

Qualitatively, the response in bone is, in general, similar to other vascular beds, even if quantitatively responses can be very different. The most surprising observation is the action of isoproterenol, which has a vasodilator effect in most vascular beds but cause significant constriction when injected into bone.[14]

Table 1.2. Summary of effects of vasoactive agents on bone.

Agent	Vascular resistance	References
Acetylcholine	↓	Driessens & Vanhoutte (1979)
Adenosine	↓	Gross *et al.* (1979)
Adrenaline	↑	Drinker & Drinker (1916)
Bradykinin	↓	Lundgaard *et al.* (1997)
Calcitonin	↑	Driessens & Vanhoutte (1981)
CGRP	↓	Lundgaard *et al.* (1997)
Endothelin	↑	Brinker *et al.* (1990); Briggs *et al.* (1998); Drescher *et al.* (2006)
Isoproterenol	↑	Brinker *et al.* (1990)
Methoxamine	↑	Brinker *et al.* (1990)
Nitric oxide	↑	Lundgaard *et al.* (1996); McCarthy *et al.* (1997)
Noradrenaline	↑	Gross *et al.* (1979); Driessens & Vanhoutte (1979); Lundgaard *et al.* (1996)
Prazosin	↓	Dean *et al.* 1992
Propranolol	↓	Dean *et al.* 1992
Rauwolszin	↓	Dean *et al.* 1992
Substance P	↓	Lundgaard *et al.* (1997)
U46619	↑	Brinker *et al.* (1990)
VIP	↓	Lundgaard *et al.* (1997)

Nitric oxide and endothelin are released from endothelial cells. Nitric oxide can be induced by fluid shear acting on the endothelium, or mediates the action of acetylcholine. The action of bradykinin is also endothelium-dependent.

1.5.3 *Endothelial-dependent vasodilation*

Although it has been established that there are many factors that control local vascular tone in bone, it is worth considering endothelial-dependent vasoreactivity in more detail, as two potent vasoactive agents produced in the endothelium, nitric oxide (vasodilator) and endothelin (vasoconstrictor), have other wide-ranging effects on bone.

1.5.3.1 *Nitric oxide in bone*

Nitric oxide (NO) is a ubiquitous signaling molecule that has many important functions in bone. It is synthesized primarily by nitric oxide synthase (NOS) from L-arginine. There are three forms of NOS — endothelial (eNOS) and neuronal (nNOS) are constitutive forms producing low levels of NO for tonic functions;[97] inducible NOS (iNOS) is upregulated and activated during inflammation, producing large amounts of NO. Shear forces produced by blood flow results in the production of NO in endothelial cells, which then effects vasorelaxation in the surrounding smooth muscle cells. NO is also released from osteocytes in response to fluid shear caused by movement of interstitial fluid.[67]

NO has both a paracrine and autocrine role in bone metabolism, modulating the activity of osteoblasts and osteoclasts.[143] NO has a concentration-dependent effect of osteoblasts. At low concentrations it stimulates mineralization; at high concentrations it inhibits osteoblast proliferation, increases osteoblast apoptosis, and increases osteoclast-mediated resorption. At appropriate concentrations, NO donors have potential therapeutic benefits in the treatment of osteoporosis.[155]

NO is highly reactive and has a short biological half-life. Therefore, although it is produced by endothelial cells in bone, it remains to be demonstrated that NO released from endothelial cells acts as a signal beyond the surrounding vascular smooth muscle.

1.5.3.2 *Endothelin in bone*

Endothelin (ET) is a potent vasoconstrictor released from vascular endothelial cells. Hypoxia has been shown to stimulate ET release, as have thrombin, angiotensin II, TGF-β, and endotoxin.[13] Although potent vasoconstrictors, it is debatable whether they play a role in moment-to-moment control of vascular tone except in situations of endothelial dysfunction.[30] ET does, however, have significant effects on osteoblasts with an important role in bone tumors.[157] ET can cause proliferation of smooth muscle cells and activation of fibroblasts.

Although ET-1is a vasoconstrictor, ET-1 has been identified in osteoclasts, osteoblasts, and young osteocytes, as well as vascular endothelial cells.[124] It plays an important role in the regulation of bone mass through stimulation of osteoblast proliferation,[131] probably through induction of IL-18 in osteoblasts,[157] and by inhibition of osteoclast motility.[1] In pathological situations, ET-1 mediates bone metastases by stimulating osteoblast proliferation and bone formation.[52] ET-1 production is increased in patients with inflammatory arthritis, and it has been proposed that the vasoconstrictive action of ET-1 in subchondral bone may contribute to the development of osteoarthritis, though both direct effects locally in subchondral bone and impairment of perfusion of articular cartilage from bone.[145]

1.5.3.3 *Endothelial function in health and disease*

There are a number of studies that now show an association between endothelial function/dysfunction and bone status. Endothelial function declines with age and this is mediated by impairment of the NOS signaling pathway; these changes may be associated with age-related loss of bone.[112] There is increasing evidence of the beneficial effects of exercise on endothelial function in bone that may counter the effects of ageing on bone.[31,35] Both studied endothelial-dependent vasoreactivity in isolated arteries supplying bone. Short-term treadmill exercise of mini-pigs produced enhancement of endothelial function, mainly through adaptations in the NOS pathway.[31] Endurance training of young and old rats showed improvement in NOS-mediated vasodilation (77% in old rats), as well as bone blood flow; peak endothelial-dependent vasodilatation correlated with trabécular bone mineral fraction.[35] Using the same model, it has also been shown that endurance exercise increases regional blood flow in bone.[130] It was estimated that the strain on the bones during the exercise was lower than the values normally assumed to provide an osteogenic stimulus, and that the data may therefore indicate a causal relationship between the vascular changes and bone density, either through the actions of NO on bone or through increases of interstitial fluid flow through bone fluid spaces driven by hydrostatic pressure. Although hydrostatic pressures are lower in magnitude than stress-generated pressures, recent computational models have suggested that the hydrostatic pressure in osteocyte lacunae is sufficient to activate osteocytes.[125]

Endothelial-dependent vasoactivity in the forearm appears to be impaired in women with osteoporosis or osteopenia. In post-menopausal Japanese women, the effect of nitroglycerin on forearm blood flow during reactive hyperaemia has been investigated.[123] Those women with osteoporosis had significantly lower response than the controls, indicating impaired endothelial function. In addition, ET-1- mediated vasoconstriction appears elevated in women with osteopenia.[94] However, although there is now accumulating evidence from both experimental and clinical studies of an association between endothelium-dependent function and bone density, the nature of the relationship needs further investigation.

1.5.4 *Autocrine and paracrine actions of bone endothelium*

The endothelium in bone does not just serve as a barrier to control solute and cellular movement and contribute to the local control of vascular tone. It has long been known that bone endothelium is a target for molecules with osteogenic actions.[24, 133] Bone endothelium is both a target for circulating hormones and local regulatory factors; vascular endothelial cells cloned from fetal bovine bone have been shown to respond to parathyroid hormone, progesterone, estrogen, insulin-like growth factors, platelet derived growth factor, basic fibroblast growth factor, and endothelial cell growth factor. In addition, endothelial cells produce potential modulators of bone activity such as fibroblast growth factor, interleukins 1 and 6, colony stimulating factors, prostacyclin, endothelin-1, and nitric oxide. A full list of chemokines, matrix molecules, cytokines, and growth factors produced by endothelial cells, osteoclasts and osteoclast precursors, and osteoblasts that may be involved in intercellular signaling can be found in a recent review.[11] Much of the evidence for this has been done using co-cultures of endothelial cells or vascular pericytes, and so there is much still to be learnt about how the potential intercellular cross-talk between bone cells and bone endothelium functions *in vivo*. Dysfunction of this aspect of endothelial activity has been implicated in pathologies of bone such as pachydermoperiostosis, osteopetrosis, rickets, inflammatory bone loss, multiple myeloma, Paget's disease, melorheostasis, Gorham-Stout disease, Klippel-Trenaunaysyndrome, and vertebral angiomatosis.[20]

1.5.5 *Coupling of bone formation and resorption*

In an adult person, bone mass is relatively constant. Bone is constantly turning over at a steady rate, with local bone resorption followed by bone formation in discrete units called bone metabolic units (BMUs). When bone mass is in a steady state, the average rate of bone resorption must equal the average rate of bone formation, but with precise temporal and spatial coordination of osteoclast and osteoblast activity within each BMU. These observations suggest that there is a mechanism that couples bone formation by osteoblasts and bone resorption by osteoclasts. Data of paracrine and autocrine actions of bone endothelium have been summarized above, and it has been argued that bone vascular endothelial cells should be considered to be part of the bone cell communication network. Following such observations, it has also been argued that the vasculature has a central role in the coupling between bone formation and resorption.[103] To summarize Parfitt's arguments: (1) bone capillaries are present at the right place and the right time; (2) vascular pericytes express many of the features of osteoblasts; (3) endothelial cells secrete potent mitogens for osteoblast activity. It was not suggested that the vasculature was the only factor involved in coupling (see Ref. 60 for a recent review), but that the vasculature could be a key contributor to the process.

1.5.6 *Action of neuropeptides in bone*

Although most innervation of bone is perivascular, and the vasoreactivity of bone has just been described, neural tissue in bone has a far more general role in bone metabolism, and nerve processes have been observed in close proximity to bone cells.[126] Genetic studies in mice have demonstrated the importance of leptin and leptin receptors in the hypothalamus in regulating bone remodeling.[42] The action of the hypothalamus is mediated by the sympathetic nervous system, and beta-blockers have a dual action of increasing bone formation and decreasing bone resorption. Both osteoblasts and osteoclasts contain receptors for CGRP, VIP, SP, and glutamate, and all these neuropeptides have effects of bone formation, bone resorption, and osteoclast formation.[88] Although these actions of the neuropeptides on bone cells have been demonstrated independently of their vasoactive effects, it is tempting to consider whether neural activity provides local coordination of bone cell activity and perfusion.

1.6 Coupling of Angiogenesis and Osteogenesis in Bone Repair and Regeneration

The physiological role of the vascular system in coupling bone formation and resorption has been described above. It has an equally important role during development repair for the formation of bone. It has often been recognized that angiogenesis preceded osteogenesis in many practical situations, and this empirical observation has led to the suggestion that the blood vessels play an active role in the process of osteogenesis, and not just a passive role of providing substrates for the process of osteogenesis.[138] Subsequent laboratory studies have given further direct support to this hypothesis. Angiogenesis precedes neo-osteogenesis, as observed and measured by Winet *et al.*[156] using a bone chamber implant and intravital microscopy.[155] Roach *et al.* suggested a chronology of interactions between the vascular system and ossification of cartilage in the epiphyses of long bones.[121] A common regulator for hypertrophic cartilage vascularization and ossification has been described.[144] A central role for VEGF in controlling mineralization during endochondral bone formation has been demonstrated.[49] An important role for angiogenesis in fracture repair has also been described.[50] Again, hypoxia is a key determinant of angiogenesis. There is limited perfusion at the fracture site, due to rupture of vessels and formation of a hematoma, resulting in a hypoxic environment. Hypoxia-inducible-factors (HIFs), discussed below, are expressed in fracture repair,[84] initiating the cascade of events associated with angiogenesis.

1.6.1 *Response of bone to hypoxia*

Hypoxia arises when there is an imbalance between oxygen delivery to a tissue provided by the circulation, and the metabolic consumption of oxygen by cells within the tissue. The response of bone to hypoxia turns out to be an extremely important mechanism in both the physiology and pathophysiology in bone, coupling angiogenesis and osteogenesis in bone development and repair.[3]

HIFs are important mediators of the effects of hypoxia on tissue. Around 100 target genes of HIFs have been identified, including VEGF, erythropoietin (EPO), iNOS, insulin like growth factor 2 (IGF-2), and endothelin-1. Under normoxic (5% or over) conditions, HIFs are rapidly degraded through hydroxylation by prolyl hydroxylase domain proteins (PHDs); however, under hypoxic conditions PHD activity decreases, and

HIFs therefore increase. This has led to the investigation of PHD inhibitors as therapeutic agents for anemia and ischemia. The actions of HIFs and PHDs are described in greater detail in a recent review.[44]

Hypoxia inducible factor 1 alpha (HIF-1α) is a key component in the coupling of angiogenesis and osteogenesis.[120] In their model, osteoblasts detect reduced levels of oxygen and nutrients and upregulate HIF-1α. HIF-1α target genes, including VEGF, are then activated. These may act directly on bone cells, or may stimulate new blood vessel formation. These vessels provide osteogenic cues and also deliver osteoblast progenitors to the site. The nature of the osteogenic signals provided by the vascular cells still need to be investigated, but PHD inhibitors are now under investigation as therapeutic agents.

An interesting clinical study has investigated the potential effects of local hypoxia on bone mineral density.[54] Patients with local systematic sclerosis were studied; volumetric bone mineral density (vBMD) was measured using peripheral quantitative CT. vBMD was measured at a juxta-articular site in the third metacarpal (a hypoxia-prone site), mid-shaft of the metacarpal, as well as proximal and mid-shaft sites in the tibia and radius. Total and trabecular vBMD were raised at the juxta-articular third metacarpal site, but not at any of the other sites, suggesting local hypoxia was stimulating bone formation.

1.6.2 *Hypoxia and the stem cell niche*

Hypoxia is thought to be a common characteristic in controlling quiescence in stem cell niches. It is therefore important to know the hypoxic state of bone marrow. Staining with pimonidazole indicated low oxygenation of vessels within the diaphysis but higher oxygenation in the metaphysis.[71] Pimonidazole is an indirect indicator of oxygenation status, and recent direct measurements of pO_2 in mouse calvaria.[129] Using two-photon phosphorescence lifetime microscopy, they found a gradient in pO_2 from vessels in the periosteum (~50 mmHg), cortical bone (~31 mmHg) and bone marrow (20.4 mm Hg); extravascular pO_2 in bone marrow was even lower (13.3 mm Hg). There was a significant concentration gradient radially away from vessels in the marrow, and also a gradient of decreasing pO_2 moving from the endosteum deeper into the marrow. It was suggested that these observations reflected the balance between supply and demand, so that even though the marrow was highly vascular, oxygen consumption is also very high in this region.[129] Although data from indirect and direct measurements of pO_2 appear contradictory, it is probable that very steep concentration gradients exist in this region, and perhaps regulation of the concentration gradient has an important physiological role.

1.6.3 *Common cellular and regulatory pathways for angiogenesis and osteogenesis*

A number of angiogenesis-stimulating factors have been described that are expressed during bone development and repair; the most important and extensively studied is VEGF, but fibroblast growth factor (FGF)[62] and placental growth factor (PlGF)[83] are also expressed. In addition to these primary factors, there are several others that act indirectly through the control of the production of angiogenic molecules; these include bone morphogenetic proteins, angiopoietin, platelet-derived growth factor and insulin-like growth factor. Matrix metalloproteinases (MMPs) are also important; these are proteolytic enzymes that produce local modification of the extracellular matrix. This is an essential precursor that facilitates angiogenesis, and contributes to the local release of angiogenic factors.[151] During fracture healing MMPs mediate vascular invasion and MMP-nil mice show persistent cartilage and no progression to bone union at the fracture site.[23]

On the cellular level, endothelial progenitor cells (EPCs) have attracted interest. They have been shown to facilitate the formation of three-dimensional pre-vascular structures in a co-culture setting with mesenchymal stem cells.[122] Furthermore, EPCs have been postulated to be utilized to enhance fracture healing[78] and to be used for tissue engineering. Reversely mesenchymal stem cells differentiated to osteoblasts have been successfully applied in patients with avascular necrosis of the hip.[48]

1.6.3.1 *Vascular endothelial growth factor (VEGF)*

VEGF, also known as vascular permeability factor, is a potent stimulator of endothelial cell proliferation both *in vivo* and *in vitro*.[68, 109] It exhibits a mitogenic and permeability-enhancing activity directed toward vascular endothelial cells;[46] other properties include the ability to induce vasodilation[70] and stimulation of hexose transport of vascular endothelium.[106] It has also been cited as a possible marker of tumor growth in some cancers notably papillary thyroid carcinoma.[66]

In bone, VEGF has been shown to play a role in development and repair processes as well as regulation of normal bone turnover.[80] These processes have a link of angiogenesis and osteogenesis in common. VEGF, usually situated in endothelial cells, will be expressed by other cells, e.g., chondrocytes, just before ingrowth of vascular capillaries.[19] VEGF is important during growth and regulates the vascular invasion into the cartilaginous anlage of the epiphysis during development of the secondary center of ossification.[36] The expression of VEGF has been shown in the epiphyseal resting cartilage prior to vascular ingrowth.[2]

Street *et al.* has measured VEGF in fracture hematoma where it has been shown to be present in large quantities.[132] The role of VEGF in fracture healing has been illustrated in a number of studies: Street showed that inhibition of VEGF activity during fracture repair would result in a decrease of angiogenesis, bone formation, and callus mineralization.[132] In more detail, Reumann *et al.* showed a sequential presence of VEGF receptors during fracture healing with specificity of VEGFR2 to callus formation.[119]

In normal bone formation VEGF is released by osteocytes in response to loading and not only stimulates blood vessel formation, but also stimulates osteoblastogenesis.[21,47,110] VEGF is expressed by periosteal-derived cells in culture[104] and a paracrine action for VEGF has been postulated for osteoblast-endothelial cell signaling.[22] VEGF has also been suggested to regulate the balance between osteoblastic and adipocyte differentiation in bone marrow mesenchymal stem cells in anon-paracrine fashion.[6] The regulation of VEGF and, therefore, bone angiogenesis by activating transcription factor 4 (ATF4), has been concluded by Zhu *et al.*[159] Mice lacking the ATF4 gene were unable to adjust to hypoxic conditions and endothelial sprouting was completely prevented during bone development. Interestingly the exposure to nicotine uncoupled angiogenesis and osteogenesis in that angiogenesis increased in response to HIF-1αbut the expression of bone morphogenetic protein 2 decreased and as a net result bone formation was impaired.[82]

The relationship of VEGF to osteogenesis has been utilized for treatment options to enhance bone formation and fracture repair: a VEGF-A gene transfer via adenovirus vectors has been successfully employed in the intact femura of white rabbits.[53] Simply using a cell-based method of gene transfer, fibroblasts transfected with VEGF were delivered to a bone defect in rabbits and the results were positive.[76] Recombinant VEGF has been equally utilized in a non-union model in rabbits,[41] more recently in a murine non-union model,[104] and in combination with BMP-4.[58]

1.6.3.2 *Other angiogenic factors*

Members of the FGF family regulate endothelial cell proliferation and migration, integrin and cadherin receptor expression, and gap junction communication.[62] FGFs are expressed during skeletal development and fracture repair. However, more work is required to understand direct and indirect pathways of FGF action on endothelial function in fracture repair.

PlGF is a VEGF homologue that binds to VEGFR-1; originally identified in the placenta, it has a far wider distribution in tissues. In bone, it mediates angiogenesis and endochondral ossification. Its expression is raised during fracture repair, and transgenic studies indicate its role in osteogenic differentiation and callus remodeling.[83]

Fracture healing requires a vascular network to maintain cell viability but also the recruitment of skeletal progenitor cells to the injury site and their successful differentiation into bone and cartilage. In addition to BMPs and VEGF, MMPs are important factors in that MMP-nil mice show persistent cartilage and no progression to bone union at the fracture site.[25]

DJ-1 is a ubiquitously expressed protein with a number of intracellular functions. It was thought also to have undefined extracellular functions, but recently it has been identified as an angiogenic factor produced by mesenchymal stem cells (MSCs). DJ-1 stimulated the differentiation of MSCs into osteoblasts, and induced angiogenesis in endothelial cells through activation of fibroblast growth factor receptor-1 signaling.[65] In a rat fracture model, extracellular application of DJ-1 enhanced bone regeneration through the formation of new vessels, an effect that was blocked with an FGFR-1 antagonist.[65]

Recently, it has been shown that microRNAs (miRNAs) have an important role in the regulation of angiogenesis. In addition, miRNAs appear to regulate chondrocyte, osteoblast, and osteoclast differentiation. Raised plasma levels of several miRNAs are found during fracture repair, and inhibition of miRNA-92a markedly enhanced angiogenesis and bone repair in a murine fracture model.[98]

1.6.4 *Bone-specific angiogenic mechanisms*

Recently, it has been shown that vascular growth in bone involves a specialized, tissue-specific form of angiogenesis. In most tissue, Notch signaling negatively controls endothelial cell proliferation; however, in bone, Notch signaling promotes endothelial cell proliferation and vessel growth.[114] Endothelium-specific genetic disruption of Notch impaired bone vessel morphology and growth, and also led to reduced osteogenesis, shortened bones, and reduced bone mass.[114] Furthermore, the newly identified capillary subtype found, type H, located within vessels, columns, and arches of mataphyseal vessels (and only otherwise found in the liver), display high proliferation rates and mediate vascular growth in bone.[71] These observations indicate a unique environment in bone for the coupling of angiogenesis and osteogenesis.

1.7 Response of Bone to Ischemia

Bone can be subject to short-term or long-term ischemia either from circulatory disturbances, or sometimes from surgical intervention (e.g., use of a tourniquet in total knee arthroplasty). Clearly, the shorter the period of ischemia the better, and although limited periods of ischemia are followed by hyperperfusion, even periods as short as a couple of hours lead to further insult through ischemia-reperfusion injury, remodeling led by decreased endothelial relaxation, increased capillary permeability, oxidant production, and leucocyte-endothelium adhesion.[43] Studies of bone have shown a similar response.[56,142]

Endothelium-dependent vasorelaxation via the L-arginine/NO pathway remains viable for up to six hours of ischemia, though vascular smooth muscle appeared viable after 12 hours of ischemia.[91] Ischemic preconditioning with short duration periods of ischemia may minimize the effects of several hours ischemia; this could be useful in situations where ischemia is planned (e.g., during surgery), but is clearly not feasible in pathological situations.

If intramedullary pressure rises too much, this can contribute to bone marrow oedema syndrome (BMOS), resulting in perhaps transient vascular compromise.[105] BMOS is identified from MRI scans by an intermediate signal on T1-weighted images, a high signal on T2-weighted images, and a hyper-intense signal in STIR images, all characteristic of an elevated water content. BMOS is associated with diseases of coagulation.

More extended periods of ischemia will lead to tissue necrosis. Corticosteroid treatment is a risk factor for the development of osteonecrosis; ET-1 constriction of the femoral epiphyseal artery is enhanced by long-term treatment though the responsiveness of other vasoactive agents was not changed, suggesting ET-1 involvement in the pathogenesis of ON.[37] At low concentrations, hydrocortisone augments vasoconstriction caused by noradrenaline, but at higher concentrations, hydrocortisone results in a dose-dependent inhibition of noradrenergic action.[37] The vascular disturbances can contribute to the development of focal areas of necrotic bone; resorption of the necrotic bone and subsequent new bone formation during this repair process can result in compromise of the mechanical integrity of bone, which can lead to problems associated with osteonecrosis.

1.8 Summary

Bone circulation plays an important role in bone physiology. The circulation is not merely a passive conduit for blood flow, but plays an active role in controlling processes in bone. At a basic science level, much now is understood about the physiological processes involved in the response of bone to hypoxia and ischemia, and the role of the circulation in various areas of bone pathology. The link between osteogenesis and angiogenesis is increasingly recognized, but this is still a rapidly expanding area. Some treatment strategies have already been based on this knowledge, and the challenge for the next few years will be to translate this understanding into novel therapeutic interventions.

References

1. Alam ASMT, Gallagher A, Shankar V, *et al.* (1992). Endothelin inhibits osteoclastic bone resorption by a direct effect on cell motility: Implications for the vascular control of bone resorption. *Endocrinology*, 130, 3617–3624.
2. Allerstorfer D, Longato S, Schwarzer C, Fischer-Colbrie R, Hayman AR, Blumer MJ (2010). VEGF and its role in the early development of the long epiphysis. *J Anat*, 216, 611–624.
3. Arnett TR, Gibbons DC, Utting JC, Orriss IR, Hoebertz A, Rosendall M, Meghji S (2003). Hypoxia is a major stimulator of osteoclast formation and bone resorption. *J Cell Physiol*, 196, 2–8.
4. Arnoldi CC, Linderholm H, Vinnerberg A (1972). Skeletal and soft tissue changes in the lower leg in patients with intracalcanean hypertension. *Acta Chir Scand*, 138, 25–37.
5. Atkinson PJ, Hallsworth AS (1982). The spatial structure of bone. In RJ Harrison and V Navaratman (eds): *Progress in Anatomy Vol 2*, Cambridge University Press, Cambridge UK.
6. Berendsen AD, Olsen BR (2014). How vascular endothelial growth factor-A (VEGF) regulates differentiation of mesenchymal stem cells. *J Histochem Cytochem*, 62, 103–108.
7. Bergula AP, Huang W, Frangos JA (1999). Femoral vein ligation increases bone mass in the hindlimb suspended rat. *Bone*, 24, 171–177.

8. Bjurholm A, Kreicbergs A, Brodin E, Schultzberg M (1988). Substance P- and CGRP-reactive nerves in bone. *Peptides*, 9, 165–171.
9. Bjurholm A (1991). Neuroendocrine peptides in bone. *IntOrthop*, 15, 325–329.
10. Brandi ML, Crescioli C, Tanini A, Frediani U, Agnusdei D, Gennari C (1993). Bone endothelial cells as estrogen targets. *CalcifTissInt*, 53, 312–317.
11. Brandi ML, Collin-Osdoby P (2006). Vascular biology and the skeleton. *Bone*, 21, 183–192.
12. Brånemark PI(1959). Vital microscopy of bone marrow in the rabbit. *Scand J Clin Lab Invest*, 11, Suppl 38.
13. Briggs PJ, Moran CG, Wood MB (1998). Actions of endothelin-1, 2, and 3 in the microvasculature of bone. *J Orthop Res*, 16, 340–347.
14. Brinker MR, Lippton HL, Cook SD, Hyman AL (1990). Pharmacological regulation of the circulation of bone. *J Bone Joint Surg*, 72-A, 964–975.
15. Brookes M (1958). The vascular anatomy of tubular bone in the rat. *Anat Rec*, 132, 25–47.
16. Brookes M, Revell WJ (1998). *Blood Supply of Bone: Scientific Aspects. London*: Springer Verlag.
17. Canas E, Terepka AR, Neuman WF (1969). Potassium and the milieu interieur of bone. *Am J Physiol*, 217, 117–120.
18. Carduso L, Fritton SP, Gailani G, Benalla M, Cowin SC (2013). A review of recent advances in the assessment of bone porosity, permeability and interstitial fluid flow. *J Biomech*, 46, 253–265.
19. Carlevaro MF, Cermelli S, Cancedda R, Descalzi Cancedda F, (2000). Vascular endothelial growth factor (VEGF) in cartilage neovascularization and chondrocyte differentiation: Auto-paracrine role during endochondral formation. *J Cell Sci*, 113, 59–69.
20. Carulli C, Innocenti M, Brandi ML (2013). Bone vascularization in normal and diseased conditions. *Front Endocrinol*, 4, 1–10.
21. Cheung WY, Liu C, Tonelli-Zasarsky RM, Simmons CA, You L (2011). Osteocyte apoptosis is mechanically regulated and induces angiogenesis in vitro. *J Orthop Res*, 29, 523–530.
22. Clarkin CE, Emery RJ, Pitsillidies AA, Wheeler-Jones CP (2008). Evaluation of VEGF-mediated signaling in primary human cells reveals a paracrine action for VEGF in osteoblast-mediated crosstalk to endothelial cells. *J Cell Physiol*, 214, 537–544.
23. Cohen J, Harris WH (1958). The three-dimensional anatomy of haversian systems. *J Bone Joint Surg*, 40-A, 419–434.
24. Collin-Osdoby P (1994). Role of vascular endothelial cells in bone biology. *J Cell Biochem*, 55, 304–309.
25. Colnot C, Thompson Z, Miclau T, Werb Z, Helm JA (2003). Altered fracture repair in the absence of MMP9. *Development*, 130, 4123–4133.
26. Cooper RR, Milgram JW, Robinson RA (1966). Morphology of the osteon. *J Bone Joint Surg*, 48-A, 1239–1244.

27. Cooper R (1968). Nerves in cortical bone. *Science*, 160, 327–328.
28. Corbett S, McCarthy ID, Batten J, Hukkanen M, Polak JM, Hughes SPF (1999). Nitric oxide mediated vasoreactivity during fracture repair. *Clin Orthop Rel Res*, 365, 247–253.
29. Crock HV (1996). *An Atlas of the Vascular Anatomy of the Skeleton and Spinal Cord.* Martin Dunitz, London.
30. Dean MT, Wood MB, Vanhoutte PM (1992). Antagonist drugs and bone vascular smooth muscle. *J Orthop Res*, 10, 104–111.
31. Delaney LE, Arce-Esquival AA, Kuroki K, Laughlin, MH (2012). Exercise training improves vasoreactivity in the knee artery. *Int J Sports Med*, 33, 114–122.
32. De Mey JGR, Vanhoutte PM (2014). End o'the line revisited: Moving on from nitric oxide to CGRP. *Life Sci*, doi: 10.1016/j/lfs.2014.04.012.
33. Dillaman RM, Roer RD, Gay DM (1991). Fluid movement in bone: Theoretical and empirical. *J Biomech*, 24(Suppl 1), 163–177.
34. Döhler JR, Hennig FF, Hughes SP (1995). Rectivity of cortical bone capillaries. Functional TEM analysis with adrenaline, ATP and insulin. *Langenbecks Arch Chir*, 380, 176–183.
35. Dominguez JM, Prisby RD, Muller-Delp JM, Allen MR, Delp MD (2010). Increased nitric oxide-mediated vasodilation of bone resistance arteries is associated with increased trabecular bone volume after endurance training in rats. *Bone*, 46, 813–819.
36. Doschak MR, Cooper DM, Huculak CN, Matyas JR, Hart DA, Hallgrimsson B, Zernicke RF, Bray RC (2003). Angiogenesis in the distal femoral chondroepiphysis of the rabbit during development of the secondary centre of ossification. *J Anat*, 203, 223–33.
37. Drescher W, Li H, Lundgaard A, Bunger C, Hansen ES (2006). Endothelin-1 induced femoral head epiphyseal artery constriction is enhanced by long-term corticosteroid treatment. *J Bone Joint Surg Am*, 88(Suppl 3), 173–179.
38. Driessens M, Vanhoutte PM (1979). Vascular reactivity of the isolated tibia of the dog. *Am J Physiol*, 236, H904–H908.
39. Driessens M, Vanhoutte PM (1981). Effect of calcitonin, hydrocortisone and parathyroid hormone on canine bone blood vessels. *Am J Physiol*, 241, H91–H94.
40. Drinker CK, Drinker KR (1916). A method for maintaining an artificial circulation through the tibia of the dog, with a demonstration of the vasomotor control of marrow vessels. *Am J Physiol*, 40, 514–521.
41. Eckardt H, Ding M, Lind M, Hansen ES, Christensen KS (2005). Recombinant human vascular endothelial growth factor enhances bone healing inan experimental nonunion model. *J Bone Joint Surg Br*, 87, 1434–1438.
42. Elefteriou F (2005). Neuronal emodelin and regulation of bone emodeling. *Cell Mol Life Sci*, 62, 2339–2349.
43. Eltzschig HK, Collard CD (2004). Vascular ischaemia and reperfusion injury. *BMJ*, 70, 71–86.

44. Fan L, Li J, Yu Z, Dang X, Wang K (2014). The hypoxia-inducible factor pathway, prolyl hydroxylase domain protein inhibitors, and their roles in bone repair and regeneration. *Bio Med Res Int*, Article ID 239356.
45. Feik SA (1993). Early periosteal changes in translation-induced bone modeling. *J Anat*, 182, 389–401.
46. Ferrara N, Davis-Smyth T (1997). The biology of vascular endothelial growth factor. *Endocr Rev*, 18, 4–25.
47. Furumatsu T, Shen ZN, Kawai A, Nishida K, Manabe H, Oohashi T, Inoue H, Ninomiya Y (2003). Vascular endothelial growth factor principally acts as the main angiogenic factor in the early stage of human osteoblastogenesis. *J Bio Chem*, 133, 633–639.
48. Gangji V, De Maertelaer V, Hauzeur JP (2011). Autologous bone marrow cell implantation in the treatment of non-traumatic osteonecrosis of the femoral head: Five year follow-up of a prospective controlled study. *Bone*, 49, 1005–1009.
49. Gerber HP, Vu TH, Ryan AM, Kowalski J, Werb Z, Ferrara N (1999). VEGF couples hypertrophic cartilage remodeling, ossification and angiogenesis during endochondral bone formation. *Nature Med*, 5, 617–618.
50. Glowacki J (1998). Angiogenesis in fracture repair. *Clin Orthop Relat Res*, 355, S82–S89.
51. Gross PM, Heistad DD, Marcus ML (1979). Neurohumoral regulation of blood flow to bone and marrow. *Am J Physiol*, 237, H440–H448.
52. Guise TA, Yin JJ, Mohammed KS (2003). Role of endothelin-1 in osteoblasticbonemetastases. *Cancer*, 97(Suppl 3), 779–784.
53. Hanley DA, Brown JP, Tenenhouse A, *et al.* (2003). Associations among disease conditions, bone mineral density, and prevalent vertebral deformities in men and women 50 years of age and older: Cross-sectional results from the Canadian multicentre osteoporosis study. *J Bone Miner Res*, 18, 784–790.
54. Heise V, Galli-Lysak I, Villiger PM, Aeberli D (2014). Increased bone mineral density at the hypoxia prone site of the juxta-articular metacarpal bone in patients with limited systemic sclerosis: A cross-sectional study. *J Musculoskelet Neuronal Interact*, 14, 189–194.
55. Hiltunen MO, Ruuskanen M, Huuskonen J, Mähönen AJ, Ahonen M, Rutanen J, Kosma VM, Mahonen A, Kröger H, Ylä-Herttuala S, (2003). Adenovirus-mediated VEGF-A gene transfer induces bone formation in vivo. *FASEB J*, 17, 1147–1149.
56. Hsieh AS, Winet H, Bao JY, Glas H, Plenk H (2001). Evidence for reperfusion injury in cortical bone as a function of crush injury ischaemia duration: A rabbit bone chamber study. *Bone*, 28, 94–103.
57. Hu M, Cheng J, Bethel N, Serra-Hsu F, Ferreri S, Lin L, Qin YX (2014). Interrelation between external oscillatory muscle coupling amplitude and in vivo intramedullary pressure related bone adaptation. *Bone*, 66, 178–181.
58. Huang YC, Kaigler D, Rice KG, Krebsbach PH, Mooney DJ, (2005). Combined angiogenic and osteogenic factor delivery enhances bone marrow stromal cell-driven bone regeneration. *J Bone Miner Res*, 20, 848–857.

59. Hukkanen M, Kontinnen YT, Santavirta S, Paavolainen P, Gu X, Terenghi G, Polak JM (1993). Rapid proliferation of calcitonin gene-related peptide-immunoreactive nerves during healing of rat tibial fracture suggests neural involvement in bone growth and remodeling. *Neuroscience*, 54, 969–979.
60. Ikeda K, Takeshita S (2014). Factors and mechanisms involved in the coupling from bone resorption to bone formation: How osteoclasts talk to osteoblasts. *J Bone Metab*, 21, 163–168.
61. Imai K, Kobayashi M, Wang J, Shinobu N, Yoshida H, Hamada J, *et al.* (1999). Selective secretion of chemotractants for haemotopoietic progenitor cells by bone marrow endothelial cells. *Br J Haematol*, 106, 905–911.
62. Javerzat S, Auguste P, Bikfalvi A (2002). The role of fibroblast growth factors in vascular development. *Trends Mol Med*, 8, 483–489.
63. Kelly PJ (1968). Anatomy, physiology and pathology of the blood supply of bones. *J Bone Joint Surg*, 50-A, 766–783.
64. Kelly PJ (1973). Comparison of marrow and cortical bone blood flow by 125I-labelled 4-iodoantityrine. *J Lab Clin Med*, 81, 497–501.
65. Kim JM, Shin JI, Cha SS, Lee CS, Hong BS, Lim S, *et al.* (2012). DJ-1 promotes angiogenesis and osteogenesis by activating FGF receptor-1 signalling. *Nat Commun*, 3, 1296.
66. Klein, *et al.* (2001). Vascular endothelial growth factor gene and protein: Strong expression in thyroiditis and thyroid carcinoma. *J Endocrinology*, 161, 41–49.
67. Klein-Nulend J, van Oers RFM, Bakker AD, Bacabac RG (2014). Nitric oxide signaling in mechanical adaptation of bone. *OsteoporosInt*, 25, 1427–1432.
68. Kondo S, *et al.* (1993). Significance of vascular endothelial growth factor/vascular permiability factor for solid growth tumours, and its inhibition in antibody. *Biochem Biophys Res Commun.* 194, pp. 1234–1241.
69. Kowalski MJ, Schemitsch EH, Kregor PJ, Senft D, Swiontowski MF (1996). Effect of periosteal stripping on cortical bone perfusion: a laser doppler study in sheep. *CalcifTissInt*, 59, 24–26.
70. Ku DD, *et al.* (1993) Vascular endothelial growth factor induces EDRF-dependent relaxation in coronary arteries. *Am. J. Physiol*, 265, H586–H592.
71. Kusumbe AP, Ramasamy K, Adams RH (2014). Coupling of angiogenesis and osteogenesis by a specific vessel subtype in bone. *Nature*, 507(7492), 323–328.
72. Langer K (1876). Über das gefäßsystem der röhrenknochenmitbeitragenzurkenntis des baues und der entwicklung des knochengewebes. *Denkschr Aked Wiss Wien*, 36, 1–5.
73. Lemon GJ, Davies DR, Hughes SPF, Bassingthwaighte JB, Kelly PJ (1980). Transcapillary exchange and retention of fluoride, strontium, EDTA, and antipyrine in bone. *CalcifTissInt*, 31, 173–181.

74. Lexer E (1904). Weitereuntersuchungenüberknochenarterien und ihrebeduutungfürkrankhaftevorgänge. *Arch Klin Chir*, 73, 481–486.
75. Li G, Bronk JT, Kelly PJ (1989). Canine bone blood flow estimated with microspheres. *J Orthop Res*, 7, 61–67.
76. Li R, Stewart DJ, von Schroder HP, Mackinnon ES, Schemitsch EH, (2009). Effect of cell-based VEGF gene therapy on healing of a segmental bone defect. *J Orthop Res*, 27, 8–14.
77. Li R, Atesok K, Nauth A, Wright D, Qamiirani E, Whyne CM, Schemitsch EH. (2011) Endothelial progenitor cells for fracture healing: a microcomputed tomography and biomechanical analysis. *J Orthop Trauma.* 26, pp. 689–692.
78. Li W, Gardenier JD, Price C, Wang LY (2010). Does blood pressure enhance solute transport in the bone lacumar-canalicular system? *Bone*, 47, 353–359.
79. Liu Y, Olsen BR (2014). Distinct VEGF functions during bone development and homeostasis *Arch ImmunolTherExp (Warsz).* PMID 24699630.
80. Lopez-Curto JA, Bassingthwaighte JB, Kelly PJ (1980). Anatomy of the microvasculature of the tibial diaphysis of the adult dog. *J Bone Joint Surg*, 62-A, 1362–1369.
81. Lundgaard A, Aalkjaer C, Holm-Nielsen P, Mulvany MJ, Hansen ES (1996). Method for assessment of vascular reactivity in bone: In vitro studies on resistance arteries isolated from porcine cancellous bone. *J Orthop Res*, 14, 962–971.
82. Ma L, Zheng LW, Sham MH, Cheung LK (2010). Uncoupled angiogenesis and osteogenesis in nicotine-compromised bone healing. *J Bone Miner Res*, 25, 1305–1313.
83. Maes C, Coenegrachts I, Stockmans I, Daci E, Luttun A, Petryk A, *et al.* (2006). Placental growth factor mediates mesenchymal cell development, cartilage turnover, and bone remodeling during fracture repair. *J Clin Invest*, 116, 1230–1242.
84. Maes C, Carmeliet G, Schipani E (2012). Hypoxia-driven pathways in bone development, regeneration and disease. *Nat Rev Rheumatol*, 8, 358–366.
85. Maltby B, Lemon GJ, Bassingthwighte JB, Kelly PJ (1982). Exchange of potassium and strontium in adult bone. *Am J Physiol*, 242, H706–H712.
86. Marenzana M, Shipley AM, Squitiero P, Kunkel JG, Rubinacci A (2005). Bone as an ion exchange organ: Evidence for instantaneous cell-dependent calcium efflux from bone not due to resorption. *Bone*, 37, 545–554.
87. Marenzana M, Chenu C (2008). Sympathetic nervous system and bone adaptive response to its mechanical environment. *J Musculoskelet Neuronal Interact*, 8, 111–120.
88. Masi L (2012). Crosstalk between brain and bone. *Clin Cases Miner Bone Metab*, 9, 13–16.
89. McCarthy ID, Hughes SPF (1986). Inhibition of bone cell metabolism increases strontium-85 uptake *CalcifTissInt*, 39, 386–389.

90. McCarthy ID, Yang L (1992). A distributed model of exchange processes within the osteon, *J Biomech*, 25, 441–450.
91. McCarthy ID, Andhoga M, Batten JJ, Mathie RT (1997). Endothelium-dependent vasodilatation produced by the L-arginine/nitric oxide pathway in normal and ischeamic bone. *Acta Orthop Scand*, 68, 361–368.
92. McCarthy ID (2005). Fluid shifts due to microgravity and their effects on bone: A review of current knowledge. *Ann Biomed Eng*, 33, 95–103.
93. Menck J, Bertram C, Lierse W, Wolter D (1992). The arterial blood supply of the tibia and practical consequences. *Langenbecks Arch Chir*, 377, 229–234.
94. Mestek ML, Weil BR, Greiner JJ, Westby CM, DeSouza CA, Stauffer BL (2010). Osteopenia and endothelin-1 mediated vasoconstrictor tone in postmenopausal women. *Bone*, 43, 542–545.
95. Moncada S, Higgs A (1993). The l-arginine nitric oxide pathway. *N Engl J Med*, 329, 2002–2012.
96. Montgomery RJ, Sutker BD, Bronk JT, Smith SR, Kelly PJ (1988). Interstitial fluid flow in cortical bone. *Microvasc Res*, 35, 295–307.
97. Morris MA, Lopez-Curto JA, Hughes SPF, An KN, Bassingthwaighte JB, Kelly PJ (1982). Fluid spaces in canine bone and marrow. *Microvasc Res*, 23, 188 200.
98. Murata K, Ito H, Yoshitomi H, Yamamoto K, Fukada A, Yoshikawa J, *et al.* (2014). Inhibition of miRNA-92a enhances fracture healing via promoting angiogenesis in a model of stabilized fracture in young mice. *J Bone Miner Res*, 29, 316–326.
99. Nelson GE, Kelly PJ, Peterson LF, Janes SM (1960). Blood supply of the human tibia. *J Bone Joint Surg Am*, 42-A, 625–636.
100. Ness J, Aronow WS (2006). Comparison of the prevalence of atherosclerotic vascular disease in postmenopausal women with osteoporosis or osteopenia versus without osteoporosis or osteopenia. *Am J Cardiol*, 97, 1427–1428.
101. Neuman WF (1969). The milieu interieur of bone: Claude Bernard revisited. *Fed Proc*, 28, 1846–1850.
102. Ogilvie CM, Lu C, Marcucio R, Lee M, Thompson Z, Hu D, Helms JA, Miclau T (2012). Vascular endothelial growth factor improves bone repair in a murine nonunion model. *Iowa Orthop J*, 32, 90–94.
103. Parfitt AM (2000). The mechanism of coupling: A role for the vasculature. *Bone*, 26, 319–323.
104. Park BW, Hah YS, Kim JR, Byun JH (2008). Vascular endothelial growth factor expression in cultured periosteal-derived cells. *Oral Surg Oral Med Oral Pathol Oral RadiolEndod*, 105, 554–560.
105. Patel S (2014). Primary bone marrow oedema syndromes. *Rheumatology*, 53, 785–792.
106. Pekala P, Marlow M, Heuvelman D, Connolly D (1990). Regulation of hexose transport in aortic endothelial cells by vascular permeability factor ad tumor necrosis factor-alpha. *J Biol Chem*, 265, 20506–20516.

107. Piekarski K, Munro M (1977). Transport mechanism operating between blood supply and osteocytes in long bones. *Nature*, 269, 80–82.
108. Pinto MR, Kelly PJ (1984). Age-related changes in bone in the dog: Fluid spaces and their potassium content. *J Orthop Res*, 2, 2–7.
109. Plouet J, Bayard F (1994). Regulations of vasculotrophin/vascular endothelial growth factor bioavailability. *Horm Res*, 42, 14–19.
110. Prasadam I, Zhou Y, Du Z, Chen J, Crawford R, Xiao Y (2014). Osteocyte induced angiogenesis via VEGF-MAPK-dependent pathways in endothelial cells. *Mol Cell Biochem*, 386, 15–25.
111. Price C, Zhou X, Li W, Wang L. (2011). Real-time measurement of solute transport within the lacunar-canalicular system of mechanically loaded bone: Direct evidence of load induced fluid flow. *J Bone Miner Res*, 26, 277–285.
112. Prisby RD, Ramsey MW, Behnke BJ, Dominguez JM, Donato AJ, Allen MR, Delp MD (2007). Ageing reduces skeletal blood flow, endothelium dependent vasodilation, and NO availability in rats. *J Bone Miner Res*, 22, 1280–1288.
113. Qin L, Mak ATF, Cheng CW, Hung LK, Chan KM (1999). Histomorphological study on pattern of fluid movement in cortical bone in goats. *Anat Rec*, 255, 380–387.
114. Ramasamy SK, Kusumbe AP, Waught L, Adams RH (2014). Endothelial Notch activity promotes angiogenesis and osteogenesis in bone. *Nature*, 507(7492), 376–380.
115. Reeve J (1978). The turnover of calcium in the exchangeable pools of bone in man and the long-term effect of a parathyroid hormone fragment. *Clin Endocrinol*, 8, 445–455.
116. Reeve J, Arlot R, Wootton R (1988). Skeletal blood flow, iliac histomorphometry, and strontium kinetics in osteoporosis: A relationship between blood flow and corrected apposition rate. *J ClinEndocrMetab*, 66, 1124–1131.
117. Reichert ILH, McCarthy ID, Hughes SPF (1995). The acute vascular response to intramedullary reaming. *J Bone Joint Surg.* 77-B, 490–493.
118. Reichert ILH (2000). The haemodynamics of reamed and undreamed intramedullary nailing. PhD thesis, University of London.
119. Reumann MK, Nair T, Strachna O, Boskey AL, Mayer-Kuckuk P (2010). Production of VEGF receptor 1 and 2 mRNA and protein during endochondral bone repair is differential and healing phase specific. *J Appl Physiol*, 109, 1930–1938.
120. Riddle RC, Khatri R, Schipani E, Clemens TL (2009). Role of hypoxia-inducible-factor 1α in angiogenic-osteogenic coupling. *J Mol Med*, 87, 583–590.
121. Roach HI, Baker JE, Clarke NM (1998). Initiation of the bony epiphysis in long bones: chronology of interactions between the vascular system and the chondrocytes. *J Bone Miner Res*, 13, 950–961.

122. Rouwkema J, Westerweel PE, de Boer J, Verhaar MC, van Blitterswijk CA (2009). The use of endothelial progenitor cells for prevascularized bone tissue engineering. *Tissue Eng Part A*, 15, 2015–2027.
123. Sanada M, Taguchi A, Higashi Y, *et al.* (2004). Forearm endothelial function and bone mineral loss in postmenopausal women. *Atherosclerosis*, 176, 387–392.
124. Sasaki T, Hong MH (1993). Endothelin-1 localisation in bone cells and vascular endothelial cells in rat bone marrow. *Anat Rec*, 237, 332–337.
125. Scheiner S, Pivonka P, Hellmich C (2013). Poromechanical stimulation of bone remodelling: A continuum micromechanics-based mathematical model and experimental validation. *Poromechanics*, V, 1867–1876.
126. Serre CM, Farley D, Delmas PD, Chenu C (1999). Evidence for a dense and intimate innervation of bone tissue, including glutamate-containing fibres. *Bone*, 25, 623–629.
127. Shim SS, Hawk HE, Yu WY (1972). The relationship between blood flow and marrow cavity pressure of bone. *Surg Gynecol Obstet*, 135, 353–360.
128. Skawina A, Litwin JA, Gorczyca J, Miodonski AJ (1994). The vascular system of human fetal long bones: A scanning electron microscope study of corrosion casts. *J Anat*, 185, 369–376.
129. Spencer JA, Ferraro F, Roussakis E, *et al.* (2014). Direct measurement of local oxygen concentration in the bone marrow of live animals. *Nature*, 508(7495), 269–273.
130. Stabley JN, Moningka NC, Behnke BJ, Delp MD (2014). Exercise training augments regional bone and marrow blood flow during exercise. *Med Sci Sports Exerc*, PMID 24658222.
131. Stern PH, Tatrai A, Semler DE, Lee SK, Lakatos P, Strielman PJ, *et al.* (1995). Endothelin receptors, second messengers and actions in bone. *J Nutr*, 125(Suppl7), 2028S–2032S.
132. Street J, Bao M, deGuzman I, Bunting S, Peale FV, Ferrara N, *et al.* (2002). Vascular endothelial growth factor stimulates bone repair by promoting angiogenesis and bone turnover. *Proc Natl AcadSci*, 99, 9656–9661.
133. Streeten EA, Brandi ML (1990). Biology of bone endothelial cells. *Bone Miner*, 10, 85–94.
134. Tami AE, Schaffler MB, Knothe Tate ML (2003). Probing the tissue to subcellular level structure underlying bone's molecular sieving function. *Biorheology*, 40, 577.
135. Tondevold E, Eriksen J, Jansen E (1979) Observations on long bone medullary pressure in relation to mean arterial blood pressure in the anaesthetised dog. *Acta Orthop Scand*, 50, 527–531.
136. Tothill P, MacPherson JN (1986). The distribution of blood flow to the whole skeleton in dogs, rabbits and rats measured with microspheres. *ClinPhysPhysiolMeas*, 7, 117–123.
137. Trias A, Fery A (1979). Cortical circulation in long bones. *J Bone Joint Surg*, 61, 1052–1059.

138. Trueta J (1963). The role of the vessels in osteogenesis. *J Bone Joint Surg*, 45-B, 402–418.
139. Trueta J (1974). Blood supply and the rate of healing of tibial fractures. *Clin Orthop Relat Res*, 105, 11–19.
140. Trueta J, Cavadias AX (1964). A study of the blood supply of long bones. *Surg Gynecol Obstet*, 118, 485–489.
141. Turner CH (1999). Site-specific skeletal effects of exercise: Importance of interstitial fluid pressure. *Bone*, 24, 161–162.
142. Urbaniak JR, Seaber AV, Chen LE (1997). Assessment of ischaemia and reperfusion injury. *Clin Orthop Relat Res*, 334, 30–36.
143. Van't Hof RJ, Ralston SH (2001). Nitric oxide and bone. *Immunology*, 103, 255–262.
144. Vu TH, Shipley JM, Bergers G, Berger JE, Helms JA, Hanahan D *et al.* (1998). MMP-9/gelatinase B is a key regulator of growth plate angiogenesis and apoptosis of hypertrophic chondrocytes. *Cell*, 93, 411–422.
145. Vukelic L, Sosa I, Cvijanovic O (2011). Correlation of endothelin-1 mRNA expression and bone structure in advanced osteoarthritis. *Med Hypoth*, 77, 927–929.
146. Wallace AL, Draper ERC, Strachan RK, McCarthy ID, Hughes SPF (1991). The effect of devascularisation upon early bone healing in dynamic external fixation. *J Bone Joint Surg*, 73-B, 819–825.
147. Wallace AL, Draper ERC, Strachan RK, McCarthy ID, Hughes SPF (1994). The vascular response to fracture micromovement. *Clin Orthop Relat Res*, 301, 281–290.
148. Wang B, Zhou X, Price C, Li W, Pan J, Wang L (2013). Quantifying load-induced solute transport and solute-matrix interactions within the osteocyte lacunar-canalicular system. *J Bone Miner Res*, 28, 1075–1086.
149. Wang L, Fritton SP, Weinbaum S, Cowin SC (2003). On bone adaptation to venous stasis. *J Biomech*, 36, 1439–1451.
150. Wang Z, Kristianto J, Ooi CY, *et al.* (2013). Blood pressure, artery size and artery compliance parallel bone size and strength in mice with differing Ece1 expression. *J Biomed Eng*, 35, 061003–3.
151. Welch RD, Johnston CE, Waldron MJ, Poteet B (1993). Bone changes associated with intraosseous hypertension in the caprine tibia. *J. Bone Joint Surg*. 75-A, 53–60.
152. Wilkes CH, Visscher MB (1975). Some physiological aspects of bone marrow pressure. *J Bone Joint Surg*, 57A, 49–57.
153. Willans SM (1989). Modelling in the analysis of ion exchange between blood and bone. PhD Thesis. University of Edinburgh.
154. Wimalawansa SJ (2007). Rationale for using nitric oxide donor therapy for prevention of bone loss and treatment of osteoporosis in humans. *Ann NY AcadSci*, 1117, 283–297.
155. Winet H (1996). The role of microvasculature in normal and perturbed bone healing as revealed by intravital microscopy. *Bone*, 19, 39S—57S.

156. Winet H, Bao JY, Moffat R (1990). Neo-osteogenesis of haversion trabeculae through a bone chamber implanted in a rabbit tibial cortex. *CalcifTissInt*, 47, 24–34.
157. Zhong X, Wang H, Huang S (2014). Endothelin-1 induces interleukin-18 expression in human osteoblasts. *Arch Oral Biol*, 59, 289–296.
158. Zhou Z, Apte SS, Soininen R, Cao R, Baaklini GY, Rauser RW, *et al.* (2000). Impaired endochondral ossification and angiogenesis in mice deficient in membrane-trype matrix metalloproteinase 1. *Proc Natl AcadSci*, 97, 4052–4057.
159. Zhu K, Jiao H, Li S, Cao H, Galson DR, Zhoa Z, *et al.* (2013). ATF4 promotes bone angiogenesis by increasing VEGF expression and release in the bone environment. *J. Bone Miner Res*, 28, 1870–1884.

CHAPTER 2

MOLECULAR TRANSPORT IN MUSCULOSKELETAL HEALTH AND DISEASE

MELISSA L. KNOTHE TATE

Professor, Graduate School of Biomedical Engineering
University of New South Wales, Sydney, Australia

ROY K. AARON

Professor of Orthopaedic Surgery
The Warren Alpert Medical School of Brown University, Providence, RI

ANITA IGNATIUS

Professor and Director, Institute of Orthopaedic
Research and Biomechanics, Ulm University, Germany

LUTZ DÜRSELEN

Professor, Institute of Orthopaedic Research and Biomechanics
Ulm University, Germany

STAN ROCKSON

Professor, Department of Cardiology
Stanford University School of Medicine, Palo Alto, CA

Cells are the living inhabitants of our organs and tissues. The layout of our organs, tissues, and their respective inhabitant cells shows the cumulative processes of patterning during development, growth, and aging, as well as the stochastic processes of proliferation and cell death throughout life. In this context, the arrangement of cells in space and in time reflects their life history. In addition, the spatiotemporal arrangement of cells provides an indicator of current and future health of our tissues and organs at any given point in time. As a fundamental tenet of surgery, cell viability depends upon the presence of patent vascular networks in cells' respective tissues and organs. Also, cells themselves provide intra- and peri-cellular communication networks across and between tissue compartments. The capacity for our tissues and organs to adapt and heal requires efficient communication between and through these cellular networks. Yet crosstalk between these networks is poorly understood. As the literally hardest tissue in the body, bone serves as the most technically challenging, exemplary model system to address this complex theme.

2.1 Introduction

Bone exhibits multiscale communication networks among osteocytes based upon the movement of pericellular fluid, ions, and nutrients through canaliculi and functional matrix pores that may serve regulatory functions to intracellular communication. In these networks, bone exhibits a molecular sieving function, effectively using different pathways to move fluid and solutes of various sizes and charge through the tissue. In a real sense, this represents an extravascular microcirculation of pericellular fluid in bone. Other tissues in and around joints participate in this fluid-based communication network.

At organ, tissue, cell, and molecular length scales, bone provides more surface area for transport of fluid and exchange and filtering of solutes, to and from the vascular and lymphatic systems, than any other organ in the body. Furthermore, barrier function is intrinsic to the maintenance of distinct, yet juxtaposed physiological environments at surfaces separating the interior and exterior milieuof bone. Addressing novel, paired computational and experimental approaches to link fluid and solute flux between different length scales in bone underscores the key role of vascular and extravascular flow in bone cells' dual role as tissue inhabitants and prototypers.

After first exemplifying experimental and computational approaches to understand molecular transport in bone, analogous approaches are then applied to the more complex, higher length scale tissue system of the knee joint. Cutting edge imaging and modeling methods are used to understand the interplay of exercise and molecular transport in the various compartments of the knee joint. These insights are finally taken to the highest length scale to understand how exercise may modulate molecular transport and communication within the organism.

2.2 Cells' Dual Role as Tissue Inhabitants and Prototypers

Cells not only generate the extracellular matrix (ECM) comprising tissues but also are the living inhabitants of the tissues that make up the organs of the human body. In short, our cells are the living component of our physical structure. Their health state is reflected in the health status of our tissues and joints and vice versa.[20,22,23] "Cells are [also] natural tissue builders,"[22] giving our tissues and organs the capacity to heal.

The integration of cell activity enables not only healing, but also tissue remodeling, and adaptation to changes in function such as mechanical loading or disuse. Although the cellular mechanisms underlying processes of healing and tissue remodeling are complex and not yet fully understood, the integration of cell activity depends on patent cellular machinery and thus cellular health. The integration also depends on cellular communication enabling navigation and coordinated activity, which in turn depend on tissue and organism health. The pericellular network provides an immediate conduit for transfer of information between cells and their matrix, as well as the vascular, lymphatic, and immune systems, which serve as bridges for further crosstalk between the tissues and organs comprising the integrated organism.[14,17,19–25]

2.3 Between Cells, Across Tissues and Organs: Molecular Transport is Central to Musculoskeletal Health and Disease

Cellular connectivity derives from prenatal developmental processes where "everything is connected from day one." Through pruning and honing of these connections, as well as through establishment and remodeling of cell-cell and cell-matrix adhesions, transport of information between cells, tissues, and organs, the musculoskeletal system takes on a higher level architecture, reflective of the boundaries of specific tissue types including muscle, bone, cartilage, meniscus, ligament, tendon, etc., all interacting with the vascular and lymphatic systems which provide major transport pathways for molecular communication.[22]

In each respective tissue of the musculoskeletal system, the pericellular fluid provides a medium through which environmental information, including mechanical forces, chemical gradients, and electrical impulses, are transmitted between and around cells, resulting in up- or down-regulation of gene expression.[14,17,19–25] Delineated by the structural network of cells, which in themselves allow for direct cell-to-cell signal transmission across tissues via intracellular signaling,[19] the contiguous pericellular fluid provides a powerful extracellular means to transfer information and modulate cellular activity. There is great impetus to elucidate the fluid environment of cells, as this knowledge could provide key insights into the mechanisms of cellular navigation and coordination during tissue remodeling and healing.

At the same time, the pericellular fluid environment abuts and is thus interdependent on the state of the solid mechanical elements of tissues, as mechanical loading of tissue causes pericellular fluid to move, much like the fluid moves when a saturated sponge is squeezed.[5,17,26] This interplay is particularly germane to the fluid environment and the structural elements of the respective tissues of the musculoskeletal system.

2.4 Approaching Molecular Transport in Musculoskeletal Health and Disease: Bone as a Case Study

Permeability through the micro- and nanoscale pericellular fluid network provides a quantitative measure of the tissue's capacity for information transfer, e.g., transport of signals and molecules via the interstitial fluid network.[16,23,31,38] Experimental measurements as well as computational predictions of tissue permeability are challenging due to the remote location of cells and their networks. Nonetheless, the state of the ECM, and in particular the extracellular or pericellular space, is recognized as a common means by which different cells from tissues as diverse as brain,[35] cartilage,[1,32,34] meniscus,[40] lymphatic tissue,[46] and bone[3] modulate and perceive their local environment.

Permeability can be predicted computationally using virtual models of cellular networks. This approach is particularly helpful to predict cellular transport efficiency across tissues and organs. Alternatively, recently developed novel rapid prototyping methods allow for measurement of permeability based on application of classical fluid dynamics to rapid prototyped physical models of pericellular networks.[23] Using state-of-the-art confocal microscopy, it is possible to get precise three-dimensional (3D), anatomical renderings of the nano-micro scale pericellular fluid space.

These data sets are then input into rapid prototyping machines, like 3D printers, to create scaled-up (by 1000x) physical models of the respective cellular networks. According to classical fluid dynamics, measurements made on these scaled-up systems yield accurate measurements of the actual microscopic system if the fluid viscosity is scaled up analogously when carrying out the experimental measures. In this way, unprecedented experimental permeability measures can be made on physical models of actual pericellular networks.

Bone tissue exhibits molecular sieving characteristics similar to the glomerulus of the kidney, where different calibers of porosity within bone, including macroscopic, vascular, pericellular, and intrinsic matrix porosity, allow for size- and charge-dependent penetration.[43] The spatial distribution and density of blood vessels and different caliber porosities, as well as intrinsic matrix properties of bone tissue, modulate interstitial fluid flow direction and magnitude and thus spatiotemporal transport properties within the organ bone.[6,41,43]

Using *in vivo* fluorescent probes of specific size and charge, the molecular sieving characteristics of bone tissue have been characterized in unloaded and mechanically loaded states. Molecules larger than approximately 67 kDa, comparable to albumin, the most prevalent carrier protein in the blood, are not transported efficiently in unloaded bone. Furthermore, application of controlled mechanical loads using a mechanical testing machine to mimic loads incurred during physiological activities, augments molecular transport through bone via load-induced fluid displacement. Specifically, using a mechanical tester to compress the forelimb of the anaesthetized rat, a fluorescent tracer is shifted from the intramedullary canal to the outside surface of the bone, with a preponderance of tracer in the periosteum after loading.[43] These studies demonstrate the effect of load-induced fluid displacements in bone from areas of higher to areas of lower pressure, much like squeezing of a saturated sponge. However, unlike a sponge that has rather permeable outside surfaces, periosteum bounds all non-articular bone surfaces.[6]

While the periosteum has often been assumed to be an impermeable boundary to bone surfaces, recent studies demonstrate the periosteum's functional barrier properties. Of particular interest for orthopaedics, at high flow rates comparable to traumatic impact loads or intramedullary reaming, periosteum exhibits increased permeability with significantly higher permeability in the bone to muscle direction than vice versa. Similarly, if the intrinsic prestress of periosteum is disrupted, e.g., through periosteal lifting or transplantation, its intrinsic permeability increases significantly and the directional-dependent characteristics dissipate.[6]

In addition, recent studies of human periosteum-derived cells demonstrate the expression of zona occludens or tight junction proteins.[7] Tight junctions between cells confer active control of molecular transport across functional barrier tissues including the blood brain barrier, the lining of the gut and lung, and the tubules of the kidney.[2,12,35] It is quite exciting to consider that bone, which provides more surface area for transport of fluid and exchange and filtering of solutes, to and from the vascular and lymphatic systems, than any other organ in the body, is bound by a functional barrier membrane that modulates molecular transport across boundaries interfacing with multiple other organ systems (blood, lymph, bone marrow, muscle, ligament, tendon).[18]

Taken together, scaled physical models and predictive virtual and stochastic computational models can be used in parallel to determine the effect of cell connectivity and transport across tissues. In this way, they provide a quantitative measure of signal transmission efficiency between cells and across tissues, as demonstrated in this case study of bone. The approach translates rapidly to other bone tissue architectures, in health and disease. For example, one can imagine applying a similar approach to understand transport in trabecular bone of the long bone metaphyses or the cranium.

2.5 Looking into the Future: Molecular Transport in Joint Health and Disease

Applied at a higher length scale, an analogous approach may yield new insights into molecular communication between different tissues and their respective cellular networks, e.g., comprising the total joint.

2.5.1 *Current state of the art and hurdles to discovery*

Similar to the understanding of bone fluid dynamics, a current stumbling block in understanding articular joint physiology in health, or clinical restoration of joint function after trauma, disease, and/or aging, is a lack of understanding of the transport mechanisms to and from the cells that constitute the living component of articular joint tissues, including cartilage, meniscus, synovium, and ligament. No longer considered to be an issue of cartilage wear and tear alone, osteoarthritis is increasingly recognized as resulting from a breakdown in cellular communication in tissues making up the complex joint architecture.

Just as in bone tissue, molecular transport among tissues of the joint provides an efficient means for communication between the cells and across tissues. Transport in, for example, cartilage, bone, meniscus, and ligament tissue has been the subject of numerous studies, yet it is surprising how few current studies address transport to and from these tissues, via the vascular system, between the bounding surfaces, or within the matrix of these respective tissues. Furthermore, the role of lymphatics in balancing transport between and across bounding membranes of these respective musculoskeletal tissues is completely unknown. This lack of knowledge may reflect contemporary subspecialization of scientific inquiry; yet it remains surprising, particularly considering the putative interactions between the tissues comprising the complex joint structure and given the significant, untapped potential of an integrative approach.

"Clinical osteoarthritis is a common final pathway secondary to many predisposing factors, most notably age, joint trauma, altered biomechanics, and obesity"[42] and is the leading cause of disability in aging adults. Loss of joint structure and function with age involves complex interactions among tissues, including cartilage, bone, meniscus, ligaments, and synovium, which together make up the complex architecture of synovial joints. It is currently not known how molecules are transported from the blood, to and between different tissue compartments within synovial joints. The beneficial effect of exercise on aging joints is also not well understood, as it appears to exert a protective effect on joint surfaces, in contrast to expected increases in wear and tear and thus joint destruction.[37,45]

As suggested by Maroudas,[34] the ECM of cartilage exhibits filtration properties and the composition of cartilage in health and disease could effectively shift the balance between transport of matrix-degrading proteolytic enzymes (of molecular weights less than 50 kDa) and their inhibitors that are transported via the blood and are "too large to penetrate into normal cartilage." Follow-on studies support this hypothesis, with an observed increase in cartilage permeability after treatment with a combination of the extracellular proteases cathepsin K (37 kDa) and collagenase (collagenase type II molecular weight is 68 kDa) but not with collagenase alone.[33] In both cartilage and bone, convective (flow-dependent) transport of interstitial fluid has been shown to augment molecular transport through tissue,[10,13,15,34,39,41,43,44] in particular enabling transport of diffusion transport-limited molecular sizes between 10 kDa and 70 kDa.[34,43] Finally, accounting for the combination of matrix binding and convective flux, "autologous... gradients" of "morphogenetic and chemotactic proteins" may enable "cells to create their own chemotactic gradients" that may modulate cellular traffic into and out of the lymphatic system.[8]

It is currently unknown whether the bounding layers of bone and cartilage (periosteum, subchondral bone, synovium) actively modulate transport into and out of tissue compartments of the joint and musculoskeletal system. The expression of ZO-1 proteins by periosteal cells[6,7] may implicate tight junctions as a means to control permeability across the periosteum, the outer bounding envelope of all bone surfaces not covered in cartilage. Furthermore, a recent study implicates the relative balance of two tight cell-cell adhesion architectures ("zippers" that seal surfaces and "buttons" that enable controlled opening of tight junctions and infiltration of lymph when pulled mechanically) as a putative means to control relative drainage of interstitial fluid via the lymphatic system, in particular during development, and during (patho)physiological processes.[46] The relative contributions of arterial and venous circulation, as well as the lymphatic circulation, to interstitial flow and molecular transport in the tissues of the musculoskeletal system are not clearly delineated.

In addition, diffusion and convection are putative transport mechanisms to and from avascular articular joint cartilage tissue,[39,41,44] although several studies have postulated the presence of small channels that physically link cartilage to the subchondral bone interface.[4] Assessment of the transport to/from and between tissue compartments via blood and interstitial fluid flow necessitates the use of an imaging modality that allows for seamless imaging of transport across organ, tissue, cellular, and molecular length scales.[9,27,31]

2.5.2 *New coupled imaging and modeling approaches*

To date, imaging modalities, including intravital imaging and high resolution multiphoton imaging, have not addressed the open questions, outlined above, in an integrated fashion, or across and between tissue compartments of the joint and length and time scales. Recent advances in *in situ* imaging of structure and function across length scales and at high spatial and temporal resolution present a unique opportunity to address this significant clinical problem.[9,27,31] Through unprecedented integration of technology and interdisciplinary approaches, molecular communication in the complex organ of a given joint can be elucidated, crossing not only disciplinary boundaries but also boundaries between tissues making up the complex knee joint.

New, cutting edge imaging methods allow for seamless imaging, from organ to tissue to cells and back, and temporal imaging during loading.[26–29] For instance, recent guinea pig studies reveal surprising findings with regard to molecular sieving properties of the respective tissues of the knee joint. Using high resolution episcopic block face imaging methods, where serial sections of cryopreserved knees are imaged and then reconstructed in 3D, it appears that the respective tissues of the knee separate molecules, delivered as a single mixed bolus to the heart, according to molecular size. In addition, the relative paucity of fluorescent molecules in muscle tissue surrounding the distal and proximal halves of the femur and knee, respectively, implicate transport from the bone to the muscle in absence of muscle pumping (the guinea pigs remain anaesthetized until the time of tissue resection).[26–29]

Longitudinal studies, including pharmaceutical and/or exercise interventions, will allow for elucidation of specific factors that may serve to prevent, reverse, or slow progression of osteoarthritis in the future. Such an approach necessitates both the capacity to apply controlled mechanical loads to the joint while imaging of molecular transport over time as well as the capacity to predict the relationship between exercise, molecular transport, and disease onset/progression/abatement.

A further new scanning electron imaging modality has enabled the first rapid throughput "Google Maps"-type images of the human hip joint, where connectivity of cells and their vascular networks can be viewed from the nanometer length scale to that of the entire hip.[30] In combination, these imaging and modeling technologies will provide a new lens through which to gain insight into multi-length and time scale structure-function relationships, within and between tissue compartments of the joint, via the venous, articular, and lymphatic systems, as well as the role of exercise and aging on molecular transport and joint physiology. In turn, these studies will provide a platform from which to promote joint health by harnessing the natural structure-function relationships of bone, cartilage, synovium, menisci, and muscle structural and fluid transport pathways.

2.6 Discussion and Future Directions

Taken to the highest length scale (the entire organism), we ultimately aim to understand how exercise (organism mobility, movement of the entire musculoskeletal system) modulates molecular transport and communication within the organismal system, for the total "pumping power" of the musculoskeletal system is likely to exceed that of the human heart. This will only be possible through a collaborative, transdisciplinary approach that leverages cutting edge imaging and modeling approaches integrated with appropriate and robust animal models and in cognizance of current and future clinical standards of care.

References

1. Alexopoulos LG, Setton LA, Guilak F (2005). The biochemical role of the chondrocyte pericellular matrix in articular cartilage. *ActaBiomater*, 1, 317–325.
2. Al-Sadi R, Boivin M, Ma T (2009). Mechanism of cytokine modulation of epithelial tight junction barrier. *Front Biosci* (landmark ed.), 14, 2765–2778.
3. Anderson EJ, *et al.* (2008). Pairing computational and scaled physical models to determine permeability as a measure of cellular communication in micro- and nano-scale pericellular spaces. *MicrofluNanoflu*, 4, 193–204.
4. Arkill KP, Winlove, CP (2008). Solute transport in the deep and calcified zones of articular cartilage. *Osteoarthritis Cartilage*, 16, 708–714.
5. Biot MA (1941). General theory of three-dimensional consolidation. *J Appl Phys*, 12, 155–164.
6. Evans S, *et al.* (2013). Periosteum, bone's "smart" bounding membrane, exhibits direction dependent permeability. *J Bone Miner Res*, 28(3), 608–617.
7. Evans S, *et al.* (2013). Solid-supported lipid bilayers as a novel platform to engineer emergence of stem cell fate and tissue architecture using periosteum derived progenitor cells, *Biomaterials*, 34, 1878–1887.
8. Fleury ME, Boardman KC, Swartz MA (2006). Autologous morphogen gradients by subtle interstitial flow and matrix interactions. *Biophys J*, 91, 113–121.
9. Freutel M, *et al.* (2013). Medial meniscal displacement and strain in three dimensions under compressive loads: MR assessment. *JMagnReson Imaging*, doi: 10.1002/jmri.24461.
10. Garcia AM, *et al.* (1996). Contributions of fluid convection and electrical migration to transport in cartilage: Relevance to loading. *Arch Biochem Biophys*, 333, 317–325.
11. Huber JD, Egleton RD, Davis TP (2001). Molecular physiology and pathophysiology of tight junctions in the blood-brain barrier. *Trends Neurosci*, 24, 719–725.
12. Knothe Tate ML (1997). Theoretical and experimental study of load-induced fluid flow phenomena in compact bone. PhD thesis, ETH (Swiss Federal Institute of Technology), Zurich.
13. Knothe Tate ML, Knothe U, Niederer P (1998). Experimental elucidation of mechanical load-induced fluid flow and its role in bone metabolism and functional adaptation, *Am J MedSci*, 316, 189–195.
14. Knothe Tate ML, Niederer P, Knothe U (1998). In vivo tracer transport through the lacunocanalicular system of rat bone in an environment devoid of mechanical loading. *Bone*, 22, 107–117.

15. Knothe Tate ML, Knothe U (2000). An ex vivo model to address transport processes and fluid flow in loaded bone. *J Biomech*, 33, 247–254.
16. Knothe Tate ML (2001). Interstitial fluid flow. In:Cowin SC, ed., *Bone Biomechanics Handbook*. New York: CRC Press.
17. Knothe Tate ML, Tami AEG, Bauer TW, Knothe U (2002). Micropathoanatomy of osteoporosis: Indications for a cellular basis of bone disease, *Adv Osteopor Fract Manage*, 2, 9–14.
18. Knothe Tate ML (2003). "Whither flows the fluid in bone?": An osteocyte's perspective, *J Biomech*, 36, 1409–1424.
19. Knothe Tate ML, *et al.* (2004). Cells in focus: The osteocyte. *Int J Biochem Cell Biol*, 36, 1–8.
20. Knothe Tate ML (2007). Multi-scale computational engineering of bones. In: Bronner F, Farach-Carson C, Mikos A, eds., *State of the Art Insights for the Future:Engineering of Functional Skeletal Tissues*. London: Springer Verlag, 141–160.
21. Knothe Tate, ML, *et al.* (2008). Mechanical modulation of osteochondroprogenitor cell fate, *Int J Biochem Cell Biol*, 40, 2720–2738.
22. Knothe Tate ML, Falls T, Atit R (2010). Engineering an ecosystem: Taking cues from nature's paradigm to build tissue in the lab and the body. *Fields Institute for Mathematics in Biology monograph series on New Perspectives in Mathematical Biology*, 57, 113–134.
23. Knothe Tate ML, Niederer P (2010). Computational modeling of extravascular fluid flow in bone. In:Suvranu D, Farshid G, Mohammad M, eds., *Computational Methods in Biomechanics*. Springer Verlag.
24. Knothe Tate ML, Tami A, Netrebko P, Milz S, Docheva D (2012). Multiscale computational and experimental approaches to elucidate musculoskeletal and ligament mechanobiology using the ulna-radius-interosseous membrane construct as a model system. *Tech Health Care*, 20, 363–378.
25. Knothe Tate ML, Aaron R, Knothe U, Zeidler D, Milz S (2014). Elucidating bone structure and function across length and time scales. Gordon Research Conference on Bones and Teeth, Galveston, January 2014.
26. Knothe Tate ML, Herynck B, Aaron R (2014). Meniscal, cartilage and subchondralbone tissue of the guinea pig knee joint exhibit molecular size selectivity after single bolus of intravitaltracer injection. Transactions of the Orthopaedic Research Society, New Orleans, March 2014.
27. Knothe Tate ML, Aaron R, Knothe U, Zeidler D, Milz S, Saidel G (2014). Hand-in-hand across length scales: Imaging and modeling of structure and function. Seventh World Congress of Biomechanics, Boston.
28. Knothe Tate ML, Zeidler D, Knothe U, Aaron R, Kark L (2014). Will seamless imaging across length scales enable modeling of multiscale structure-function relationships? IMAG MSM Consortium Meeting, NIH Bethesda.
29. Knothe Tate ML, *et al.* (2015). Engineering and commercialization of human-device interfaces, from bone to brain. *Sci Transl Med*, (in press).
30. Knothe U, *et al.* (2015). Rapid throughput, seamless imaging of human hip joint tissue across length scales to elucidate emergent structure-function

relationships. Transactions of the Orthopedic Research Society, Las Vegas, 40, 1121.

31. Korhonen RK, *et al.* (2006). Collagen network of articular cartilage modulates fluid flow and mechanical stresses in chondrocyte. *Biomech Model Mechanobiol*, 5, 150–159.
32. Lotke PA, Granda JL (2005). Alterations in the permeability of articular cartilage by proteolytic enzymes. *Arthritis Rheum*, 15, 302–308.
33. Maroudas A (1976). Transport of solutions through cartilage: Permeability to large molecules. *J Anat*, 122, 335–347.
34. Mitchell LA, *et al.* (2011). Differential effects of claudin-3 and claudin-4 on alveolar epithelial barrier function. *Am J Physiol Lung Cell Mol Physiol*, 301, L40–L49.
35. Nicholson C, Tao L (1993). Hindered diffusion of high molecular weight compounds in brain extracellular microenvironment measured with integrative optical imaging. *Biophys J*, 65, 2277–2290.
36. Penninx BWJH, *et al.* (2001). Physical exercise and the prevention of disability in activities of daily living in older persons with osteoarthritis. *Arch Intern Med*, 161, 2309–2316.
37. Piekarski K, Munro M (1977). Transport mechanism operating between blood supply and osteocytes in long bones. *Nature*, 269, 80–82.
38. Quinn TM, Kocian P, Meister JJ (2000). Static compression is associated with decreased diffusivity of dextrans in cartilage explants. *Arch Biochem Biophys*, 384, 327–334.
39. Sanchez-Adams J, Wilusz RE, Guilak F (2013). Atomic force microscopy reveals regional variations in the micromechanical properties of the pericellular and extra cellular matrices of the meniscus. *J Orthop Res*, 31, 1218–1225.
40. Shafieyan Y, *et al.* (2014). Diffusion of MRI and CT contrast agents in articular cartilage under static compression. *Biophys J*, 107, 485–492.
41. Sokolove J, Lepus CM (2013). Role of inflammation in the pathogenesis of osteoarthritis: Latest findings and interpretations. *Ther Adv Musculoskelet Dis*, 5, 77–94.
42. Tami A, Schaffler MB, Knothe Tate ML (2003). Probing the tissue to subcellular level structure underlying bone's molecular sieving function. *Biorheology*, 40, 577–590.
43. Torzilli PA, *et al.* (1983). Movement of interstitial water through loaded articular cartilage. *J Biomech*, 16, 169–179.
44. Valderrabano V, Steiger C (2011). Treatment and prevention of osteoarthritis through exercise and sports. *J Aging Res*, Article ID 374653.
45. Yao LC, *et al.* (2012). Plasticity of button-like junctions in the endothelium of airway lymphatics in development and inflammation. *Am J Pathol*, 180, 2561–2575.
46. mechbio.org, last accessed on May 10, 2015.

Part 2

Techniques of Measurement of Bone Circulation

CHAPTER 3

THE MICROSPHERE METHOD FOR INVESTIGATING BONE BLOOD FLOW

HERMANN ANETZBERGER

Orthopädische Gemeinschaftspraxis am OEZ, Munich, Germany

CHRISTOF BIRKENMAIER

Department of Orthopaedics, Physical Medicine and Rehabilitation
Ludwig-Maximilian-University Munich, Grosshadern Campus,
Munich, Germany

Bone tissue possesses the particular capacity to adapt to prevalent mechanical stress during the entire life span.[108] This requires continuous bone remodeling, which in turn depends on an adequate supply of nutrients and oxygen via the vascular system. It would hence be expected, that pathological conditions that entail anabolic or catabolic processes of the skeleton (e.g., fracture healing, osteoporosis, chronic regional pain syndrome, osteonecrosis, and arthrosis) would result in alterations of bone blood flow.

In 1691, the Englishman Clopton Havers described how blood vessels enter long bones and, once inside, subdivide into the bone marrow. He theorized at that time that the contraction of small glands inside the bone marrow releases a nutritional fluid, which then is distributed inside the bone by means of small canals.[47] These canals soon became known as Haversian canals.

However, despite the fact that the importance of blood supply for bone growth and bone healing was already established by the 19th century, it would take another 100 years for knowledge about the vascular architecture of bone to be significantly augmented.

The introduction of new methods such as the Spalteholz technique,[91] microangiography[57,100] by means of injection with Indian ink,[18] or the injection of plastics[109] allowed for a detailed investigation of the arterial and venous blood supply as well as of the capillary system of bone. The arterial supply of long bones is comprised of several vascular systems. In the diaphyseal region, one or two nutritional arteries enter the bone via the nutritional foramina. They subdivide and supply predominantly the diaphyseal bone and the bone marrow.[19] Inside the marrow, the nutritional arteries form a sinusoid capillary network.[98] In the metaphyseal and epiphyseal regions of a long bone, multiple arteries of varying caliber enter from the periarticular vascular network also by means of canals.[2,79,99]

During growth, the physis forms a barrier between these two capillary systems, whereas after the completion of growth, multiple anastomoses are formed. This leads to epiphyseal and meta-physeal arteries providing up to 40% of a long bone's perfusion. They supply the subchondral plate, the subarticular trabeculae and the cancellous bone of the metaphysis.[98,99] Periosteal vessels also contribute to bone vascular supply by mainly perfusing the cortical bone and by forming anastomoses with vessels from the marrow space.[28,99] Within the bone tissue, blood vessels run within the Haversian canals and within the Volkmann canals with both of these systems being interconnected.[37] Within the marrow space, the capillary network consists of sinusoid vessels (analog to the liver sinusoids) that drain into collecting veins. From these, the venous blood is carried via so-called emissary veins that penetrate the bone cortex in immediate proximity to a nutritional artery.[28,99] The venous blood from the epiphysis and metaphysis is regionally collected and drained via epi- and metaphyseal veins. The periosteal venous complex is connected to the collecting vein as well as to intramuscular and interfascicular veins. Fig. 3.1 schematically displays the blood supply of a long bone.

Knowledge of bone hemodynamics is essential for the understanding of physiological and pathological processes.[65] This is underscored by the fact that under physiological conditions, total skeletal perfusion reaches 10% of cardiac output (CO) in rabbits.[1,88] It is the goal of this chapter to provide an overview of the current knowledge of bone perfusion with specific consideration of the microsphere method.

3.1 The Microsphere Method

Whereas the vascular architecture of bone in general is well understood, there are only few experimental studies that examine intraosseushemodynamics. One reason for this situation lies in the considerable technical

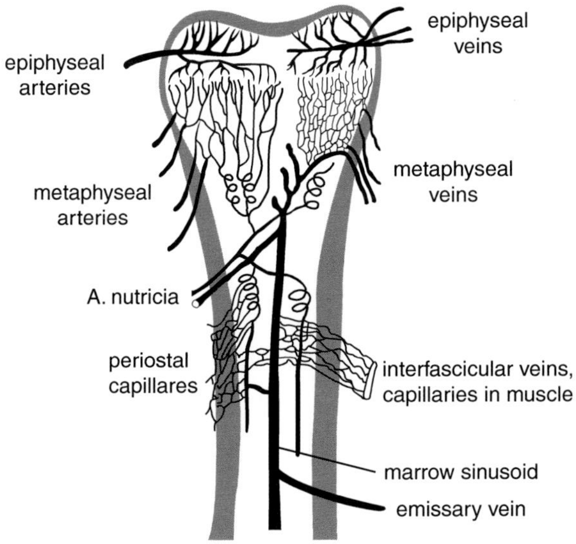

Fig. 3.1. Vascular organization of a long bone (according to Brookes, 1998).

difficulty in performing perfusion measurements within such a complex vascular architecture and within the dense bone tissue. The microsphere method (MS-method) probably represents the most suitable tool for the measurement of regional bone blood flow (RBBF). Rudolph and Heymann introduced the use of radioactive microspheres (RM) for the measurement of regional organ blood flow in 1967.[80] This method is based upon the principle that microspheres (MS) that were injected into the left ventricle are homogeneously distributed within the blood stream because of the turbulent flow within the ventricle. MS are distributed with the blood into the periphery and become lodged in the precapillary bed of all organs due to the larger diameter of microspheres than of the capillary vessels. Because of the homogenous distribution of the microspheres in the arterial blood, the number of MS within a certain tissue volume is proportional to the organ perfusion. About one year later, this method was improved upon by the addition of the technique of arterial reference sampling.[30,54,64,69] During and after the injection of the MS, arterial blood is sampled by means of a precision pump with a known withdrawal rate. As a result, a virtual reference organ with a known perfusion is generated. At the end of the experiment the number of MS in the reference blood samples and in the tissue samples were determined indirectly by counting the radioactivity or measuring the fluorescence intensity. The blood flow of the organ of interest can be calculated as follows:

$$\text{Blood Flow}_{\text{organ}} = \frac{\text{withdrawal rate}_{\text{Harward pump}} * \text{number MS}_{\text{organ sample}}}{\text{number MS}_{\text{reference sample}}} \tag{3.1}$$

The underlying principle is schematically explained in Fig. 3.2. Once this method had been introduced, regional blood flow was tested by means of RM for applicability and validated for various organs by a large number of experiments.[11, 22, 29, 64, 106] The radioactivity of the spheres entails several disadvantages. Beyond the health hazards for the laboratory personnel and considerable time consumption (continuous monitoring for radioactivity in the laboratory, proper disposal of contaminated experimental tissues),

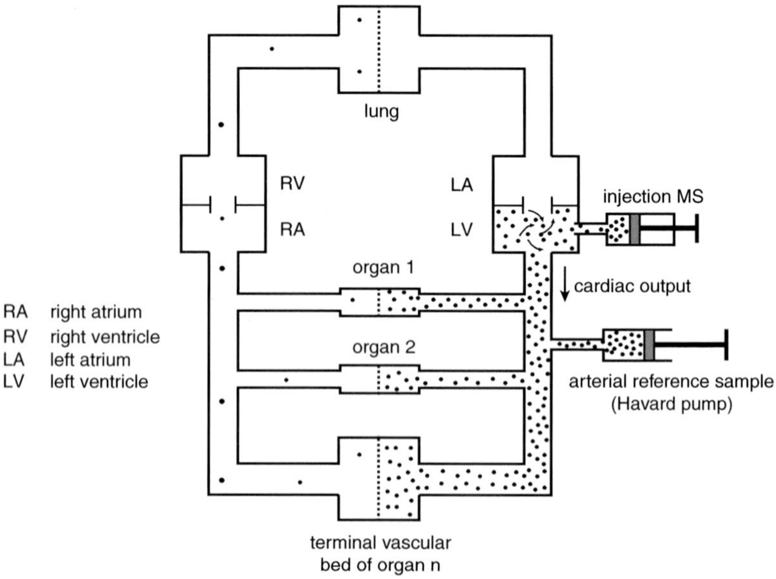

Fig. 3.2. Schematic drawing of the microsphere method.
Microspheres are injected into the left ventricle. Because of the turbulent flow, they will be homogenously distributed within the arterial blood. From the left ventricle, MS are traveling with the blood stream into the periphery and are trapped due to their bigger diameter in the capillary system. Only 1–4% of MS are shunting through the capillary bed, but become trapped in the capillary bed of the lung. During and after the injection of the spheres, arterial blood is sampled by means of a Harvard pump with a known withdrawal rate. Blood flow in an organ can then be calculated from the respective number of spheres contained in the organ and in the arterial reference sample.

the use of RM also is rather costly (approved laboratories, correct disposal of contaminated objects, special equipment for radioactivity monitoring).

Another disadvantage is the limited usability of RM in long-term experiments based on a short half-life of the employed isotopes and on the finding that isotopes may dissociate from the microspheres during the experiments and hence lead to erroneous results.[101]

These disadvantages implied a clear need for non-radioactive indicators to be used with such MS. Hale *et al.* introduced colored MS that led to valid measurements in comparison to RM.[43] Because of the toxicity of the solvent required to extract the dye from the MS and because of the high time consumption for the necessary processing, this technique in the end could not replace the RM method.

In 1993, Glenny *et al.* introduced fluorescent microspheres (FM) and validated these in comparison to RM.[38] The key advantage of FM lies in the fact that they exhibit a characteristic excitation and emission (light) spectrum, which in turn enables the exact determination of the intensity of each particular fluorescent dye by use of a fluorescence spectrophotometer. Initially, time consumption with this method was still comparatively high and methodical errors during sample processing proved to be another problem. In 1999, the Institute for Surgical Research at the LMU Munich was successful in developing a dedicated filtration system (sample processing unit: SPU), which allowed for a complete recovery of MS from blood and tissue samples.[74] Completely automated sample processing further increased precision and reliability of the FM method while at the same time drastically reducing the required time.[93] The superiority of the FM method versus colored MS or RM has since been established in numerous experiments on heart, lungs, kidneys, muscle, spleen, and brain[38, 72, 73, 83, 84, 94, 101] and eventually also in bone.[6–10]

The predominant advantages of using the MS method by means of FM as opposed to other techniques are:

- The measurement of RBBF can be performed minimally invasively and without direct manipulation of the bone itself.
- Heterogeneity of blood flow within a long bone can be studied.
- The absolute blood flow within an organ can be calculated by using arterial reference sampling, which in turn permits for the comparison of the blood flow between different regions of the same long bone and between right and left sides in paired bones.

- The use of the MS technique allows for the measurement of cardiac output (CO) during the injection, which is of relevance for the correct interpretation of the absolute blood flow values and can be calculated as:

$$\text{Cardiac output} = \frac{\text{withdrawal rate}_{\text{Harvard pump}} * \text{number MS}_{\text{injected}}}{\text{number MS}_{\text{reference sample}}} \tag{3.2}$$

- Methodological errors can easily be controlled for by simultaneously injecting two different microsphere species.
- The blood flow values of other organs can be determined simultaneously. Knowledge of blood flow in other organs like lung or kidneys is essential to exclude methodological errors due to inadequate mixing or shunting of the spheres.

The application of this method for measuring bone blood flow requires that its inherent limitations are well understood and that potential sources of error are excluded. In order to achieve highly precise and valid measurements, the following recommendations regarding experimental setup and error limitation should be followed:

- Aprerequisite for the valid application of the MS method is a homogenous distribution of the MS within the blood.[104] Injection of the MS into the left ventricle guarantees such a homogenous distribution because of the predominantly turbulent flow within the left ventricle.[16, 20, 22, 59] In our experiments, we ascertained a correct position of the injection catheter before each individual injection by means of obtaining the typical left ventricular pressure curve. A symmetrical distribution of MS between both kidneys can be used as an additional parameter because of the typically symmetrical perfusion of both kidneys.[16] In none of the experiments performed did we observe a difference between the blood flow values of the left and the right kidneys.
- Stochastic errors may occur because of too low a number of MS in tissue samples or in the arterial reference samples.[21, 22] The number of MS in a tissue sample is dependent upon the specific hemodynamic conditions, the regional organ blood flow, the size of the tissue samples, and the number of MS injected. Depending on sample size, in a rabbit at least 1 million MS per kg body weight (BW) should be used.[6] We developed a standardized dissection scheme for humerus, femur, and tibia in rabbits (Fig. 3.3) and we were able to demonstrate that most bone samples contained in excess of 400 MS. Only both femoral condyles, both distal

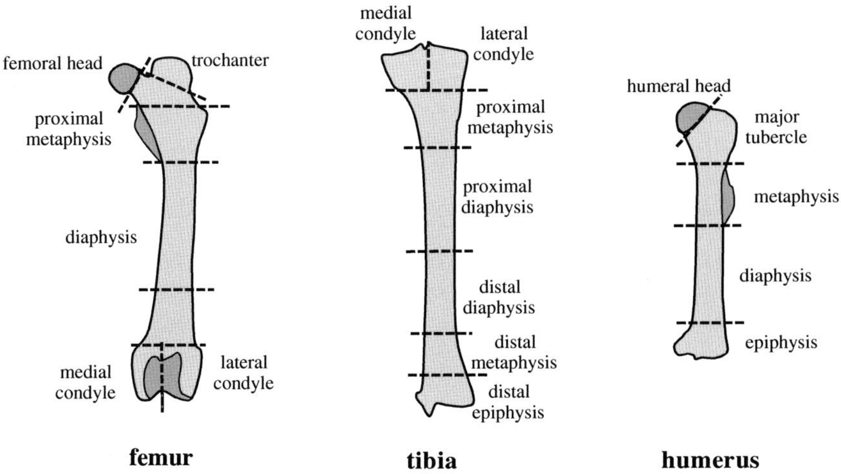

Fig. 3.3. Dissection scheme.

tibialdiaphyses and both distal tibialmetaphyses contained fewer MS, but still a minimum of 150 MS each, which according to other authors' results still yields reliable measurements.[71]

- Since the method is based on the principle that all injected MS are being lodged in the capillary bed of an organ, none or only a minimal proportion of these MS should reach the venous circulation by means of arterio-venous anastomoses. Should, in fact, a significant number of MS bypass the targeted capillary bed, an underestimation of the real bone perfusion would be the result. This potential source of error can be quantified independent of the MS diameter and by the determination of the so-called shunt rate. In bone, the shunt rate with MS with a diameter of 15 μm is typically between 1 and 4%.[39,41,42,45,46,66] Even though the shunt rate of MS with a diameter of 15 μm is low, recirculation from other organs such as the gastrointestinal tract or the soft tissue in general could lead to an overestimation of the real organ perfusion. Since MS with a diameter of 15 μm are typically completely caught in the lung's capillary bed, this source of error appears to be negligible.[11,54,104] An increase in lung perfusion with repeated measurements could therefore be an indirect indicator for a high shunt rate. We observed an increase in lung perfusion neither in short-term nor in long-term experiments despite an up to six-fold injection with 1×10^6 MS/kg BW, which also argues against the existence of a relevant shunting of MS.[10]

- The blood flow measurement of an organ depends significantly upon the hemodynamic situation at the moment of MS injection. Arterial pressure and CO therefore need to be known for a correct interpretation of the measured blood flow values and CO should be determined during the experiment.[11] The number of MS in the source suspension may vary after repeated aliquotingdespite adequate shaking, vortexing, and ultrasonication.[6] As a consequence, the specific number of MS injected should be measured from a separate reference aliquot for each injection.
- A potentially relevant influence of the injected MS upon the hemodynamic situation in the experimental animal has been investigated in numerous studies and was uniformly found to be nonexistent.[22,24,29,54,58,59] We observed no compromise of the macrohemodynamical parameters in any of our experiments despite injections of up to 21×10^6 MS/kg BW.[10]
- There also appears to be no appreciable compromise of the local bone microcirculation as a result of the partial embolization of the precapillary vascular bed. On the one hand, the total number of blocked capillaries remains very small. On the other hand, it has been shown in one study employing intravitalmicroscopy, that the embolization of arterioles and capillaries by MS leads to an immediate opening of collateral vessels, which renders a relevant effect of such embolizations onto the local microcirculation improbable.[44] We also observed a perfect consistency of results when employing simultaneous injection of MS for RBBF-measurements in short-term as well as in long-term experiments, virtually excluding a relevant effect of these embolizations upon the local hemodynamics.
- In order to reduce a systematic error induced by a loss of indicator dye during sample processing in our experiments, we utilized an automated robotic system with an SPU for the isolation of FM from tissue and blood samples.[74,93] In contrast to other organs, the usage of FM in bone requires a decalcification process to be used prior to further tissue processing. We have shown that such a decalcification process does not adversely affect the fluorescence characteristics of the FM.[6]
- Faulty arterial reference blood sampling also might be the source of a methodical error. Typically, such blood draws are performed via a catheter in the abdominal aorta, the carotid artery, or the auricular artery. The location of these catheters does not introduce a methodical error.[10,22,92] The reference blood draw must begin simultaneous to the MS injection and must be continued until oneminute after the end of the

MS injection.[11] When drawing more than three samples, we recommend a sampling speed of 1.76 ml/min, since above 3.54 ml/min, an influence on the macrohemodynamics is possible as a result of hypovolemia.

By means of validation studies, we have been able to establish the MS method using FM in combination with arterial reference blood draws as being a precise and reliable technique for measuring RBBF. The evaluation of methodological errors was performed under stable hemodynamicconditions[5] as well as under induced hypovolemia.[5] The mean methodological error (meanRD_{meth}) was calculated according to the method described by Zwissler *et al.*[112] from the absolute blood flow values (ml/min/100g) obtained by simultaneously injecting MS:

$$RD_{meth} = \frac{\text{standard deviation}}{\text{mean}} \tag{3.3}$$

$$\text{mean}RD_{meth} = \sqrt{\frac{\sum RD_{meth}^2}{n}}, \tag{3.4}$$

where n is number of tissue samples

$$RD_{meth} = \sqrt{\frac{1}{n}}, \tag{3.5}$$

where n is number of MS in tissue samples

$$RD_{meth}^2 = RD_{count}^2 + RD_{theo}^2, \tag{3.6}$$

where RD_{count} is measurement error.

For the use of FM, the methodological error was found to be $7.5 \pm 1.5\%$. The methodological error (RD_{meth}) consists of the theoretical error (RD_{theo}) and the measurement error (RD_{count}), which originates from the quantification of fluorescence or radioactivity, respectively. The theoretical error was comparable for all types of MS. The real measurement error (composed of the methodical and the theoretical errors) was lowest with the use of FM ($3.6 \pm 3.2\%$) as compared to RM ($5.7 \pm 4.7\%$). Since the absolute number of MS in different body regions varies dependent on tissue volume and blood flow, the methodical error (RD_{meth}) pertaining to each tissue sample was calculated against the number of MS in the tissue sample. The upper limit of the 95% confidence interval (CI) of the coefficient of variation was 9.6% for bone samples containing between 151 and 250 MS for both, FM and RM. When tissue samples contained more than 384 MS per sample, the upper limit of the 95% CI was at 6.2% for FM (Fig. 3.4) and at 8.6% for RM.

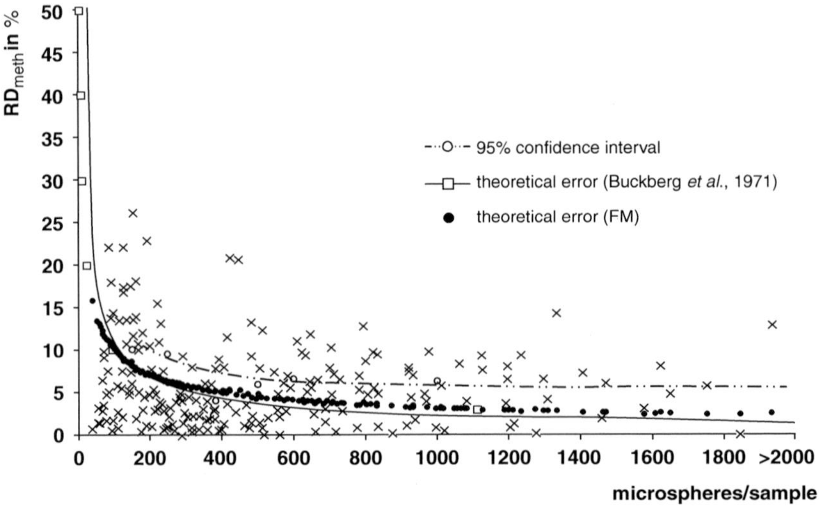

Fig. 3.4. Methodological error of the FM method is dependent of the number of MS within the tissue sample ($n = 240$). The x-axis shows the number of MS per sample whereas the y-axis shows the mean methodical error in percent. In addition, the theoretical error (according to Buckberg *et al.*, 1971) as well as the real theoretical error and the lower limit of the 95% confidence interval are displayed.

In order to compare the *intra* methodological as well as the *inter* methodological reliability of the FMS method, we compared the blood flow values that were obtained by simultaneously injecting differently labeled MS according to the method of Bland and Altmann.[17] The comparison of simultaneously measured blood flow values yielded highly concordant results, under constant hemodynamic conditions as well as under hypotension.[7,8] In rabbits, valid measurements can be performed even after the injection of a total of 15×10^6 MS. We were also able to demonstrate that valid bone blood flow values can be obtained with the MS method in long-term experiments.[9] Figures 3.5 and 3.6 display the relative blood flow values after the simultaneous injection of two different FM species, calculated by means of a regression analysis and according to the method of Bland and Altmann.[17]

3.2 Bone Blood Flow Studies

3.2.1 *Heterogeneity of bone blood flow*

Under constant hemodynamic conditions in rabbits, the mean blood flow is approximately 14 ml/min/100g in the humerus, approximately

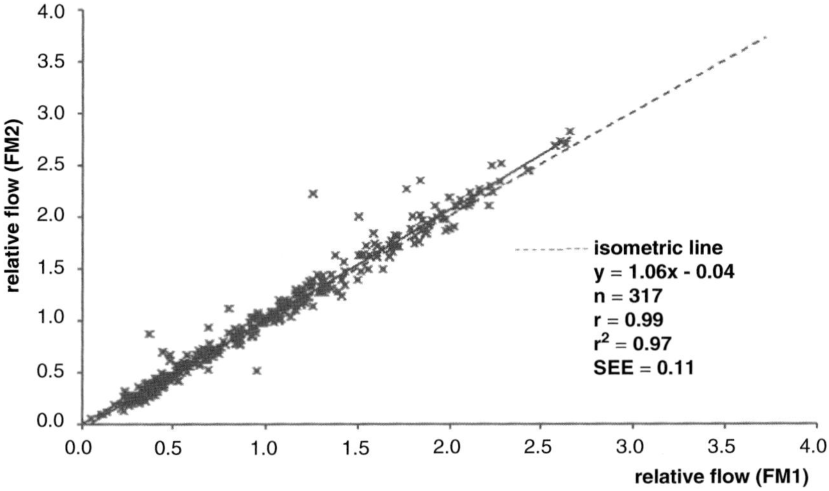

Fig. 3.5. Regression analysis of relative flow values of each bone sample obtained by simultaneous injection of microspheres. The solid line represents the slope of linear relationship; the dotted line is the isometric line ($y = 1x + 0$).

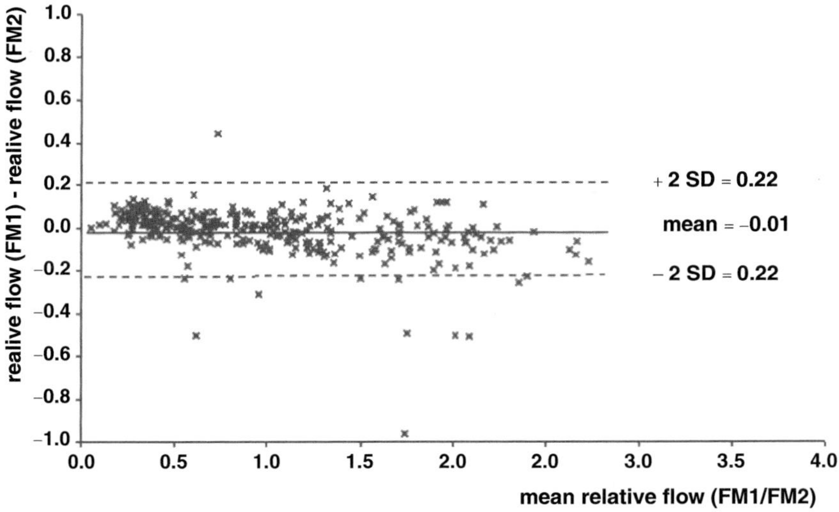

Fig. 3.6. Comparison of relative flow values of each bone sample obtained by simultaneous injection of microspheres according to Bland and Altman. The data show uniform distribution of scatter above and below zero and a mean difference of 0.00 ± 0.11 (mean $\pm$ SD); the solid line represents mean difference and the dotted line ± 2 standard deviation.

11 ml/min/100g in the femur, and approximately 7 ml/min/100g in the tibia.[7,88] One possible reason for this difference could be a different arteriovenous pressure gradient or a different peripheral vascular resistance. Previous works already have suggested that regional blood flow varies between different regions within a long bone.[25,55,87] We therefore studied the RBBF distribution of the long bones and found that RBBF within the humerus was highest in the greater tubercle (about 24 ml/min/100g) followed by the metaphysis (about 20 ml/min/100g). The lowest RBBF values were observed in the diaphysis and in the distal epiphysis (about 9 ml/min/100g). Within the femur, the highest RBBF values were measured in the femoral neck (about 20 ml/min/100g) whereas the femoral condyles were significantly less perfused (about 6 ml/min/100g). In the femoral head, the greater trochanter, and the metaphysis, RBBF varied between 8 ml/min/100g and 14 ml/min/100g. Within the tibia, the highest RBBF values were observed in the proximal metaphysis (about 13 ml/min/100g) and medial and lateral tibialcondyle (about 11 ml/min/100g), whereas the lowest values were found in the distal epiphysis and the epiphysis (about 3 ml/min/100g). The RBBF distribution (heterogeneity) within a long bone remained identical under constant and under altered hemodynamic conditions. It is well known that RBBF shows variability between individuals. We were able to demonstrate that there are no side differences by comparing blood flow values of right- and left-sided bone samples from identical regions of humerus, femur, and tibia under constant and various hemodynamic conditions. This observation is in keeping with the results of many other investigators.[1,23,34,39,55,66,77,89,92] Because of interindividual variance, we recommend comparing the corresponding left- and right-sided regions in experimental settings, since this practice permits sensitive detection of even small alterations in RBBF. By using such intraindividual comparisons, the number of experimental animals can also be reduced significantly. Figure 3.7 shows the heterogeneity of RBBF in long bones.

3.2.2 *Autoregulation of bone blood flow*

Organ perfusion predominantly depends upon systemic perfusion pressure, even though many organs possess the ability to self-regulate their perfusion within certain limits. This physiological mechanism was first described by Bayliss in 1902 and provides the maintenance of organ perfusion under varying systemic blood pressure conditions.[15] The ability of an organ to maintain its perfusion at a constant level was later termed "autoregulation"

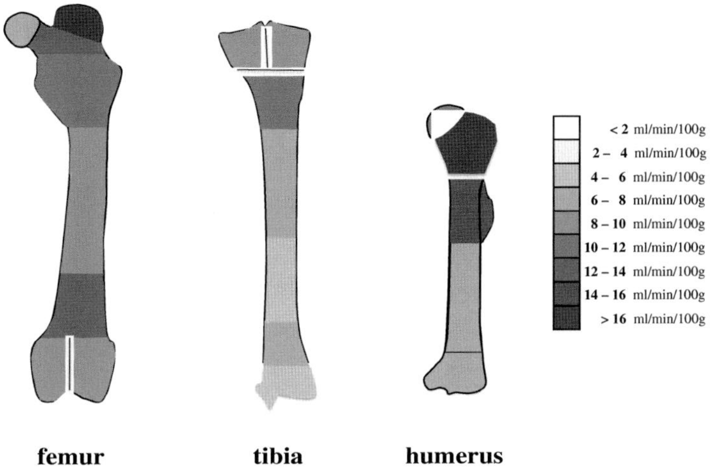

Fig. 3.7. Heterogeneity of RBBF in long bones.

and was first found in the kidney.[76] The same mechanism was subsequently found in other organs, for example the brain and the intestine.[61,63] There are different possibilities to achieve autoregulation of organ perfusion: myogenic, metabolic, tissue pressure, local neural control, and in the kidney tubuloglomerular feedback.[53] For the control of bone perfusion, neurogenic, hormonal, and metabolic influences have been found in addition to perfusion pressure.[25,27,34,41,86,97] In several hemodynamic studies, a drop in bone perfusion was observed with hemorrhagic shock.[81,111] Even though a local regulation of bone perfusion via the smooth muscle cells within the walls of the nutritional arteries appears possible,[32,96] an autoregulation mechanism for bone has not been found yet. Since bone does not only fulfill a supportive function but also is the main hematopoietic organ, an autoregulation mechanism would make sense. Hemorrhagic shock leads to an impairment of the bone marrow and a functional reduction of the erythropoietic cell line[62,78] whereas osteoblasts and osteoclasts are considerably ischemia-resistant.[65] In the context of a validation study, we observed that bone perfusion remained unchanged under moderate hypotension, whereas severe hypotension led to a drop in perfusion.[7] In order to test this hypothesis, the mean arterial pressure was lowered in steps from 100 mm Hg to 30 mm Hg by removing blood from the circulation. The hemodynamic parameters measured during this experiment showed the typical reaction of the organism to acute hypovolemic shock. While the heart rate slightly increased and the CO remained constant between 100 and 80 mm Hg of arterial pressure, CO dropped significantly by about 45% of baseline starting from mean arterial pressures (MAP) of 60 mm Hg.

As a control for this experimental setup, we measured the perfusion of both kidneys. Renal blood flow remained constant despite lowering the MAP from 100 mm Hg to 80 mm Hg. Only further lowering of the MAP to 60, 40, and 30 mm Hg resulted in a reduction of renal perfusion with the curve reflecting the typical features of an autoregulation mechanism (Fig. 3.8).

We observed the same phenomenon in bone. Bone perfusion remained stable under moderate hypotension (lowering of MAP from 100 to 80 mm Hg) and only a further lowering of MAP to below 60 mm Hg resulted in a statistically significant reduction of the perfusion in the humerus, the femur, and the tibia. Figure 3.9 shows the blood flow in the tibia during arterial hypotension.

These observations represent an extension of preexisting knowledge. Michelsen stated that the arteries supplying the bone possess only weak autoregulatory potential.[68] This opinion was founded on the observation that increasing perfusion pressure led to an increase in blood flow and in intramedullary pressure. Since these experiments were performed by

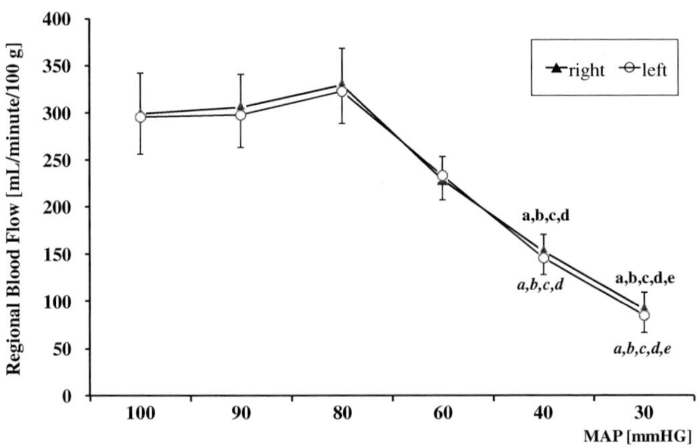

Fig. 3.8. Blood flow in ml/min/100g of the kidney under hypotension, ($n = 8$, mean $\pm$ SEM). a: significantly different to 100 mm Hg MAP; b: significantly different to 90 mm Hg MAP; c: significantly different to 80 mm Hg; d: significantly different to 60 mm Hg MAP: e: significantly different to 40 mm Hg. Roman print: left, italic print: right.

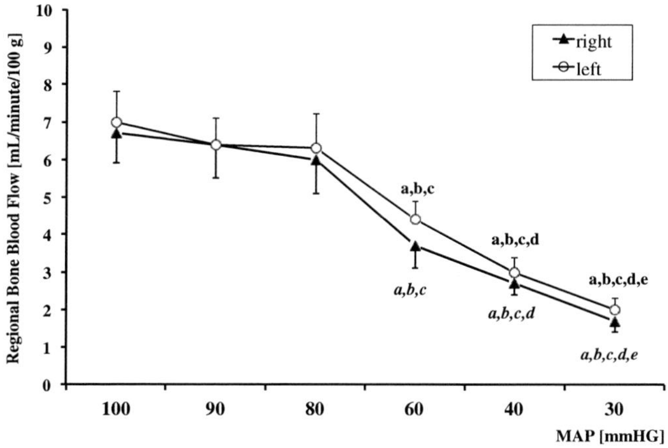

Fig. 3.9. RBBF in ml/min/100g of the tibia under hypotension, ($n = 8$, mean $\pm$ SEM). a: significantly different to 100 mm Hg MAP; b: significantly different to 90 mm Hg MAP; c: significantly different to 80 mm Hg; d: significantly different to 60 mm Hg MAP; e: significantly different to 40 mm Hg. Roman print: left, italic print: right.

directly measuring blood flow through the nutritional artery, manipulation influences of the surgical preparation are probable and hence the value of these results regarding the autoregulatory capacity of bone perfusion is limited. It appears obvious that the regulation of the wall tone of intraosseus vessels regulates perfusion. This is supported by the observation that the peripheral vascular resistance decreased when lowering the MAP from 100 to 80 mm Hg. A constant blood supply to the bone is maintained by vasodilation.

The same applies for each region within a long bone. Despite lowering the MAP from 100 to 80 mm Hg, regional perfusion remains constant. Starting from a MAP of 60 mm Hg, there is a significant reduction in bone blood flow for all regions. There are no particularly vulnerable regions in which RBBF would decrease with minimal reductions in MAP. These observations support the hypothesis that the perfusion of the different regions of a long bone is controlled by one common mechanism.[103] We were able to demonstrate for the first time, that bone perfusion possesses an autoregulatory mechanism. With slight changes in arterial blood pressure (moderate hypotension), bone perfusion can be held constant, independent of systemic blood pressure. Under severe hypotension (shock), there is a linear reduction in perfusion, which is dependent on the perfusion pressure.

3.2.3 *Local cooling reduces bone blood flow*

In order to reduce pain and swelling, it is common practice to apply ice onto acute soft tissue injuries. Cooling slows down the local metabolism, reduces energy consumption and cell damage, and also slows down nerve conduction speed.[12,31] The consequences of cooling on the perfusion of the skin are especially well investigated. Cooling of the skin initially leads to rapid vasoconstriction, mediated by cold receptors that, beyond a centripetal signal transmission, cause a local release of no repinephrine from sympathetic nerve endings leading to vasoconstriction. Non-neuronal mechanisms cause a transient vasodilation at the early stages of a cold stimulus, but with continued cold exposure, vasoconstriction, also mediated by non-neuronal mechanisms, supersedes this vasodilation. This vasoconstriction is caused by a blockage of the nitric oxide (NO)pathway.[48,51,52,56,95,110] There are no previous studies, however, that focus on the effects of cooling on the perfusion of muscle and bone. We therefore studied the effects of incrementally lowering the surrounding temperature from 32°C to 2°C on the perfusion of bone and muscle tissues.[102] To achieve this, the hind leg of an experimental animal was placed in a water bath, which then was cooled down step by step by the addition of ice and with the non-cooled contralateral side being used as a control. We measured the blood flow in both femora, both tibiae, both gastrocnemius muscles, and both anterior tibial muscles. The measured intramuscular temperature was on average about 3 degrees higher than the temperature of the water bath; the MAP and CO were constant throughout the experiments, thus excluding macrohemodynamical influences on our results. Cooling caused a significant reduction in femoral and tibial perfusion within the regions of the femur that were completely covered by the water bath exhibiting a statistically significant reduction in RBBF between 51% (distal metaphysis) and 88% (lateral condyle). In contrast to these observations, the perfusion of the proximal femur (femoral head, femoral neck, and greater trochanter) increased during the course of the experiment whereas the perfusion of the proximal metaphysis remained constant and the perfusion of the diaphysis and the distal metaphysis decreased slightly. We interpret the increase in perfusion in the uncooled, proximal regions of the femur as possibly being the effect of a reflex vasodilation. The tibia and all regions within the tibia, in contrast, showed a linear decrease in perfusion and we did not observe any particularly vulnerable regions within the femur and the tibia (Fig. 3.10). This constant decrease in perfusion most likely is the result of a vasoconstriction of intraosseus vessels. The

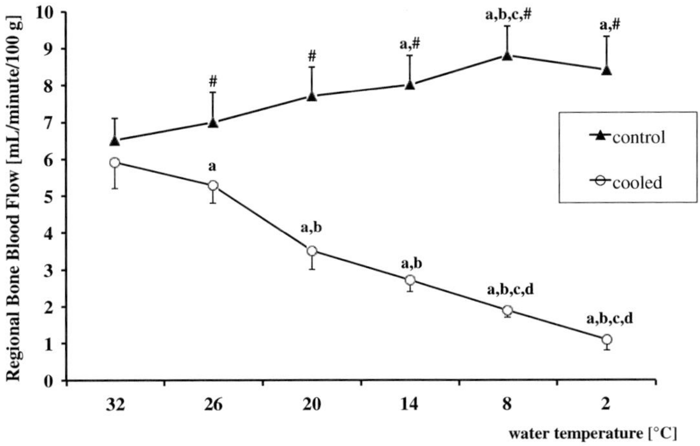

Fig. 3.10. RBBF in ml/min/100g of the tibia with local cooling, (n = 6, mean ± SEM). a: significantly different to 32°C; b: significantly different to 26°C; c: significantly different to 20°C; d: significantly different to 14°C; e: significantly different to 8°C; #: significant difference between control and treated specimens.

perfusion of the uncooled contralateral control extremity increased during the experiment, which is most likely the result of a reflex counter regulation (vasodilation). The underlying mechanism, however, remains poorly understood and deserves further investigation. Our findings match those from studies on skin perfusion.[13, 14, 36, 52] Local cooling dramatically reduces bone perfusion and hence represents a simple method for a reduction of both pain and bleeding.

Blood flow in the anterior tibial muscle was 7 ml/min/100g and remained nearly constant despite cooling 32°C to 20°C. Further lowering of the water temperature led to a significant increase in perfusion to 8 ml/min/100g. Muscle perfusion in the cooled extremity and the control extremity initially remained identical, but exhibited a statistically significant difference starting from a water temperature of 26°C. Blood flow in the anterior tibial muscle of the control extremity was between 7.8 ± 0.7 and 5.7 ± 0.4 ml/min/100g. During the second and the third measurement (26° and 20°C water temperature), there were transient, but statistically significant, drops in muscle perfusion, after which perfusion remained constant again (Fig. 3.11). The changes in perfusion of the gastrocnemius muscle under cooling conditions show identical curves.

Our results demonstrate that muscle and bone tissues respond differently to local cooling. In contrast to bone, muscle responds with increased

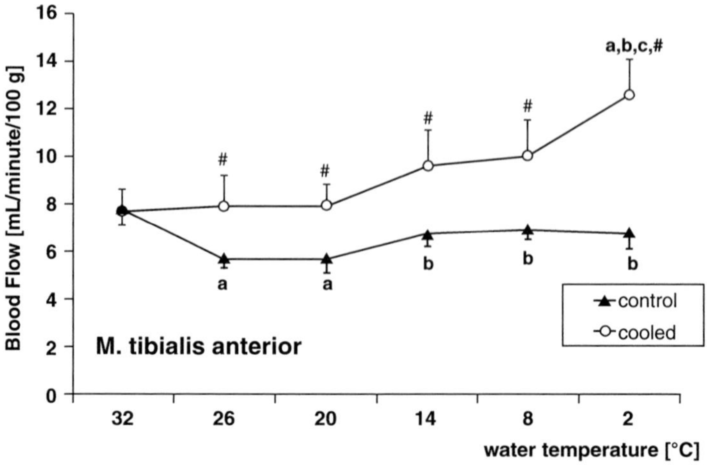

Fig. 3.11. Regional blood flow in ml/min/100g in the anterior tibial muscle under cooling, ($n = 6$, mean $\pm$ SEM). a: Significantly different to 32°C; b: Significantly different to 26°C; c: Significantly different to 20°C; d: Significantly different to 14°C; e: Significantly different to 8°C, #: significant difference between control and cooled extremities.

perfusion despite increased cooling. This observation suggests that local perfusion is regulated via complex mechanisms. Two different models could explain the fact that muscle perfusion was upregulated in our experiments while bone perfusion was simultaneously reduced. One explanation could be a vasoconstriction of large vessels supplying both, muscle and bone combined with a concomitant dilation of the muscle vasculature. Alternatively, vasodilation of these large, more proximal vessels combined with vasoconstriction of the bone vasculature and vasodilation of the muscle vasculature could explain our results. The recruitment of non-perfused capillaries is a possible additional phenomenon. Since the MS method employed in our studies does not provide data on the regulation of vascular wall tone, this work cannot further clarify the vasomotor mechanisms upon which these phenomena are based. The increased muscle perfusion, however, protects this tissue, which is rather sensitive toward cold-induced ischemia, and it may also aid in maintaining core body temperature under hypothermic conditions.

3.2.4 *Effects of tourniquet application on bone and muscle blood flow*

Tourniquets are routinely employed during musculoskeletal procedures in order to reduce blood loss and improve visibility. These pneumatic cuffs are typically inflated to a pressure of up to 300 mm Hg on the upper extremity, and to a pressure of up to 500 mm Hg at the lower extremity. The upper acceptable limit of ischemia time lies between two and three hours[26, 33, 35, 90] with the risk of a reperfusion injury correlating with the duration of ischemia and the inflation pressure.[49, 60, 107] However, these pressure and time limits are based on clinical experience rather than scientific studies and post-operative complications do occur with much shorter ischemia times. The interruption of arterial perfusion by inflating a tourniquet immediately reduces the blood supply to the tissues and impairs the venous drainage. This initiates the phase of primary ischemia with a slowing of the blood flow and with a concomitant impairment of drainage, hence increasing the intracapillary pressure. Cell damage combined with tissue edema is the direct result and cell sludge causes microembolism, in turn promoting the release of cytotoxic metabolites and endotoxins. This further impairs venous drainage and increases the risk of deep vein thrombosis while the acidic metabolites arising during ischemia lead to tissue acidosis and increase the risk for tissue damage even further.[70] Once the tourniquet is released, the reperfusion of the extremity is characterized by an abnormally high vascular permeability and a vasodilation of small vessels, leading to a fluid shift into the extravascular space. Platelets and white blood cells that have been activated during ischemia adhere to the endothelium and further disturb the microcirculation. This phenomenon is called the "no-reflow phenomenon" or secondary ischemia. The second phase of reperfusion begins about one week after these events with a neovascularization of the damaged tissue.[49]

These damages caused by ischemia are summarized under the term "post-tourniquetsyndrome" and have been studied predominantly in muscle and nervous tissue.[105] Its typical complications are swelling, pain, a reduced wound healing capacity, necroses, and functional impairment of muscles and nerves.[82] The risk of a hemarthrosis after an arthroscopy is also increased, depending on the duration of the tourniquet time.[85] Even though the pathophysiological knowledge about ischemia can, to a certain extent, be transferred from other organs to bone tissue, several questions remain unanswered. We studied the early reperfusion phase in bone and muscle tissue using the MS method. In white New Zealand rabbits, a tourniquet was applied to one thigh for 60 minutes in group 1 and for 120 minutes in group 2. During ischemia and after release of the tourniquet, perfusion was measured in both tibiae and in both gastrocnemius and tibial muscles. During ischemia, the tibia received almost no perfusion with less than 0.5 ml/min/100g. In group 1, one minute after tourniquet release, perfusion

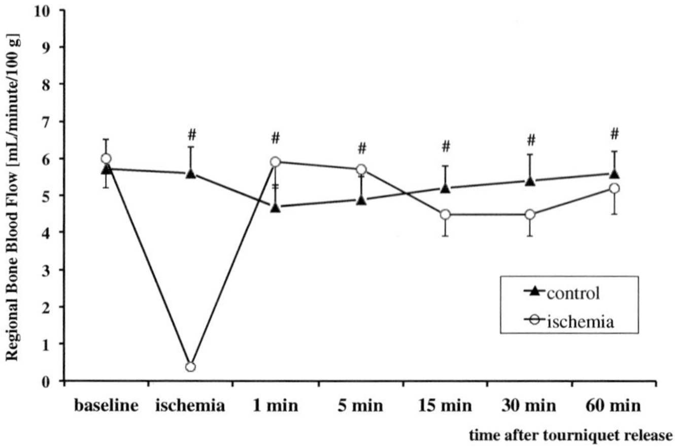

Fig. 3.12. Regional blood flow of the tibia after 60 minutes tourniquet ($n = 6$, mean ± SEM); # indicates a significant difference between control and treated tibia.

increased significantly and was about 1 ml/min/100g higher than that of the control side without tourniquet. Subsequently, blood flow was reduced again and onwards from 15 minutes after tourniquet release until the end of the experiment, it remained by about 1 ml/min/100g lower than in the control side (Fig. 3.12). The same observation was made within the individual bone regions. While perfusion normalized in group 1 after 15 minutes, it remained elevated by 2 ml/min/100g in comparison to the control side even after 90 minutes in group 2 (Fig. 3.13).

In group 1, blood flow in the gastrocnemius muscle was around 12 ml/min/100g before inflating the tourniquet and dropped to 0.6 ml/min/100g with the tourniquet inflated. After tourniquet release, perfusion immediately increased 3.5-fold to 40 ml/min/100g with a subsequent continuous normalization to the starting value within 15 minutes. The control side exhibited constant perfusion during the course of the experiment and the tibial muscle behaved similarly to the gastrocnemius muscle (Fig. 3.14).

After 120 minutes of ischemia (group 2), the post-ischemia increase in perfusion was much more pronounced. Muscle perfusion increased six-fold immediately with tourniquet release, after which it continuously dropped to reach the values of the control side again after 90 minutes (Fig. 3.15). The results of this study demonstrate that a tourniquet duration of two hours already leads to very relevant alterations in the microcirculation

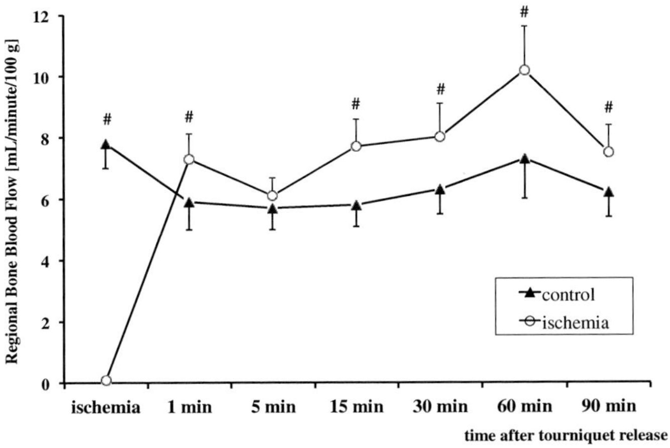

Fig. 3.13. Regional blood flow of the tibia after 120 minutes tourniquet ($n = 7$, mean $\pm$ SEM); # indicates a significant difference between control and treated tibia.

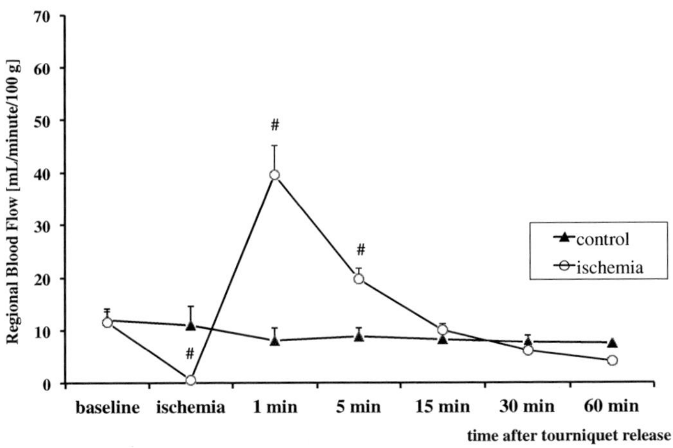

Fig. 3.14. Regional blood flow of the M. gastrocnemius after 60 minutes tourniquet, ($n = 6$, mean $\pm$ SEM), # indicates a significant difference between control and treated M. gastrocnemius.

of bone and muscle tissue. After the release of a tourniquet, there is significant hyperperfusion, which is more pronounced in muscle than it is in bone and with longer ischemia leading to a longer and more pronounced hyperperfusion. These alterations in perfusion play an important role in the pathogenesis of the reperfusion syndrome. As a result of the

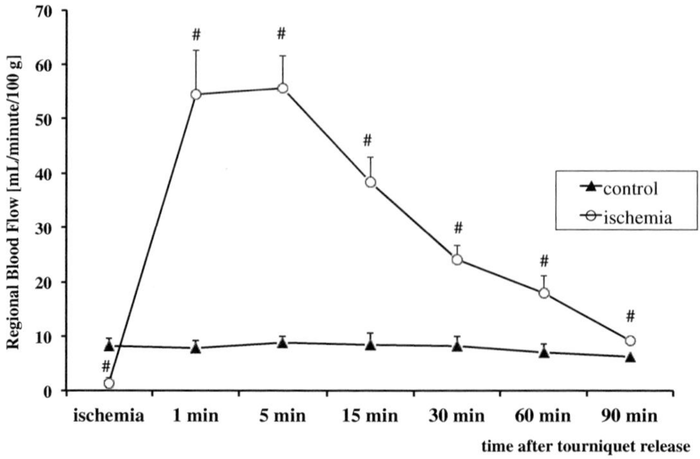

Fig. 3.15. Regional blood flow of the M. gastrocnemius after 120 minutes tourniquet, ($n = 6$, mean $\pm$ SEM), # indicates a significant difference between control and treated M. gastrocnemius.

increased endothelial permeability after ischemia, there is the chance that this increased perfusion leads to a progressive extravasate which in turn can further impair the already compromised microcirculation and eventually lead to a post-tourniquet syndrome.

3.2.5 *The relevance of bone blood flow in the pathogenesis of osteoarthritis*

Early during the development of osteoarthritis (OA), structural changes in the subchondral bone can be observed as well as bone marrow edema and micronecroses.[50] A reduction in trabecular thickness and in the thickness of the subchondral layer has been observed in early stages of OA,[67] whereas in more progressed stages an increased thickness of the subchondral layer is the result of adaptive changes, in response to an altered biomechanical loading situation.[3,4,75] These morphological changes and the fact that the subchondral bone plate is well perfused,[32] lead to the suspicion that processes such as hyperemia and angiogenesis might play key roles in the development of OA.[89] Figure 3.16 shows a fluorescent microscopic view of an FM lodged in the capillary bed of the subchondral bone plate. We studied the relevance of bone perfusion in a long-term experiment and by employing a meniscectomy model for the induction of OA. The meniscectomy was performed by means

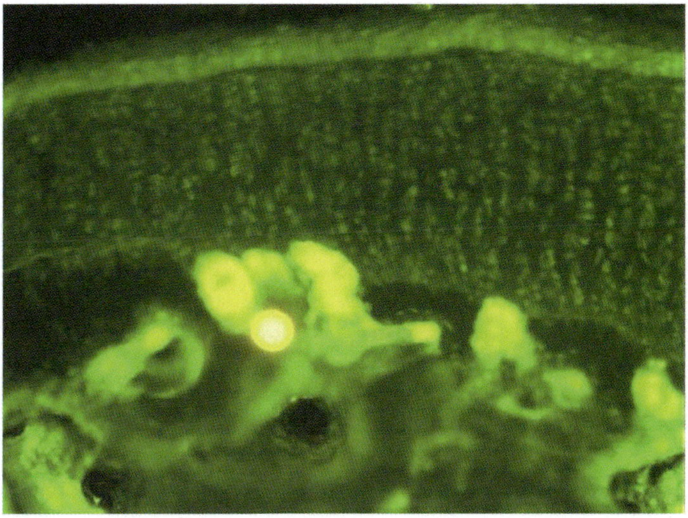

Fig. 3.16. Fluorescent microscopic view of histological bone sections of tibial subchondral bone plate (magnification 10 ×).

of a mini arthrotomy and the regional bone flow was measured at defined time points thereafter. During the complete experiment, the rabbits were kept in large-animal containers with access to open space. There were no changes in body weight in any of the three experimental groups, which indicates that the procedure was tolerated well. One week after meniscectomy, all animals were back to full, unimpaired loading of the treated limbs.

All measurements were performed under constant physiological conditions. As early as one week after meniscectomy, the RBBF close to the joint increased significantly in comparison to the untreated control side. This significant increase was observed until the seventh post-operative week, but a (not statistically significant) tendency toward increased perfusion was maintained until the end of the observation period. The time course of RBBF in the medial tibial plateau after meniscectomy is displayed graphically in Fig. 3.17. In tibial regions distant to the joint and in the humeri, RBBF was equal between sides at all times.[9] This confirms the findings by Shymkiw *et al.*, who observed an increased bone blood flow in the femoral condyles of rabbits up to the 48th post-operative week, after resecting the anterior cruciate ligament for the purpose of OA induction.[89] They also found a significant reduction in periarticular bone density and concluded from these observations, that the increase in perfusion was linked to the

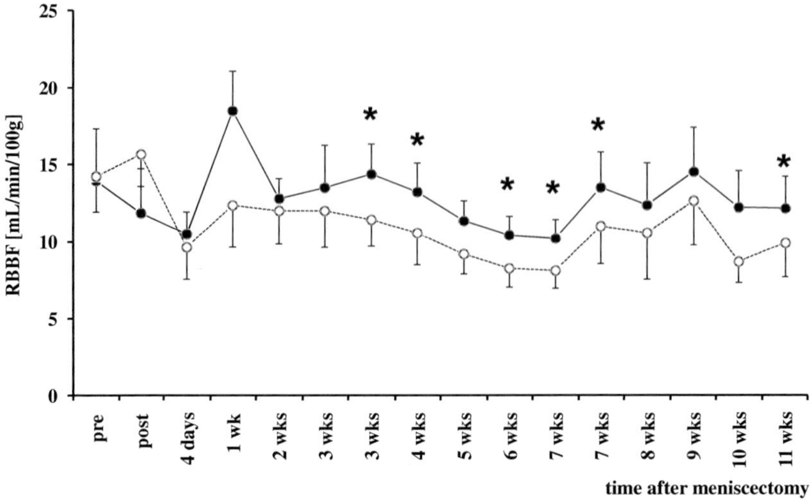

Fig. 3.17. Regional bone blood flow (RBBF) after meniscectomy. Pre: before meniscectomy; post: immediately after meniscectomy; wks: weeks; ∗ indicates a statistically significant difference versus the untreated control side.

structural changes in the subarticular bone, induced by the altered biomechanical loading conditions. A direct influence of the meniscectomy procedure as a reason for these changes appears unlikely, since Gross *et al.* were able to exclude an increased perfusion after sham operations.[40] Long-term studies are required to better understand the relevance of bone perfusion under both physiological and pathological conditions. Our investigations demonstrate that the FM method is reliable for long-term studies and that it delivers reliable data. We observed an increase in regional blood flow in the tibial plateau and in the femoral condyles, indicating that changes in regional bone perfusion are a crucial step in the development of OA.

3.2.6 *Clinical relevance of bone blood flow studies and future research meniscectomy*

Our data demonstrate that the MS method in combination with reference sampling and when using FM is the method of choice when measuring regional bone blood flow. The perfusion of a long bone is heterogeneous with the RBBF in the epiphysis and in the metaphysis being distinctly higher than in the diaphysis and with a gradual decrease toward the periphery.

We were able to show that bone perfusion is subject to an autoregulatory mechanism, which allows maintenance of constant bone perfusion during moderate changes in blood pressure.

Severe hypotension leads to a linear decrease in bone perfusion and the absolute amount of bone and muscle perfusion is temperature-dependent.

Cooling leads to a decrease in bone perfusion while it causes an increase in muscle perfusion. This observation could be interpreted as a protective mechanism, since muscle is very sensitive to hypoperfusion. However, it can also be seen as a regulatory mechanism for the stabilization of the core temperature under hypothermic conditions.

Our experiments demonstrate that the use of a tourniquet for the commonly recommended one-and two-hour time limits causes considerable alterations in the microcirculation of bone and muscle tissues. An increase in the duration of the ischemia leads to a stronger and a longer-lasting hyperperfusion once the tourniquet is released. After meniscectomy, there is an increase in RBBF in proximity to the affected joint which indicates that the structural changes in the subchondral bone that take place with the beginning of OA also are related to hyperperfusion.

After establishing and validating the MS method for short-term and long-term animal experiments, it is now possible to investigate the importance of bone perfusion in various pathological and physiological conditions of the skeletal system.

Acknowledgments

Our biggest thanks go to Professor Konrad Messmer, the former head of the Institute for Surgical Research at the LMU Munich. All studies were performed in this institution. Without his guidance, his mentorship, this research would not have been possible.

References

1. Aalto K, Slätis, P (1984). Blood flow in rabbit osteotomies studied with radioactive microspheres. *Acta Orthop Scand*, 55, 637–639.
2. Albrektsson T (1985). Microvascular anatomy and function of bone. *Acta Orthop Scand*, 56, 167–168.
3. Anetzberger H, Mayer A, Glaser C, Lorenz S, Birkenmaier C, Müller-Gerbl M (2014). Meniscectomy leads to early changes in the mineralization distribution of subchondral bone plate, *Knee Surg Sports Traumatol Arthrosc*, 22, 112–119.

4. Anetzberger H, Metak G, Scherer MA, Putz R, Müller-Gerbl M (1995). Anpassung der subchondralen Knochenplatte nach Meniskektomie als Folge einer Änderung der Spannungsverteilung. *Osteologie*, 4, 224–232.
5. Anetzberger H (2004). Messung der regionalen Knochendurchblutung mit Hilfe fluoreszierender Mikrosphären. Validierung und Etablierung der Methode am Knochen im Akut- und Langzeitversuch. *Habilitationsschrift.*
6. Anetzberger H, Thein E, Walli AK, Messmer K (2003). Determination of RBBF by means of fluorescent microspheres using an automated sample processing procedure. *Eur Surg Res*, 35, 337–345.
7. Anetzberger H, Thein E, Becker M, Walli, AK, Messmer K (2003). Validity of fluorescent microspheres method for bone blood flow measurement during intentional arterial hypotension. *J Appl Physiol*, 95, 1153–1158.
8. Anetzberger H, Thein E, Becker M, Zwissler B, Messmer K (2004). Microspheres accurately predict RBBF. *Clin Orthop*, 424, 253–265.
9. Anetzberger H, Thein E, Löffler G, Messmer K (2004). Fluorescent micrsophere method is suitable for chronic bone blood flow measurement: Along-term study after meniscectomy in rabbits. *JAppl Physiol*, 96, 1928–1936.
10. Anetzberger H, Thein E, Maier M, Birkenmaier C, Messmer K (2004). Fluorescent microspheres are reliable for serial bone blood flow measurements. *Clin Orthop*, 427, 241–248.
11. Archie JPJ, Fixler DE, Ullyot DJ, Hoffman JI, Utley JR, Carlson EL (1973). Measurement of cardiac output with and organ trapping of radioactive microspheres. *J Appl Physiol*, 35, 148–154.
12. Arrica M, Bissonnette B (2007). Therapeutic hypothermia. *Semin Cardiothorac Vasc Anesth*, 11, 6–15.
13. Bailey SR, Eid AH, Mitra S, Flavahan S, Flavahan NA (2004). Rho kinase mediates cold-induced constriction of cutaneous arteries: Role of alpha2C-adrenoceptor translocation. *Circ Res*, 94, 1367–1374.
14. Bailey SR, Mitra S, Flavahan S, Flavahan NA (2005). Reactive oxygen species from smooth muscle mitochondria initiate cold-induced constriction of cutaneous arteries. *Am J Physiol Heart Circ Physiol*, 289, 243–250.
15. Bayliss WM (1902). On the local reaction of the arterial wall to changes of internal pressure. *J Physiol (Lond.)*, 28, 220–231.
16. Bhattacharya J, Beilin LJ (1980). Left ventricular cannulation for microsphere estimation of rabbit renal blood flow. *Am J Physiol*, 238, 736–739.
17. Bland JM, Altman DG (1986). Statistical methods for assessing agreement between two methods of clinical measurement. *Lancet,*1, 307–310.
18. Brookes M, Helal B (1968). Primary arthritis, venous engorgement and osteogenesis. *J Bone Joint Surg Br*, 50, 493–504.
19. Brookes M, Revell, WJ (1998). *Blood Supply of Bone.* Berlin, Heidelberg, New York: Springer Verlag, 1–3, 7–22, 136–141, 210–265.
20. Buckberg GD (1975). Studies of regional coronary flow using radioactive microspheres. *Ann Thorac Surg*, 20, 46–51.

21. Buckberg GD, Kattus AAJ (1973). Factors determining the distribution and adequacy of left ventricular myocardial blood flow. *Adv Exp Med Biol*, 39, 95–113.
22. Buckberg GD, Luck JC, Payne DB, Hoffman JI, Archie JP, Fixler DE (1971). Some sources of error in measuring regional blood flow with radioactive microspheres. *J Appl Physiol*, 31, 598–604.
23. Bünger C, Bulow J, Hjermind J, Harving S (1983). Haemodynamics of the juvenile dog knee in relation to increased venous outlet resistance. *Pflügers Arch*, 399, 129–133.
24. Consigny PM, Verrier ED, Payne BD, Edelist G, Jester J, Baer RW, Vlahakes GJ, Hoffman JI (1982). Acute and chronic microsphere loss from canine left ventricular myocardium. *Am J Physiol*, 242, H392–H404.
25. Cumming JD (1962). A study of blood flow to bone and marrow by a method of venous effluent collection. *J Physiol (Lond.)*, 162, 13–20.
26. Daehlback LO, Rais O (1966). Morphologic changes in striated muscle following ischemia:Immediate postischemic phase. *Acta Chir Scand*, 131, 430–440.
27. Davis RF, Jones, LC, Hungerford DS (1987). The effect of sympathectomy on blood flow in bone:Regional distribution and effect over time. *J Bone Joint Surg Am*, 69, 1384–1390.
28. De Bruyn PP, Breen PC, Thomas, TB (1970). The microcirculation of the bone marrow. *Anat Rec*, 168, 55–68.
29. Dole WP, Jackson DL, Rosenblatt JI, Thompson WL (1982). Relative error and variability in blood flow measurements with radiolabeled microspheres. *Am J Physiol*, 243, H371–H378.
30. Domenech RJ, Hoffman JIE, Noble MIM, Saunders KB, Henson JR, Subijanto S (1968). Total and regional coronary blood flow measured by radioactive microspheres in conscious and anesthetized dogs. *Circ Res*, 25, 581–596.
31. Drinkwater E (2008). Effects of peripheral cooling on characteristics of local muscle. *Med Sport Sci*, 53, 74–88.
32. Duncan CP, Shim SS (1977). The autonomic nerve supply of bone:An experimental study of the intraosseous adrenergic nervi vasorum in the rabbit. *J Bone Joint Surg Br*, 59, 323–330.
33. Egkher E, Freund R, Kroitzsch U, Wielke B (1986). Blood pressure-dependent, process-controlled hemostasis to minimize tourniquet syndrome. *Unfallchirurgie*, 12, 200–203.
34. Ferrell WR, Khoshbaten A, Angerson WJ (1990). Responses of bone and joint blood vessels in cats and rabbits to electrical stimulation of nerves supplying the knee. *J Physiol*, 431, 677–687.
35. Flatt AE (1972). Tourniquet time in hand surgery. *Arch Surg*, 104, 190–192.
36. Freedman RR, Sabharwal SC, Moten M, Migaly P (1992). Local temperature modulates alpha 1- and alpha 2-adrenergic vasoconstriction in men. *Am J Physiol*, 263, 1197–1200.
37. Frick H, Leonhardt H, Starck, D (1992). *Taschenlehrbuch der gesamten Anatomie Band 1*. Georg Thieme Verlag(Stuttgart, New York), 15–21.

38. Glenny RW, Bernard S, Brinkley M (1993). Validation of fluorescent-labeled microspheres for measurement of regional organ perfusion. *J Appl Physiol*, 74, 2585–2597.
39. Gregg PJ, Walder DN (1980). Regional distribution of circulating microspheres in the femur of the rabbit. *J Bone Joint Surg Br*, 62, 222–226.
40. Gross TS, Damji AA, Judex S, Bray RC, Zernicke RF (1999). Bone hyperemia precedes disuse-induced intracortical bone resorption. *J Appl Physiol*, 86, 230–235.
41. Gross PM, Heistad DD,Marcus ML (1979). Neurohumoral regulation of blood flow to bones and marrow. *Am J Physiol*, 237, H440–H448.
42. Gross PM, Marcus ML, Heistad DD (1981). Measurement of blood flow to bone and marrow in experimental animals by means of the microsphere technique. *J Bone Joint Surg Am*, 63, 1028–1031.
43. Hale SL, Alker KJ, Kloner RA (1988). Evaluation of non radioactive, colored microspheres for measurement of regional myocardial blood flow in dogs. *Circulation,* 78, 428–434.
44. Hales JRS, King RB, Fawcett AA (1979). Observations on the validity of using "NEN-TRAC"microspheres for measuring organ blood flow. *Pflügers Arch*, 379, 295–296.
45. Hansen ES, He SZ, Hjortdal VE, Kjolseth D, Soballe K (1992). Distribution of blood flow in normal and arthritic joints: Role of arteriovenous shunting studied in growing dogs. *Am J Physiol*, 262, H38–H46.
46. Hansen ES, Hjortdal VE, Kjolseth D, He SZ, Hoy K, Soballe K, Bünger C (1991). Arteriovenous shunting is not associated with venous congestion in bone:Knee tamponade studied with 15-microns and 50-microns microspheres in immature dogs. *Acta Orthop Scand*, 62, 268–275.
47. Havers C (1691). *Osteologia Nova, or some New Observations of the Bones.* Communicated to the Royal Society in several disorders (London, England).
48. Hodges GJ, Zhao K, Kosiba WA, Johnson JM (2006). The involvement of nitric oxide in the cutaneous vasoconstrictor response to local cooling in humans. *J Physiol (Lond.)*, 573, 849–857.
49. Hsieh AS, Winet H, Bao JY, Glas H, Plenk H (2001). Evidence for reperfusion injury in cortical bone as a function of crush injury ischemia duration: Arabbit bone chamber study. *Bone*, 28, 94–103.
50. Imhof H, Breitenseher M, Kainberger F, Trattnig S (1997). Degenerative joint disease: Cartilage or vascular disease? *Skeletal Radiol*, 26, 398–403.
51. Johnson JM, Kellogg DL Jr (2010). Local thermal control of the human cutaneous circulation. *J Appl Physiol*, 109, 1229–1238.
52. Johnson JM, Yen TC, Zhao K, Kosiba WA (2005). Sympathetic, sensory, and nonneuronal contributions to the cutaneous vasoconstrictor response to local cooling. *Am J Physiol Heart Circ Physiol*, 288, 1573–1579.
53. Johnson PC (1986). Autoregulation of blood flow. *Circ. Res*, 59, 483–495.
54. Kaihara S, Van Heerden PD, Migita T, Wagner HNJ (1968). Measurement of distribution of cardiac output. *J Appl Physiol*, 25, 696–700.

55. Kane WJ (1968). Fundamental concepts in bone-blood flow studies. *J Bone Joint Surg Am*, 50, 801–811.
56. Kellogg DL Jr (2006). In vivo mechanisms of cutaneous vasodilation and vasoconstriction in humans during thermoregulatory challenges. *J Appl Physiol*, 100, 1709–1718.
57. Kelly PJ, Janes JM, Peterson LFA (1959). The effect of arterio-venous fistulae on the vascular pattern of the femora of immature dogs: Amicroangiographic study. *J Bone Joint Surg Am*, 41, 1101–1108.
58. Kleen M, Zwissler B, Schosser R, Messmer, K (1996). Determination of regional pulmonary blood flow with systemically injected nonentrapped microspheres. *J Appl Physiol*, 81, 695–706.
59. Kobrin I, Kardon MB, Oigman W, Pegram BL, Frohlich ED (1984). Role of site of microsphere injection and catheter position on systemic and regional haemodynamics in rat. *Am J Physiol*, 247, H35–H39.
60. Kokki H, Vaatainen U, Penttila I (1998). Metabolic effects of a low-pressure tourniquet system compared with a high-pressure tourniquet system in arthroscopic anterior crucial ligament reconstruction. *Acta Anaesthesiol Scand*, 42, 418–424.
61. Larsen B, Lassen NA (1979). Regulation of cerebral blood flow in health and disease. *Adv Neurol*, 25, 7–22.
62. Liang L, Xu G, Zhang Y, Chen W, Li J, Liang T (2010). Resuscitation with hydroxyethyl starch solution prevents bone marrow mononuclear apoptosis in a rat trauma-hemorrhagic shock model. *J Trauma*, 68, 655–661.
63. Lundgren O (1989). Autoregulation of intestinal blood flow: Physiology and pathophysiology. *J Hypertens Suppl*, 7, 79–84.
64. Makowski EL, Meschia G, Droegemüller W, Battaglia FC (1968). Measurement of umbilical arterial blood flow to the sheep placenta and fetus in utero. Distribution to cotyledons and the intercotyledonary chorion. *Circ Res*, 23, 623–631.
65. McCarthy I (2006). The physiology of bone blood flow: A review. *J Bone Joint Surg Am*, 88, Suppl 3, 4–9.
66. McGrory BJ, Moran CG, Bronk J, Weaver AL, Wood MB (1994). Canine bone blood flow measurements using serial microsphere injections. *Clin Orthop*, 303, 264–279.
67. Messner K, Fahlgren A, Ross I, Andersson B (2000). Simultaneous changes in bone mineral density and articular cartilage in a rabbit meniscectomy model of knee osteoarthrosis. *Osteoarthritis Cartilage*, 8, 197–206.
68. Michelsen, K (1968). Haemodynamics of the bone marrow circulation. *Acta Physiol Scand*, 73, 264–280.
69. Neutze JM, Wyler F, Rudolph AM (1968). Use of radioactive microspheres to assess distribution of cardiac output in rabbits. *Am J Physiol*, 215, 486–495.
70. Ostman B, Michaelsson K, Rahme H, Hillered L (2004). Tourniquet-induced ischemia and reperfusion in human skeletal muscle. *Clin Orthop Relat Res*, 418, 260–265.

71. Polissar NL, Stanford DC, Glenny RW (2000). The 400 microsphere per piece "rule" does not apply to all blood flow studies. *Am J Physiol Heart Circ Physiol*, 278, H16–H25.
72. Powers KM, Schimmel C, Glenny RW, Bernards CM (1999). Cerebral blood flow determinations using fluorescent microspheres: Variations on the sedimention method validated. *J Neurosci Methods*, 87, 159–165.
73. Prinzen FW, Glenny RW (1994). Developments in non-radioactive microsphere techniques for blood flow measurement. *Cardiovasc Res*, 28, 1467–1475.
74. Raab S, Thein E, Harris AG, Messmer K (1999). A new sample-processing unit for the fluorescent microsphere method. *Am J Physiol*, 276, H1801–H1806.
75. Radin EL, Rose RM (1986). Role of subchondral bone in the initiation and progression of cartilage damage. *Clin Orthop*, 213, 34–40.
76. Rein H (1931). Vasomotorische regulationen. *Ergebn Physiol*, 32, 28–72.
77. Revell WJ, Brookes M (1994). Haemodynamic changes in the rat femur and tibia following femoral vein ligation. *J Anat*, 184, 625–633.
78. Robinson Y, Matenov A, Tschoke SK, Weimann A, Oberholzer A, Ertel W, Hostmann A (2008). Impaired erythropoiesis after haemorrhagic shock in mice is associated with erythroid progenitor apoptosis in vivo. *Acta Anaesthesiol Scand*, 52, 605–613.
79. Rogers WM, Gladstone H (1950). Vascular foramina and arterial supply of the distal end of the femur. *J Bone Joint Surg Am*, 32, 867–874.
80. Rudolph AM, Heymann MA (1967). The circulation of the fetus in utero. Methods for studying distribution of blood flow, cardiac output and organ blood flow. *Circ Res*, 21, 163–184.
81. Rutherford RBS, Kaihara S, Schwentker EP, Wagner HN Jr (1968). Regional blood flow in hemorrhagic shock by the distribution of labeled microspheres. *Surg Forum*, 19, 14–15.
82. Saunders KC, Louis DL, Weingarden SI, Waylonis GW (1979). Effect of tourniquet time on postoperative quadriceps function. *Clin Orthop Relat Res*, 143, 194–199.
83. Schimmel C, Frazer D, Glenny RW (2001). Extending fluorescent microsphere methods for regional organ blood flow to 13 simultaneous colors. *Am J Physiol Heart Circ Physiol,* 280, H2496–H2506.
84. Schimmel C, Frazer D, Huckins SR, Glenny RW (2000). Validation of automated spectrofluroimetry for measurement of regional organ perfusion using fluorescent microspheres. *Comput Methods Programs Biomed*, 62, 115–125.
85. Sherman OH, Fox JM, Snyder SJ, Del Pizzo W, Friedman MJ, Ferkel RD, Lawley MJ (1986). Arthroscopy "no-problem surgery":An analysis of complications in two thousand six hundred and forty cases. *J Bone Joint Surg Am*, 68, 256–265.
86. Shim SS, Copp DH, Patterson FP (1966). Bone blood flow in the limb following complete sciatic nerve section. *Surg Gynecol Obstet*, 123, 333–335.

87. Shim SS (1968). Physiology of blood circulation of bone. *J Bone Joint Surg Am*, 50, 812–824.
88. Shim SS, Copp DH, Patterson FP (1967). An indirect method of bone blood-flow measurement based on the bone clearance of a circulating bone-seeking radioisotope. *J Bone Joint Surg Am*, 49, 693–702.
89. Shymkiw RC, Bray RC, Boyd SK, Kantzas A, Zernicke RF (2001). Physiological and mechanical adaptation of periarticular cancellous bone after joint ligament injury. *J Appl Physiol*, 90, 1083–1087.
90. Solonen KA, Tarkkanen L, Narvanen S, Gordin R (1968). Metabolic changes in the upper limb during tourniquet ischaemia:A clinical study. *Acta Orthop Scand*, 39, 20–32.
91. Spalteholz KW (1914). Über das Durchsichtigmachen von menschlichen und tierischen Präparaten und seine theoretischen Bedingungen: Nebst Anh.: Über Knochenfärbung, 2., erw. Aufl., (Hirzel S., Leipzig, Deutschland).
92. Syftestad GT,Boelkins JN (1980). Effect of hemorrhage on blood flow to marrow and osseous tissue in conscious rabbits. *Am J Physiol*, 238, H360–H364.
93. Thein E, Raab S, Harris AG, Messmer K (2000). Automation of the use of fluorescent microspheres for the determination of blood flow. *Comput Methods Programs Biomed*, 61, 11–21.
94. Thein E, Raab S, Harris AG, Kleen M, Habler O, Meisner F, Messmer K (2002). Comparison of regional blood flow values measured by radioactive and fluorescent microspheres, *Eur Surg Res*, 34, 215–223.
95. Thompson-Torgerson CS, Holowatz LA, Flavahan NA, Kenney WL (2007). Cold-induced cutaneous vasoconstriction is mediated by Rho kinase in vivo in human skin. *Am J Physiol Heart Circ Physiol*, 292, 1700–1705.
96. Thurston T (1982). Distribution of nerves in long bones as shown by silver impregnation. *J Anat*, 143, 719–728.
97. Tondevold E, Bulow J (1983). Bone blood flow in conscious dogs at rest and during exercise. *Acta Orthop Scand*, 54, 53–57.
98. Trueta J (1963). The role of the vessels in osteogenesis. *J Bone Joint Surg Br*, 45, 402–418.
99. Trueta J, Harrison MHM (1953). The normal vascular anatomy of the femoral head in adult man. *J Bone Joint Surg Br*, 35, 442–461.
100. Tucker FR (1949). Arterial supply to the femoral head and its clinical importance. *J Bone Joint Surg Br*, 31, 82–93.
101. Van Oosterhout MF, Prinzen FW, Sakurada S, Glenny RW, Hales JR (1998). Fluorescent microspheres are superior to radioactive microspheres in chronic blood flow measurements. *Am J Physiol*, 275 H110–H115.
102. Venjakob AJ, Vogt S, Stöckl K, Tischer T, Jost PJ, Thein E, Imhoff AB, Anetzberger H (2013). Local cooling reduces RBBF. *J Orthop Res*, 31, 1820–1827.
103. Vogt S, Venjakob AJ, Stöckl K, Tischer T, Jost PJ, Imhoff AB, Thein E, Anetzberger H (2013). Evidence of an autoregulatory mechanism of RBBF at hypotension. *Arch Orthop Trauma Surg*, 133, 1233–1241.

104. Wagner HN Jr, Rhodes BA, Sasaki Y,Ryan JP (1969). Studies of the circulation with radioactive microspheres. *Invest Radiol*, 4, 374–386.
105. Wakai A, Winter DC, Street JT, Redmond PH (2001). Pneumatic tourniquets in extremity surgery. *J Am Acad Orthop Surg*, 9, 345–351.
106. Warren DJ, Ledingham JGG (1974). Measurement of cardiac output distribution using microspheres:Some practical and theoretical considerations. *Cardiovasc Res*, 8, 570–581.
107. Winet H, Hsieh A, Bao JY (1998). Approaches to study of ischemia in bone. *J Biomed Mater Res*, 43, 410–421.
108. Wolff J (1892). *Das Gesetz der Transformation der Knochen.* Berlin, Deutschland: Verlag A Hirschwald.
109. Wray JB, Lynch C (1959). The vascular response to fracture of the tibia in the rat. *J Bone Joint Surg Am*, 41, 1143–1148.
110. Yamazaki F, Sone R, Zhao K, Alvarez GE, Kosiba WA, Johnson JM (2006). Rate dependency and role of nitric oxide in the vascular response to direct cooling in human skin. *J Appl Physiol*, 100, 42–50.
111. Yu W, Shim SS, Hawk HE (1972). Bone circulation in hemorrhagic shock:An experimental study. *J Bone Joint Surg Am*, 54, 1157–1166.
112. Zwissler B, Schosser R, Weiss C, Iber V, Weiss M, Schwickert C, Spengler P, Messmer K (1991). Methodological error and spatial variability of organ blood flow measurements using radiolabeled microspheres. *Res Exp Med (Berl.)*, 191, 47–63.

CHAPTER 4

LASER DOPPLER FLOWMETRY

SETH O'DONNELL, SCOTT RITTERMAN

Rhode Island Hospital, Department of Orthopaedic Surgery
The Warren Alpert Medical School of Brown University, Providence, RI

LEE RUBIN

Assistant Professor of Orthopaedic Surgery
Division of Adult Reconstruction
The Warren Alpert Medical School of Brown University, Providence, RI

4.1 Introduction

Blood flow is a fundamental property of cellular, tissue, and organ metabolism. Homeostasis of skeletal microcirculation is central to bone metabolism, calcium balance, fracture repair, bony response to stress, and the osseous integration of implantable prostheses. Additionally, pathological alteration in normal skeletal blood flow has important clinical consequences. While osteonecrosis of the hip is a well-known ischemic phenomenon leading to degenerative joint disease, osteoarthritis may have an ischemic origin as well.[13]

Laser Doppler flowmetry (LDF) is a technique developed over 30 years ago to allow invasive and non-invasive measurement of blood flow within tissue. Initially used by Stern to measure blood flow in human skin and rodent renal tissues, the technology has demonstrated ease of use and reproducible results for both real-time dynamic and steady state monitoring of biological tissues when compared to other methods of blood flow measurement.[33, 34, 39] Its development and application has been detailed by Swiontkowski, an early proponent of LDF use in orthopaedic surgery.[37]

4.2 Physiology

LDF relies on the Doppler shift phenomenon to measure relative changes in microvascular circulation. Light is emitted by a helium-neon gas or near-infrared semiconductor laser that is absorbed and scattered by the tissues under the probe (Fig. 4.1). Back-scattered (reflected) light is measured by one or more photodetectors. Movement of red blood cells within the microcirculation under the field of study leads to alterations in the signal amplitude being reflected back to the photodetector(s). The alteration in the frequency of the signal represents the Doppler shift and allows for signal processing to occur. (Moor Instruments [Internet]) Fredriksson *et al.* provides an excellent in-depth review of the theory behind LDF.[6]

Swiontkowski *et al.* (1986) demonstrated utility of the technique and offered comparison with established methods of blood flow measurement, concluding that easy-to-use LDF had several advantages over established microsphere techniques.[39] Standefer *et al.* evaluated the ability of four different techniques to detect ischemic events in juvenile pigs. When comparing LDF to fiber optic pressure, piezoelectric pressure, and the partial

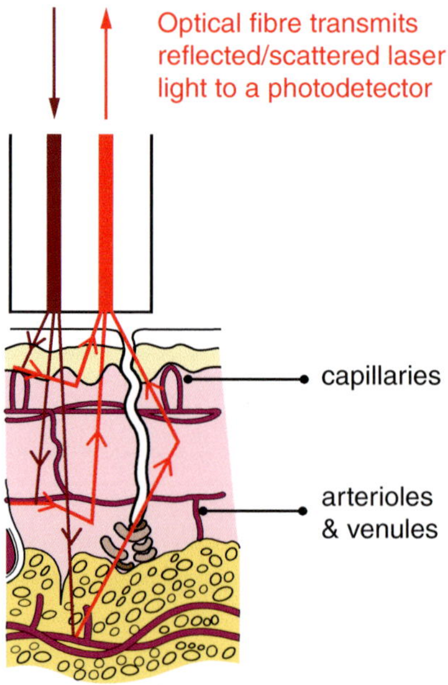

Fig. 4.1. Principle of laser Doppler flowmetry. Reprinted with permission from Moor Medical.

pressure of oxygen, they found that all methods recognized ischemic events. However, the time required for 50% reduction in oxygenation differed, with LDF noted to be the fastest although subject to motion artifact.[31]

LDF measurements are relative and measured in blood perfusion units, or flux, which is proportional to the velocity and concentration of RBCs within the tissues studied. No constant or baseline values have been identified for human tissues; therefore, LDF is best used to measure the response of the microcirculation in a tissue under varying physiological circumstances. Vegter's 1991 canine work sought to demonstrate a relationship between increased intracapsular pressure and decreased hip blood flow. While LDF flux values were shown to be highly reproducible, with increased pressure impacting femoral head blood flow in both juvenile and adult dogs, this study further demonstrated the great variability in LDF flux measurements within the same animal and between animals.[40]

4.3 Devices

Multiple devices and probes have been developed for different applications. With current manufacturers including Perimed (www.perimed-instruments.com), Moor (us.moor.co.uk), and BioPac (www.biopac.com), the specific probe design allows for unique tissue measurements. Probes may be invasive or non-invasive and often are custom designed for the intended application. Exact positioning and stability is vital to decrease motion artifact caused by the instrument, observer, or subject. As the probes can be highly sensitive to movement of the user, patient, or device, a critical effort at limiting the *in situ* movement of a given probe is essential to obtaining quality data for analysis and is facilitated through specialized stands, holders, guides, or sutures. Probes may be used with direct application or through endo- or arthroscope portals. Bone probes (Fig. 4.2) generally require a pre-drilled hole to decrease motion artifact. Long term implantable probes are also available for use.[23] Limitations in the penetration, absorption, and reflection of laser light as well as probe design and signal processing generally result in an area of study limited to less than 2mm depth and a 2.5 mm area.

4.4 Clinical Applications

In the orthopaedic literature, LDF has been frequently used to evaluate the changes in blood flow to the femoral head under varying physiologic

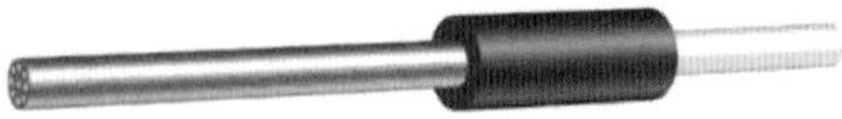

Fig. 4.2. Standard bone probe, VP7BS, Moor Instruments. Diameter is 3.3 mm, standard needle length is 100 mm, with a range of 30–150 mm. http://us.moor.co.uk/i/products/66/157_xl.png. Reprinted with permission.[17]

and iatrogenic stresses. In the adult, most blood supply to the femoral head comes from the medial femoral circumflex artery which ascends on the ventral side of the short external rotators and pierces the hip capsule posteriorly and inferiorly on the femoral neck.[3,43] Perforating vessels then enter the hip joint capsule to supply the femoral head with blood. This tenuous blood supply is at risk of disruption during femoral neck fracture and surgical or traumatic hip dislocation, and secondary to any process resulting in a hip joint effusion which itself may cause a pressure-based occlusion of the terminal penetrating arterioles supplying oxygenation to the femoral head.

LDF offers a minimally invasive way to monitor blood supply throughout a surgical procedure. Before any surgical manipulation, a baseline measurement of red blood cell flux must be obtained. Age, systemic illness limiting perfusion (e.g., lupus, sickle cell anemia, and inflammatory vasculitis), vasoactive drugs, environmental conditions, type of anesthesia, and hemodynamic status can influence baseline values. Prior studies have demonstrated that values differ between and within patients to such an extent that comparisons are possible only in the relationship of normal to pathologic within the same patient.[25,38] Comparison of the baseline measurement to a measurement at any point throughout the surgical procedure can alert the surgeon to any changes in femoral head microcirculation which may require further action.

The Swiontkowski group also demonstrated early clinical utility of LDF while evaluating osteonecrosis of the femoral head.[35] This work provided a mechanism for direct measurement of subchondral bone blood flow and demonstrated that articular cartilage, due to its low blood flow, did not impede penetration of laser Doppler. Although results within patients had a wide variation, they were reproducible and measurements in areas of collapse were found to be significantly lower than normally perfused areas in the same patients.[38]

4.4.1 *Fractures and osteotomies*

Beck's group found that increased intracapsular pressure in human subjects caused loss of pulsatile LDF signal, which subsequently returned with aspiration of joint, suggesting that monitoring before, during, and after decompression of fracture hematoma or other effusion will demonstrate adequate decompression and return of femoral head blood flow.[4]

In cases of planned rotational proximal femoral osteotomy for avascular necrosis (AVN) of the femoral head, ensuring that the intact articular surface is at least 1/3 of the total head area is important for successful outcomes. Standard studies, including x-ray, CT scan, and MRI are not sensitive in this regard. In a series by Fukuoka, these modalities failed to demonstrate the full extent of a lesion up to 25% of the time. The margin of necrotic tissue was unable to be identified by MRI in 5% of patients.[7] Laser speckle, a form of flowmetry, was used as an adjunct to MRI to increase the accuracy of necrotic area size determination. Necrotic margins were evident in a subset of hips (approximately 5% of those studied) that were not revealed with MRI or surgical evaluation of the collapse. A major downside to laser speckle, compared to other forms of LDF, is that dislocation of the femoral head was necessary to obtain the flow map.

4.4.2 *Surgical approaches*

The effect of surgical approach to the hip on femoral head perfusion has been evaluated. Khan's group looked at femoral head blood flow following posterolateral and posterior (transgluteal) approaches. Using cefuroxime concentration in bone as an indirect indicator, their data indicated significantly more damage to blood flow with posterolateral approach.[12] Additional study demonstrated decreased blood flow following posterior approach for hip resurfacing arthroplasty; however, intraoperative comparison to the anterolateral approach using LDF failed to demonstrate significant differences.[19] This work is in contrast to more recent work which used LDF to demonstrate up to a 40% reduction in blood flow with the posterior approach.[1] A modified posterior approach for hip resurfacing was shown to preserve femoral head oxygenation using a gas electrode.[32] The clinical relevance of these studies is questionable as follow-up study demonstrated no significant difference in blood flow at one year using SPECT-CT scan in a small sample size.[2]

Zlotorowicz *et al.* (2013) demonstrated the development of AVN in 10 out of 35 patients with a fracture/dislocation of the hip, two of whom were without any blood flow to the femoral head following reduction as assessed by CT angiography.[43] Previous study monitoring femoral head blood flow during planned surgical subluxation or dislocation of the hip demonstrated decreased blood flow when the posterior femoral neck was allowed to rest on the posterior acetabulum. LDF demonstrated a return of signal not only when the hip was moved out of extreme positions but also when reduced. Following reduction, LDF demonstrated reduced signal amplitudes (when compared to baseline values) for up to 30 minutes.[24] Precise, real-time measurement of blood flow allows meticulous surgical care to avoid maneuvers that jeopardize blood flow to the fragile femoral head.

4.4.3 *Arthroplasty*

Two groups have looked at the impact of patellar blood flow on anterior knee pain following total knee arthroplasty. The study demonstrated that while flexion does decrease flow, medial arthrotomy has minimal impact on patellar blood flow and diminished blood flow was not significantly related to anterior knee pain.[10,14] Hupel's group evaluated perfusion of the proximal femur at four stages during both cemented and uncemented Total Hip Arthroplasty (THA). Although blood flow was reduced in both groups, the greatest change occurred during pressurized cementing of the femoral component.[11]

4.4.4 *Soft tissues*

LDF also has non-bony orthopaedic roles and has been used as an adjunct during surgical release of the carpal tunnel. Seiler *et al.* demonstrated the relative ischemia of the median nerve in carpal tunnel syndrome using LDF.[30] With adequate release of the transverse carpal ligament, what was random flow at the site of median nerve compression became synchronous with the pulse. These findings were correlated with improvement in the patient's symptoms.

LDF has been used arthroscopically during rotator cuff surgery to demonstrate decreased labral blood flow in type I SLAP lesions.[9] It has also been used to show decreased flow in diseased rotator cuff injury. Levy's findings demonstrated decreased flow in areas of impingement and hyperemia at the edges of tears with an inability to demonstrate the theoretical "critical zone" of hypoperfusion in a normal cuff.[18]

Perhaps the greatest area of recent clinical attention has been the use of LDF in oral maxillary facial surgery in prediction of osteoradionecrosis, the osseointegration of dental implants, and monitoring perfusion of the mandible or maxilla during reconstructive deformity procedures.

Irradiated bone has a high incidence of AVN and poor osseointegration of dental implants. Work by Verdonck's group has validated that blood flow in the mandible can be assessed by LDF at the time of implant placement.[42] Kokovic evaluated the role of perfusion at sites of planned dental implants and evaluated implant stability, and proposed that LDF was a potentially useful adjunct in predicting future implant stability.[15]

The role of blood flow in LeFort osteotomies has been evaluated with LDF and demonstrated multisegmental maxillary osteotomies result in significant reduction in blood flow.[16] Although long-term outcomes were not reported, LDF was used as a successful adjunct demonstrating real-time flow monitoring. Sato *et al.* looked at three month outcomes following LeFort osteotomies. Using LDF they demonstrated that increased pulpal blood flow on postop day one resulted in increased pulpal sensation at three months and potentially could be used as an indicator to predict healing.[29]

Capsaicin, a compound derived from chili peppers, has been used as an oral anesthetic. LDF has been used to study if changes occur in oral blood flow after topical application in humans. Patients treated solely with capsaicin had a significant increase in oral blood flow; those treated with topical lidocaine in addition to capsaicin had decreased blood flow to the gingival mucosa.[41]

4.5 Limitations

LDF is not without limitations. In their critical review Obeid *et al.* highlight many of the common pitfalls.[25] LDF provides a *relative* measure of blood flow in tissue, and given the wide variability in microcirculation (both within and between individuals) current LDF use is limited to monitoring responses at specific physiologic sites. No standard "normal" values exist for human bone blood flow. All measurements are relative and able to be compared only to measurements at the same site, in the same individual. The conversion to an electrical signal must correct for artifact and often involves algorithms to average signals to provide a continuous "representative" measure of blood flow. Many studies evaluating blood flow have small patient sample sizes and recommend additional study.

Motion is a common and substantial source of artifact that has resulted in improved techniques, including probes that can be sutured in place, specialized probe holders, and stabilizing techniques such as directly drilling into bone. As probes have become smaller to decrease this "noise," the volume and depth of tissue examined has also become smaller, again limiting interpretation. Artifact is also introduced when the probe is not placed perpendicular to the tissue being studied, thus skewing the emitted and reflected light on the photoreceptors. This can result in artificially low readings.[7]

Reduction of motion artifact can be facilitated though specialized probe designs; however, these techniques may prevent an otherwise non-invasive procedure. A small hole is drilled into the anterosuperior femoral head/neck junction. Through this small opening, the LDF bone probe is placed and values obtained.

The measured values (in BPU or flux) obtained during LDF do not carry units of flow but are instead relative BPU. Calibration with each use is essential to provide an accurate measurement of relative blood flow within the tissue of study. The lack of generalizability and standard measurement values among individuals again limits its utility to changing physiological circumstances within one individual and probably limits its widespread use in general.

Although LDF has demonstrated utility, it may not be available for general use given the cost and necessary equipment (e.g., application-specific probes) required for such monitoring. Rubin *et al.* sought an alternative for blood flow measurement and demonstrated a technique for "direct intraosseous pressure" monitoring using a 2-mm drill hole, a rigid spinal needle, and an arterial pressure monitor attached to the anesthesia monitor.[28] While not as scientifically advanced as using LDF, this alternative can be created as needed from on-hand, basic equipment in nearly any operating theater as needed. Madhuri *et al.* demonstrated a similar technique to address the concern of price and access to LDF.[21]

4.6 Future Directions

Laser Doppler flowmetry has been established as a reproducible method to evaluate local blood flow with non-invasive and minimally invasive techniques. A variety of clinical and laboratory studies have established a baseline utility while recommending future studies for continued development.

LDF is perhaps best applied clinically to bones in order to specifically evaluate regional microcirculations notorious for suffering vascular insults. Examples include the scaphoid, talus, and femoral head. Study of osseointegration of prostheses and implants has also shown benefit. Intraoperative evaluation of bony fragments in cases of severe trauma potentially can guide the extent of debridement and decrease the risk of infection.[36] Phisitkul *et al.*, evaluating talar blood flow using either medial or two-incision approach for triple arthrodesis in cadaveric specimens, recommended further studies with real-time intraoperative laser Doppler. The subsequent publication recommended contrast MRI; however, LDF provides distinct advantages to contrast MRI as it can be done in real time, including intraoperatively during provocative maneuvers.[26] Other methods, such as Doppler ultrasound and vibrometry, have been investigated as non-invasive methods of blood flow measurement. Graif demonstrated these can be useful tools in the assessment of hip vascularity; however, additional study and validation with LDF should be made.[8] Dahl's group has used Doppler ultrasound with vibrometry to demonstrate experimental osseointegration of total ankle arthroplasty components, and it is possible that future work will provide more solid clinical data.[5]

Animal models have been used in laboratory settings to further the study of skeletal perfusion during aging and following endocrine insults.[27] Macdonald *et al.* recently used a scanning form of laser Doppler to demonstrate a two-dimensional map of blood flow and neovascularization in a rat fracture model. While furthering the work of Matsumoto *et al.*, they were able to demonstrate rebound vascularization about a fracture following initial decreased profusion.[20, 22] Murnaghan utilized LDF in a murine model to evaluate impedance of blood flow secondary to non-steroidal anti-inflammatory drug use in the setting of fractures. This technique reveals additional roles for experimental investigation to evaluate and examine the impact various noxious stimuli, medications, and interventions have on bones with a tenuous blood supply at baseline.[23] Future utilization of LDF in patients with risk factors which may predispose them to delayed union (including tobacco use, diabetes, immunosuppression, anemia, and malnutrition) could potentially guide treatment and use of supportive measures to encourage healing.

4.7 Conclusions

Laser Doppler flowmetry has been shown to be a useful adjunct when evaluating blood flow in bone. Though limitations exist, LDF has been validated when compared to other methods of blood flow measurement. It has been established as a repeatable, real-time instrument to assess blood flow with non-invasive techniques that do not alter the physiology of the studied tissues in both clinical and laboratory settings.

References

1. Amarasekera HW, Costa ML, Foguet P, Krikler SJ, Prakash U, Griffin DR (2008). The blood flow to the femoral head/neck junction during resurfacing arthroplasty: A comparison of two approaches using Laser Doppler flowmetry. *J Bone Joint Surg Br*, 90, 4, 442–445.
2. Amarasekera HW, Roberts P, Costa ML, Parsons N, Achten J, Griffin DR, Williams NR (2012). Scintigraphic assessment of bone status at one year following hip resurfacing: Comparison of two surgical approaches using SPECT-CT scan. *Bone Joint Res*, 1(5), 86–92.
3. Beaulé PE, Ganz R, Leunig M (2008). Blood flow to the femoral head and hip resurfacing arthroplasty. *Der Orthopäde*, 37(7), 659–666.
4. Beck M, Siebenrock KA, Affolter B, Nötzli H, Parvizi J, Ganz R (2004). Increased intraarticular pressure reduces blood flow to the femoral head. *Clin Orthop Relat Res*, 424, 149–152.
5. Dahl MC, Kramer PA, Reinhall PG, Benirschke SK, Hansen ST, Ching RP (2010). The efficacy of using vibrometry to detect osteointegration of the Agility total ankle. *J Biomech,* 43(9), 1840–1843.
6. Fredriksson I, Fors C, Johansson J (2007). Laser Doppler flowmetry: Atheoretical framework. Department of Biomedical Engineering, Linkoping University.
7. Fukuoka S, Hotokebuchi T, Jingushi S, Fujii H, Sugioka Y, Iwamoto Y (1999). Evaluation of blood flow within the subchondral bone of the femoral head: Use of the laser speckle method at surgery for osteonecrosis. *J Orthop Res,* 17(1), 80–87.
8. Graif M, Schweitzer ME, Nazarian L, Matteucci T, Goldberg BB (1998). Color Doppler hemodynamic evaluation of flow to normal hip. *J Ultrasound Med*, 17(5), 275–280.
9. Hashiuchi T, Sakurai G, Takakura Y, Inoue K, Kumai T, Tanaka Y (2014). Superficial blood flow of the superior labrum associated with rotator cuff tear using laser Doppler flowmeter. *J Orthop Sci*, 19(3), 424–428.
10. Hempfing A, Schoeniger R, Koch PP, Bischel O, Thomsen M (2007). Patellar blood flow during knee arthroplasty surgical exposure: Intraoperative monitoring by laser Doppler flowmetry. *J Orthop Res,* 25(10), 1389–1394.

11. Hupel TM, Schemitsch EH, Aksenov SA, Waddell JP (2000). Blood flow changes to the proximal femur during total hip arthroplasty. *Can J Surg,* 43(5), 359–364.
12. Khan A, Yates P, Lovering A, Bannister GC, Spencer RF (2007). The effect of surgical approach on blood flow to the femoral head during resurfacing. *J Bone Joint Surg Br*, 89(1), 21–25.
13. Kiaer T, Pedersen NW, Kristensen KD, Starklint H. (1990). Intra-osseous pressure and oxygen tension in avascular necrosis and osteoarthritis of the hip. *J Bone Joint Surg Br*, 72(6), 1023–1030.
14. Kohl S, Evangelopoulos DS, Hartel M, Kohlhof H, Roeder C, Eggli S (2011). Anterior knee pain after total knee arthroplasty: Does it correlate with patellar blood flow? *Knee Surg Sports Traumatol Arthrosc,* 19(9), 1453–1459.
15. Kokovic V, Krsljak E, Andric M, Brkovic B, Milicic B, Jurisic M, Rahman MM, Hämmerle CHF (2014). Correlation of bone vascularity in the posterior mandible and subsequent implant stability: Apreliminary study. *Implant Dentistry,* 23(2), 200–205.
16. Kretschmer WB, Baciut G, Baciut M, Zoder W, Wangerin K (2009). Changes in bone blood flow in segmental LeFort I osteotomies. *Oral Surg Oral Med Oral Pathol Oral Radiol Endod,* 108(2), 178–183.
17. Laser Doppler Monitor: Moor Instruments: http://us.moor.co.uk/product/moorvms-ldf-laser-doppler-monitor/1, last accessed on July 9, 2014.
18. Levy O, Relwani J, Zaman T, Even T, Venkateswaran B, Copeland S (2008). Measurement of blood flow in the rotator cuff using laser Doppler flowmetry. *J Bone Joint Surg Br,* 90-B, 7, 893–898.
19. Lorenzen ND, Stilling M, Ulrich-Vinther M, Trolle-Andersen N, Prynø T, Søballe K, Birke-Sørensen H (2013). Increased post-operative ischemia in the femoral head found by microdialysis by the posterior surgical approach: Arandomized clinical trial comparing surgical approaches in hip resurfacing arthroplasty. *ArchOrthop Trauma Surg,* 133(12), 1735–1745.
20. Macdonald W, Shefelbine SJ (2013). Characterising neovascularisation in fracture healing with laser Doppler and micro-CT scanning. *Med Biol Eng Comput*, 51(10), 1157–1165.
21. Madhuri V, Dutt V, Samuel K, Gahukamble AD (2011). Intra-operative femoral head vascularity assessment: An innovative and simple technique. *Indian J Orthop*, 45(3), 231–235.
22. Matsumoto T, *et al.* (2008). Fracture induced mobilization and incorporation of bone marrow-derived endothelial progenitor cells for bone healing. *J Cell Physiol*, 215(1), 234–242.
23. Murnaghan M, Li G, Marsh DR (2006). Nonsteroidal anti-inflammatory drug-induced fracture nonunion: an inhibition of angiogenesis? *J Bone Joint Surg Am*, 88(Suppl 3), 140.
24. Nötzli HP, Siebenrock KA, Hempfing A, Ramseier LE, Ganz, R (2002). Perfusion of the femoral head during surgical dislocation of the hip: Monitoring by laser Doppler flowmetry. *J Bone Joint Surg Br*, 84(2), 300–304.
25. Obeid AN, Barnett NJ, Dougherty G, Ward G (1990). A critical review of laser Doppler flowmetry. *J Med Eng Technol.* 14(5), 178–181.

26. Phisitkul P, Haugsdal J, Vaseenon T, Pizzimenti MA (2013). Vascular disruption of the talus: Comparison of two approaches for triple arthrodesis. *Foot Ankle Int*, 34(4), 568–574.
27. Roche B, Vanden-Bossche A, Normand M, Malaval L, Vico L, Lafage-Proust MH (2013). Validated laser Doppler protocol for measurement of mouse bone blood perfusion: Response to age or ovariectomy differs with genetic background. *Bone*, 55(2), 418–426.
28. Rubin LE, Galante NJ, Smith BG, DeLuca PA (2008). Direct intraosseous pressure monitoring of the femoral head during surgery for slipped capital femoral epiphysis. *Orthopedics*, 31(7), 663–666.
29. Sato M, Harada K, Okada Y, Omura K (2003). Blood-flow change and recovery of sensibility in the maxillary dental pulp after a single-segment Le Fort I osteotomy. *Oral Surg Oral Med Oral Pathol Oral Radiol Endod,* 95(6), 660–664.
30. Seiler JG, Milek MA, Carpenter GK, Swiontkowski MF (1989). Intraoperative assessment of median nerve blood flow during carpal tunnel release with laser Doppler flowmetry. *J Hand Surg*, 14(6), 986–991.
31. Standefer KD, Pierce WA, Sucato DJ, Kim HKW (2012). Detecting a disruption of blood flow to the femoral head after ischemic injury using fourdifferent techniques: Apreliminary study. *J Pediatr Orthop,* 32(1), 75–80.
32. Steffen RT, De Smet KA, Murray DW, Gill HS (2011). A modified posterior approach preserves femoral head oxgenation during hip resurfacing. *J Arthroplasty*, 26(3), 404–408.
33. Stern MD, Bowen PD, Parma R, Osgood RW, Bowman RL, Stein JH (1979). Measurement of renal cortical and medullary blood flow by laser-Doppler spectroscopy in the rat. *The American Journal of Physiology*. 236, 1 (Jan. 1979), F80–87.
34. Stern MD, Lappe DL, Bowen PD, Chimosky JE, Holloway GA, Keiser HR, Bowman RL (1977). Continuous measurement of tissue blood flow by laser-Doppler spectroscopy. *Am J Physiol*, 232(4), H441–H448.
35. Swiontkowski M, Tepic S, Ganz R, Perren SM (1986). Laser Doppler flowmetry for measurement of femoral head blood flow: Experimental investigation and clinical application. *Helvetica Chirurgica Acta*, 53(1–2), 55–59.
36. Swiontkowski MF (1989). Criteria for bone debridement in massive lower limb trauma. *Clin Orthop Relat Res*, 243, 41–47.
37. Swiontkowski MF (1991). Laser Doppler flowmetry: Development and clinical application. *Iowa Orthop J*, 11, 119–126.
38. Swiontkowski MF, Ganz R, Schlegel U, Perren SM (1987). Laser Doppler flowmetry for clinical evaluation of femoral head osteonecrosis: Preliminary experience. *ClinOrthop Relat Res,* 218, 181–185.
39. Swiontkowski MF, Tepic S, Perren SM, Moor R, Ganz R, Rahn BA (1986). Laser Doppler flowmetry for bone blood flow measurement: Correlation with microsphere estimates and evaluation of the effect of intracapsular pressure on femoral head blood flow. *J Orthop Res*, 4(3), 362–371.

40. Vegter J, Klopper PJ (1991). Effect of intracapsular hyperpressure on femoral head blood flow. Laser Doppler flowmetry in dogs. *Acta Orthop Scand*, 62(4), 337–341.
41. Verdickt GM, Abbott PV (2001). Blood flow changes in human dental pulps when capsaicin is applied to the adjacent gingival mucosa. *Oral Surg Oral Med Oral Pathol Oral Radiol Endod*, 92(5), 561–565.
42. Verdonck HWD, Meijer GJ, Kessler P, Nieman FH, de Baat C, Stoelinga PJW (2009). Assessment of bone vascularity in the anterior mandible using laser Doppler flowmetry. *Clin Oral Implants Res*, 20(2), 140–144.
43. Zlotorowicz M, Czubak J, Caban A, Kozinski P, Boguslawska-Walecka R (2013). The blood supply to the femoral head after posterior fracture/dislocation of the hip, assessed by CT angiography. *Bone Joint J*, 95-B(11), 1453–1457.

CHAPTER 5

ENGINEERING AND CLINICAL ASPECTS OF PHOTOPLETHYSMOGRAPHY

ROY K. AARON

Professor, Orthopaedic Surgery
The Warren Alpert Medical School of Brown University, Providence, RI

OUSSAMA FADIL

School of Engineering
Brown University, Providence, RI

JENNIFER RACINE

Department of Orthopaedics
The Warren Alpert Medical School of Brown University, Providence, RI

DOMENICO PACIFICI

Assistant Professor, School of Engineering
Brown University, Providence, RI

5.1 Introduction

Photoplethysmography (PPG) is a non-invasive optical technique that can be used to measure the real-time variation of clinically relevant physiologic parameters and extract physiological information from living organisms. In this chapter, we present experimental evidence demonstrating the effectiveness of PPG using multiple wavelengths, provide examples of clinically relevant applications, particularly the detection of oxygen content and blood flow in bone, and discuss the basic physics and engineering aspects of light-matter interactions that make PPG possible. PPG takes advantage of complex light-matter interactions occurring when light at visible or near-infrared wavelengths impinges upon, and interacts with, human tissues or organs.[3, 19] The basic principle of PPG is that real-time changes of certain physiological parameters can affect physical processes governing the interaction of light with complex media (such as blood, skin, bone), causing a measurable, modulated variation in the fraction of light that is either reflected and/or transmitted.

PPG has been used to study a number of biological tissues and organs in preclinical animal and human models including cardiovascular, lung, skin, muscle, and bone.[2,9,22,26] Its primary use has been to assess blood flow-related phenomena.[9,22] The features of PPG that contribute to its clinical utility are that it is non-invasive and that the AC component of the pulse wave is synchronous with the cardiac cycle. Essentially, PPG can detect blood volume changes in the circulatory system of several organs including capillary beds and, therefore, its clinical utility to date has been largely in circulatory diagnostics with a prime example being pulse oximetry.[2] The simplest interpretation of the PPG waveform defines its applicability for circulatory measurements. The rising edge of the pulse (anacrotic) reflects systole and the declining edge (catacrotic) reflects diastole and wave reflections.[2] Red, or near infrared wavelengths, are often chosen for the PPG light source since they are most compatible with the absorption spectra of blood and facilitate measurements of blood flow and blood volume.[2,16]

5.2 PPG Measurements of Bone Circulation and Oxygen Content

Physiological measurements of circulation and oxygenation non-invasively in bone have been technically difficult. Currently, techniques that measure perfusion in soft tissues are not clinically applicable to bone since they cannot penetrate it (Doppler ultrasound), are invasive (laser Doppler and contrast MRI), or are destructive (fluorescent microspheres). Invasive techniques are unsuitable to screen for the presence of disease and cannot be used repeatedly to monitor responses to treatment. Laser Doppler flowmetry has a shallow penetration depth, typically around 1 mm, which limits its applicability to bone blood flow measurements without invasive probe placement or surgery. The ideal technique would be completely non-invasive and inexpensive enough to be used in a variety of clinical settings. Other techniques include photoacoustic imaging (PAI) and electrical impedance tomography (EIT). PAI uses non-ionizing lasers to generate a photoacoustic response and can reflect biological chromophores by optical absorbance.[12,31] EIT uses low frequency alternating currents to derive physiological information from the measurement of tissue conductivity. Both PAI and EIT have limitations in specificity and spatial field of view.

Bone is particularly suitable for optical imaging techniques because it is transparent to near infrared light (800–1100 nm). Many diseases involving bone exist in which measurement or imaging of function, particularly perfusion and oxygen content, would be highly advantageous. Some of these conditions are metastatic cancer, osteoporosis, osteoarthritis, and trauma, all diseases of substantial prevalence. In each case, disease initiation or progression depends upon changes in normal blood flow. Therefore, the assessment of blood flow (perfusion) represents an opportunity for early diagnosis, staging and disease characterization, planning treatment, and following response to therapy. Understanding the time dynamics and spatial distribution of perfusion also offers the opportunity to gain insight into the pathogenesis of these conditions and, therefore, to design new treatments.

PPG typically relies on few electronic components, e.g., a light emitting diode (LED) and a photodetector (PD), to record physiological changes related to blood circulation through light-matter interaction. PPG has been used to measure blood flow in human skin, muscle, and bone, but has not been applied extensively to monitor human bone diseases. The use of PPG in the context of bone blood flow measurement is heavily dependent upon the choice of appropriate wavelengths for the discrimination of intraosseous and intracutaneous blood flow. An adequate choice has to take into account the different optical properties of bone and skin at several wavelengths as well as their effects on light propagation in the tissues.

Preliminary studies of the optical properties of bone have shown that it is nearly transparent to light in the near-infrared spectral range (800–1100 nm), thus providing a "biological window" for measuring blood flow. PPG takes advantage of this unique biological window to transcutaneously and non-invasively make several measurements of the interior of bone. Blood flow measurements by PPG also depend upon light absorption by blood and this absorption is different for oxygenated and deoxygenated hemoglobin. At a wavelength of ∼808 nm, known as an isosbestic point, the absorption coefficients for oxygenated and deoxygenated hemoglobin are the same, enabling determination of total hemoglobin concentration irrespective of oxygen saturation levels[13] (Fig. 5.1). Using different wavelengths, below and above the isosbestic point, the oxygenated and deoxygenated hemoglobin concentrations can be determined independently, permitting measurements of venous and arterial blood flow. A notable application is the determination of oxygen content and circulation in human brain made possible by the fact that bone is translucent in the 800–1,100 nm range.[10,15]

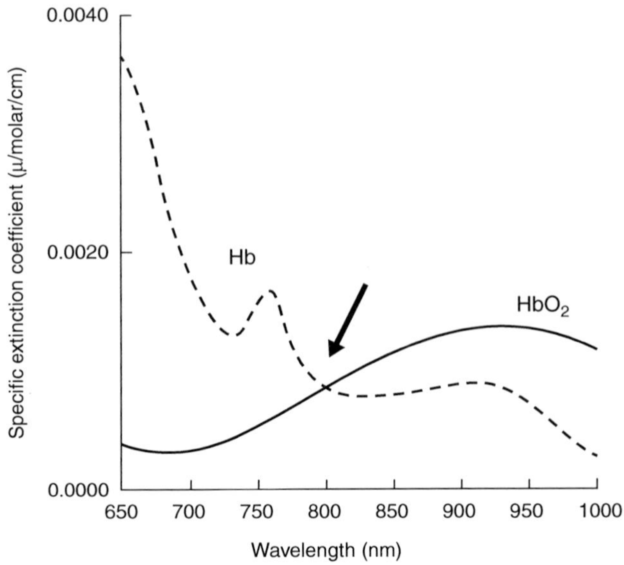

Fig. 5.1. Absorption spectra of hemoglobin.[9]

Light with $\lambda < 600\,\text{nm}$ only penetrates about 1–2 μm and can be used to measure skin blood flow and develop a subtraction algorithm to improve sensitivity to bone perfusion.

5.3 Physiology of Multispectral PPG

To test the feasibility of PPG for real-time measurement of blood flow, preliminary studies have been performed using a simple PPG optrode consisting of two LEDs with different wavelengths (532 nm and 850 nm, respectively) and a PD placed at a fixed separation distance from both LEDs. Figure 5.2 shows the use of two LEDs with wavelengths selected to preferentially sample the skin (green light) and arterial (infrared light) blood perfusion. The red light beam is able to penetrate deeper than the green beam into the tissue, thus enabling characterization of circulation beneath several tissue layers.

Figure 5.3 shows an example of a typical PPG oscilloscope waveform originating from detection and processing of diffuse reflectance from the two wavelengths at separate time intervals. Both the green and infrared signals can be used to infer the heart rate of the patient (in this case, 67.4 beats per minute). However, the two signals differ substantially in their rise and

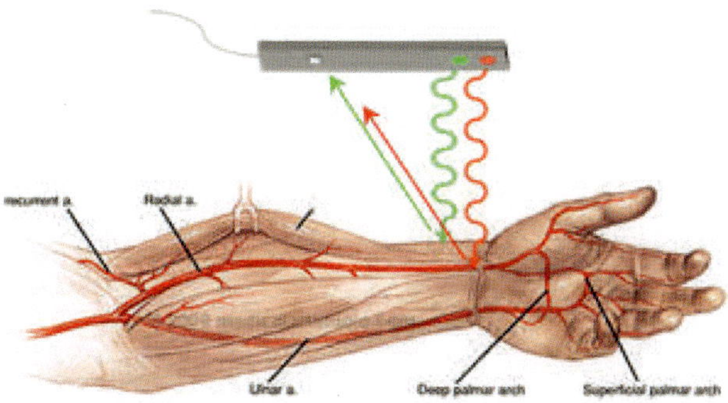

Fig. 5.2. Two-color photoplethysmography (PPG) for detection of radial pulse as well as skin (green arrow) versus artery (red arrow) blood flows. The optrode is in contact with the skin, recording the superficial diffuse reflectance at each wavelength.

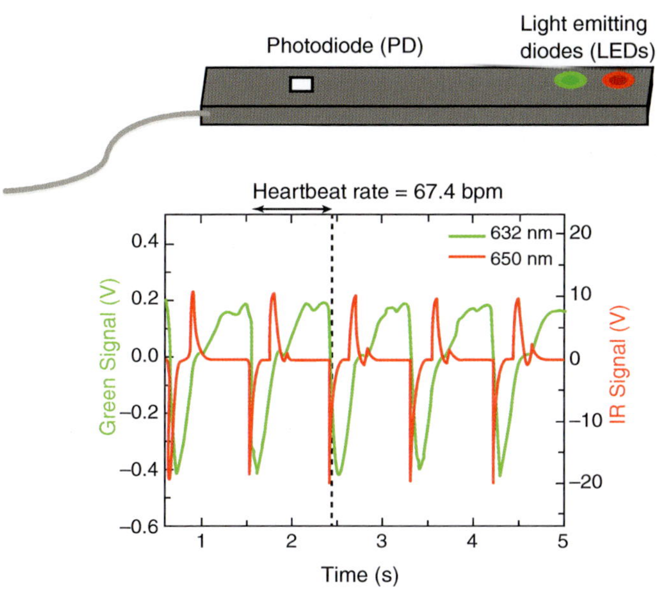

Fig. 5.3. Measurement of heartbeat rate and blood flow using two light beams originating from LEDs with different wavelengths in the visible (green line, $\lambda = 532\,\text{nm}$) and in the near-infrared (NIR, red line, $\lambda = 850\,\text{nm}$). The "green" light beam samples the first superficial layers of the skin, thus detecting capillary skin blood flow, while the "red" light beam penetrates deeper into the tissue and is therefore able to sample the artery blood flow.

decay times, with the green signal showing a slower response time while the red one shows a much faster response time. This difference arises from the fact that the two LEDs are sampling different regions. The red LED can access the arterial flow directly (therefore leading to a faster modulation of the light intensity upon interaction with arterial blood flow), while the green LED, being characterized by a shallower penetration depth, can only sample the superficial tissue layers and give information on the skin blood flow. As can be seen from Fig. 5.3, the green signal lags behind the red one, suggesting that there is a physiological delay between the vascular and skin perfusion. Moreover, the green signal shows slower rise and decay times, most likely indicative of the slower transit of blood through the skin capillary bed.

Figure 5.4 displays an experiment in which arterial blood flow is occluded at time $t = 2$ seconds. Blood flow is then monitored in realtime for both skin (green) and artery (red) perfusion. The signal originating from the arterial blood flow (red) ceases almost immediately while the signal originating from interaction of light with skin blood flow shows a much slower decay time, due to a slower, measurable flow rate of skin perfusion. Both signals have finite, measurable time constants.

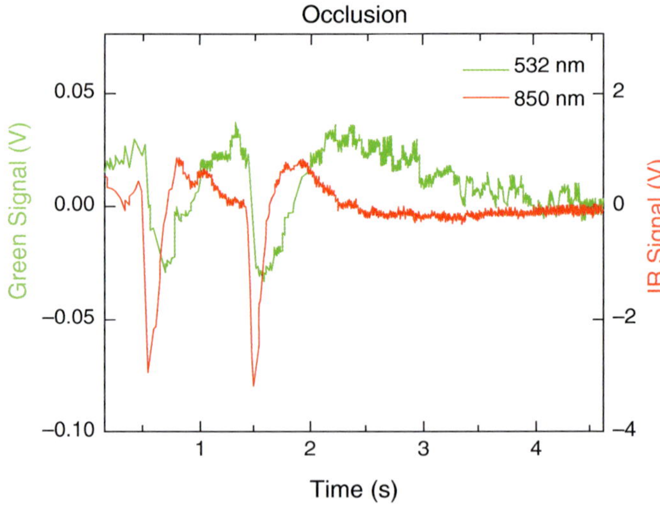

Fig. 5.4. Two-color PPG experiment showing detection of blood flow "occlusion maneuver" at $t = 2$ s, as well as estimate of different time-constants for blood flow suppression in skin (slower, green line) and radial artery (faster, red line).

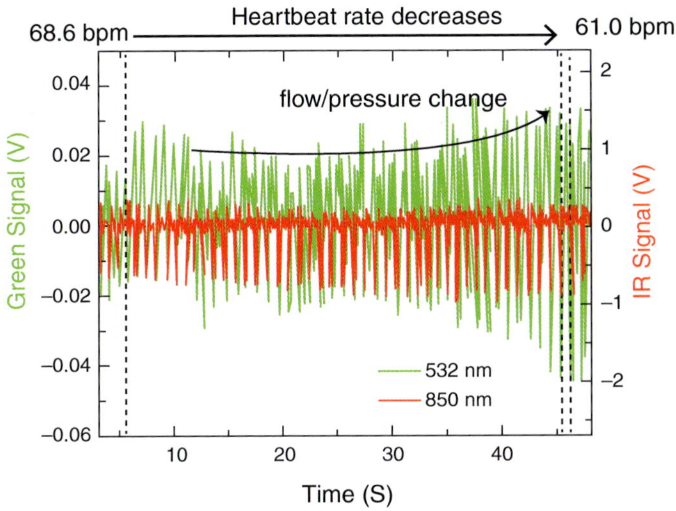

Fig. 5.5. PPG experiment showing variation of blood flow/pressure during a Valsalva maneuver.

Another experiment has attempted to quantify the perfusion changes occurring with a Valsalva maneuver. The two-color PPG experiment reported in Fig. 5.5 shows the ability of the PPG to quantify the heart rate change (in this case a decrease by ∼10%), as well as changes in the skin and arterial blood flow caused by a physiological response induced by the maneuver.

The preliminary experiments and results reported in Figs. 5.2–5.5 demonstrate the potential of two-color PPG as a quantitative technique for measurements of heart rate, blood flow, and real-time changes of blood perfusion in a human subject.

5.4 Optical and Engineering Aspects of PPG

5.4.1 *Introduction to light-matter interaction*

PPG as an optical technique is based on inferring information on a complex medium based on its interaction with the incident light beam generated, for example, by a light emitting diode.[23] In order to get a better sense of the potential as well as the limits of the technique, it is important to get a sense of the fundamental nature of these interactions. To this end, we adopt the quantized picture of light as a collection of elementary particles, named photons, incident upon a complex medium such as human skin or tissue. Each photon will interact with the medium according to the following physical processes:

(a) *Reflection*

As the photon travels from the source and hits the boundary between air and tissue, or between any two layers, it can simply bounce off the surface. In optics this is referred to as reflection. Reflection can be divided into specular and diffuse, the ratio between the two depending on whether the sample surface is more or less polished.

(b) *Transmission*

Alternatively, if the photon is not reflected, it can penetrate through the surface and into the tissue and, if no further interactions take place along its path, it will propagate undisturbed and be eventually transmitted through the back surface of the thick complex medium. Depending on the physical properties of the tissue, a larger or smaller fraction of light will penetrate in the tissue.

(c) *Scattering (single and multiple)*

If the photon is able to penetrate into the medium, as it travels through the tissue/organ, it may collide with other molecules or particles with dimensions smaller, equal, or larger than the wavelength of the incident light. As a result of one (single scattering) or several (multiple scattering) elastic collisions, the initial direction of propagation of the transmitted photon can be significantly altered while its energy (color) will remain unchanged. Depending on the specific tissue and/or material, the photon will change its direction of propagation more or less frequently. For uniform, isotropic media and flat interfaces, the photon will propagate in a straight line due to the lack of scattering events. The tissue properties will also affect how abrupt is this change in direction determining the distribution of scattering angles.

(d) *Absorption*

A photon propagating in a complex medium may suddenly stop moving within the object, or from the perspective of an external observer, disappear, giving up its energy to excite molecules (such as water, hemoglobin, etc.) or vibrational modes in the system (heat). In practice, the photon is absorbed and its energy converted into heat, more often than not, or electronic excitations of molecules or solids. Different tissues/materials will have different "affinity" to absorb photons, captured by their absorption coefficient, a wavelength-dependent physical quantity.

(e) *Fluorescence*

As a consequence of light absorption, a fraction or all of the absorbed energy could be reconverted into a propagating photon that will generally have different direction and color. This process leads to the emission of light from the medium. Typically, the probability for this emission to occur is low, and it can be enhanced by injecting specific fluorescent molecules (such as GFP — green fluorescent protein, or RFP — red fluorescent protein) or properly designed fluorescent beads. Detection of the fluorescence signal may contain useful information about the underlying tissue/organ.

Broadly speaking, PPG takes advantage of a large number of these individual events (a)–(e) occurring and amounting to measurable signals, either in transmission and/or in reflection mode. For example, a series of scattering events can lead to a significant fraction of the incident photons being sent back toward the surface and resulting in a measurable light intensity signal at the sample surface, if the photons are able to escape the surface and not be subject to total internal reflection.

In practice, a clinician is concerned with measuring changes in physiological quantities (blood flow, saturation level, heart rate, etc.) and can rely on two factors to this end, namely:

(1) *Changes in the optical properties of the complex medium caused by varying physiological parameters*

Intuitively speaking, if one is to measure a change in the PPG signal, there has to be an underlying change in the optical properties of the medium light is interacting with. For example, an increased blood volume will result in greater absorption of photons at those wavelengths where the absorption coefficients of oxy- and deoxyhemoglobin are high. Notably, if a physiological event doesn't result in a change in optical properties, it can't be detected by PPG. To complicate things, there could also be artifacts in the detected PPG signal determined by the interference of external parameters that may affect the observed light-matter interaction without being directly related to the physiological changes under investigation. For example, slight motions of the patient's head and statistical fluctuations of the incident ambient light can affect contactless PPG. Moreover, several physiological parameters may cause similar variations to PPG signals — being for example responsible for identical changes in the optical properties of the tissue under investigation — thus resulting in results that are indistinguishable using PPG.

(2) *Experimentation with multiple wavelengths*

It is important to note that the abovementioned optical properties and physical processes ruling the light-matter interaction are wavelength-dependent; meaning light of different frequencies or colors will behave differently in the same tissue. Here we unveil a powerful aspect of PPG that is far from being fully exploited by current devices and research. Although two physiologically distinct tissue samples have the same properties at a certain wavelength, they can be distinguished by exploiting their potential difference in optical properties at a different wavelength, or at multiple wavelengths at once. A device that operates in this fashion is "multispectral" and can take advantage of wavelengths that are beyond the visible range.

Models that aim to simulate light propagation in tissues, and Monte Carlo simulation in particular, often take an approach that is analogous to the thought experiment presented in this section. In general, Monte Carlo simulations exploit the fact that the behavior of random systems can be approximated by analyzing the results of multiple trials, treated individually and independently. Someone interested in knowing how likely a certain coin is to fall heads can simply take the coin under inspection, flip it multiple times, count the number of heads, and divide by the total number of trials.

In optics, Monte Carlo simulations aim to predict the interaction of light — represented as a collection of multiple, virtually identical photons — with matter by examining how each individual photon will interact, deterministically, with the complex medium.[11] Each photon is initialized with a certain weight and propagated through the medium in successive steps.[30] At each step the photon weight is decreased (absorption) and its direction of propagation changed (scattering) according to the optical properties of the medium. After multiple runs, one can gain significant information such as the aggregate photon energy deposited at a certain location (for radiation therapy) or the angle at which photons are reflected through the surface (for optical tomography). The photon weight can be used to estimate the light intensity that will be measured if light is actually shone onto a material that has the same optical properties as the one used in the simulation.

5.4.2 *Theoretical aspects of PPG*

PPG is a specific example of the well-documented problem of the interaction of light with complex media. The problem can be broken down into two complementary aspects. The first, called "the forward problem", aims to infer the light distribution within a certain media, given the optical properties of the latter.[8,25] The second, referred to as "the inverse problem," intends to infer optical properties of some media given the light distribution it exhibits.[17,24,29] Often, as is the case in PPG, the full light distribution is hard to measure and one has to resort to the yet more complicated task of inferring optical parameters based on some local intensity measure.

In the case of PPG, the forward problem would translate into determining some function of the light distribution — in this case, light intensity at the surface — based on the optical parameters of the complex medium — that is, the tissue under inspection. While PPG doesn't require a solution to the forward problem (given that the quantity of interest, light intensity, is already observed), understanding the latter provides some insight as to how, and why, PPG works. From an engineering point of view, any medium can be abstracted into optical properties that characterize the interaction of the medium with light as a function of wavelength, and this interaction will determine the measured spectral transmittance and reflectance.[1] In general, three parameters are sufficient to fully characterize the propagation of light in tissue:[29]

(1) The absorption coefficient records the attenuation in intensity experienced by light per unit distance traveled through the medium. More specifically, it is known that light intensity decays exponentially with respect to distance traveled in the medium. The scattering coefficient records the exact rate of decay. Alternatively, the absorption coefficient can be interpreted as the inverse of the average distance traveled by the photon before being absorbed. In other words, the larger the absorption coefficient, the smaller the distance the photon will travel in the material on average.
(2) The scattering coefficient expresses the degree to which light is deflected as it travels through a medium. By analogy with the absorption coefficient, the scattering coefficient can be viewed as the inverse of the average distance traveled by a photon before its path is altered.
(3) The anisotropy factor represents the average angle at which light is scattered.

Given this abstraction of media into optical properties, one can have more informed insight as to the mechanism by which PPG operates. As light is shone onto human skin, it will undergo absorption and scattering before being fully absorbed or being reflected at the surface. The heart of PPG as a measurement technique resides in the fact that optical parameters change as a function of physiological parameters.[27] The relationship between the scattering coefficient and the medium under study doesn't have a closed-form solution and can depend on the geometry of the medium as much as on its composition. Nonetheless, it is still the case that a change in a biological parameter affects optical constants and yields a different light response.

As such, the signal recorded by a PPG device is thought to be mainly affected by four physiological factors:[14,20] (1) shape and movement of the vessel walls, (2) red blood cells' orientation, (3) blood volume, and (4) oxygenation level of the hemoglobin. By isolating the effect of each factor on optical properties one can predict the intensity of light with a satisfying precision. The problem PPG aims to solve, however, lies elsewhere.

Based on the observed intensity of light with conventional photo detectors, either in reflection or transmission mode, or both for some applications, what are the underlying optical parameters, and eventually the underlying physiological quantities of interest? In this particular concept of the problem, we distinguish two regimes, the *continuous regime* and the *periodic regime*, each requiring a different approach.

In the continuous regime, the PPG device returns the measurement of the average reflected light intensity as a function of wavelength. Constant measurements are useful in determining relatively stable physiological properties and more particularly blood saturation levels.[28] In the case of blood, the main species to be detected are oxyhemoglobin HbO_2, deoxyhemoglobin Hb, and water H_2O.[32] The extinction coefficients of these species are known and tabulated. Finally, the absorption coefficient can be obtained from intensity measurements returned by the PPG probe. Finding the concentration of oxyhemoglobin and deoxyhemoglobin is a multilinear regression problem requiring intensity measurements at three wavelengths. Often, the problem is simplified by assuming a constant water concentration (80% on average) and taking measurements at just two wavelengths.

In the periodic regime, the PPG measures a varying light density from which periodic information such as rate of bone blood flow can be extracted.[22] In this application, however, measurements of scattering coefficients are harder to obtain with a PPG probe, and it is harder to find a closed-form relationship between hemodynamic parameters and optical parameters. It is for these reasons that various papers present different interpretations as to the factors affecting the intensity of the periodic PPG signal.

5.5 Clinical Applications of PPG

There are two operational configurations of PPG: *transmission*, where the tissue sample is placed between the light source and the detector, and *reflection*, or adjacent, where the light source and detector are placed sidebyside.[2] The depth of penetration is a function of wavelength, distance between light source and detector, and optical qualities of tissue including absorbance and scattering. Depths of 1 cm from the skin surface are easily achievable. The PPG signal is unaffected by variations in Hgb saturation at the isosbestic point (800–805 nm). The shape of the pulse wave is said to reflect changes in perfusion of the peripheral arterial bed but this assertion has been challenged and data is insufficient for clinical precision.

PPG has been used to monitor a variety of physiological parameters in the clinical setting including heart rate, blood oxygen saturation, cardiac output, and arterial compliance. Used in the transmission mode, the most common clinical application is pulse oximetry. This exploits the synchrony of the pulse wave with the cardiac cycle and, by configuring wavelengths on either side of the isosbestic point for hemoglobin, can determine oxygen saturation. It is now standard for monitoring during anesthesia.[18] Attempts have been made to extract from the PPG waveform, characteristics of the cardiac cycle such as cardiac output and stroke volume based upon the Windkessel model. Clinical devices are available to estimate cardiac output, stroke volume, and aortic blood flow based upon the model, but the precision of the Windkessel model is debated. Applications to peripheral arterial disease have been limited by lack of sensitivity and specificity due to alterations in vascular compliance, pressure, and flow rates that have not been completely defined.

Other applications besides cardiovascular have been reported, including skin and muscle.[4, 26] Of particular interest are studies of bone blood flow.[5, 22] Naslund used PPG in the reflection mode with wavelengths of 560 nm for skin and 804 nm for bone.[22] This study recorded PPG signals with conditions of venous and arterial occlusion and demonstrated the ability of PPG to record pulse waves under variable blood flow conditions. Subsequent studies demonstrated an increase in patellar blood flow of 61% after high-intensity muscle contraction compared to an increase of 22% after lower-intensity work ($P < 0.001$).[21] PPG has also been used to characterize post-ischemic reperfusion in bone.[6] Monte Carlo simulation demonstrates that determination of oxygen saturation was robust. Subsequent studies quantified orthostatically imposed circulatory responses in bone.[7]

Clinical applications for bone remain to be developed and are limited largely by calibration and the construction of algorithms relating voltage to blood flow. However, developments in non-invasive optical imaging are rapid and PPG should be a clinically useful tool for measurement of bone circulation. Acquisition of circulatory information in bone is especially important since it is associated with development, growth, and senescence of the skeleton. Measurement of blood flow and oxygen content would be highly advantageous for disease states of high prevalence involving bone including metastatic cancer, osteoporosis, osteoarthritis, and avascular necrosis. In skeletal trauma and reconstruction, the determination of viable from non-viable tissue is of extreme importance. The debridement of non-viable bone is often critical to control of infection, healing of bone, and the provision of healthy recipient beds for bone grafts. The assessment of bone viability can also guide treatment decisions regarding internal fixation or prosthetic replacement of proximal humeral and femoral fractures and in fractures with precarious circulation such as scaphoid and talus. Negative pressure therapy for open extremity wounds in now a standard of care; however, the effects on bone blood flow are unknown. The non-invasive assessment of blood flow (perfusion) with PPG represents an opportunity for early diagnosis, staging and disease characterization, enhanced clinical decision making, and following response to therapy. Understanding the time dynamics and spatial distribution of perfusion also offers the opportunity to gain insight into the pathogenesis of these conditions and, therefore, to design new treatments.

5.6 Conclusions

PPG is one of several non-invasive imaging techniques that can be used to extract physiological information from living organisms. PPG has been used to study a variety of biological tissues including cardiovascular, pulmonary, skin, muscle, and bone. It is particularly applicable to assessing circulatory phenomena including blood flow volume and rate, and oxygenation. Bone is particularly suitable for optical imaging techniques such as PPG because it is transparent to near-infrared light. In a number of disease states including osteoarthritis, osteoporosis, and bone metastases, disease initiation or progression depends upon changes in normal circulation. Therefore, the assessment of perfusion represents an opportunity for early diagnosis and disease characterization, planning treatment, and following response to therapy.

Studies of the optical properties of bone have demonstrated that it is nearly transparent to light in the near-infrared spectral range, providing a biological window for measuring blood flow. Using a variety of wavelengths, oxygenated blood can be separated from deoxygenated blood, permitting assessment of oxygen content and saturation. Applications to a number of disease states and conditions are currently under development.

References

1. Aizu Y, Maeda T, Kuwahara T, Hirao T (eds.) (2011). Spectral reflectance fitting based on Monte Carlo simulation using a multi-layered skin tissue model. *Proc. SPIE* 8088, Diffuse Optical Imaging III, 80880P. doi:10.1117/12.889626.
2. Allen J (2007). Photoplethysmography and its application in clinical physiological measurement. *Physiol Meas*, 28(3), R1–R39.
3. Anderson RR, Parrish JA (1981). The optics of human skin. *J Invest Dermatol*, 77(1), 13–19.
4. Bergstrand S, Lindberg LG, Ek AC, Linden M, Lindgren M (2009). Blood flow measurements at different depths using photoplethysmography and laser Doppler techniques. *Skin Res Technol*, 15(2), 139–147.
5. Binzoni T, Blanchi S, Fasel JH, Bounameaux H, Hiltbrand E, Delpy D (2002). Human tibia bone marrow blood perfusion by non-invasive near infrared spectroscopy: A new tool for studies on microgravity. *J Gravit Physiol*, 9(1), P183–184.
6. Binzoni T, Leung T, Hollis V, Bianchi S, Fasel JH, Bounameaux H, *et al.* (2003). Human tibia bone marrow: Defining a model for the study of haemodynamics as a function of age by near infrared spectroscopy. *J Physiol Anthropol Appl Human Sci*, 22(5), 211–218.
7. Binzoni T, Leung TS, Courvoisier C, Giust R, Tribillon G, Gharbi T, *et al.* (2006). Blood volume and haemoglobin oxygen content changes in human bone marrow during orthostatic stress. *J Physiol Anthropol*, 25(1), 1–6.
8. Boas D, Culver J, Stott J, Dunn A (2002). Three dimensional Monte Carlo code for photon migration through complex heterogeneous media including the adult human head. *Optics Express*, 10(3), 159–170.
9. Challoner AV, Ramsay CA (1974). A photoelectric plethysmograph for the measurement of cutaneous blood flow. *Phys Med Biol*, 19(3), 317–328.
10. Ferrari M, Giannini I, Sideri G, Zanette E (1985). Continuous non invasive monitoring of human brain by near infrared spectroscopy. *Adv Exp Med Biol*, 191, 873–882.
11. Flock ST, Wilson BC, Patterson MS (1989). Monte Carlo modeling of light propagation in highly scattering tissues. II: Comparison with measurements in phantoms. *IEEE Trans Biomed Eng*, 36(12), 1169–1173.
12. Grinvald A, Lieke E, Frostig RD, Gilbert CD, Wiesel TN (1986). Functional architecture of cortex revealed by optical imaging of intrinsic signals. *Nature*, 324(6095), 361–364.

13. Horecker B (1943). The absorption spectra of hemoglobin and its derivatives in the visible and near infra-red regions. *J Biol Chem*, 148, 173–183.
14. Jespersen LT, Pedersen OL (1986). The quantitative aspect of photoplethysmography revised. *Heart Vessels*, 2(3), 186–190.
15. Jobsis FF (1977). Noninvasive, infrared monitoring of cerebral and myocardial oxygen sufficiency and circulatory parameters. *Science*, 198(4323), 1264–1267.
16. Jones DP (1987). Medical electro-optics: Measurements in the human microcirculation. *Physics in Technology*, 18(2), 79.
17. Kumar YP, Vasu RM (2004). Reconstruction of optical properties of low-scattering tissue using derivative estimated through perturbation Monte-Carlo method. *J Biomed Optics*, 9(5), 1002–1012.
18. Kyriacou PA (2006). Pulse oximetry in the oesophagus. *Physiol Meas*, 27(1), R1–R35.
19. Mannheimer PD (2007). The light-tissue interaction of pulse oximetry. *Anesthesia and Analgesia*, 105(6 Suppl), S10–S17.
20. Mateus J, Hargens AR (2012). Photoplethysmography for non-invasive in-vivo measurement of bone hemodynamics. *Physiol Meas*, 33(6), 1027–1042.
21. Naslund J, Naslund S, Lundeberg E, Lindberg L, Lund I (2011). Bone blood flow is influenced by muscle contractions. *J Biomed Sci Eng*, 4(7), 490.
22. Naslund J, Pettersson J, Lundeberg T, Linnarsson D, Lindberg LG (2006). Non-invasive continuous estimation of blood flow changes in human patellar bone. *Med Biol Eng Comput*, 44(6), 501–509.
23. Patterson MS, Chance B, Wilson BC (1989). Time resolved reflectance and transmittance for the non-invasive measurement of tissue optical properties. *ApplOptics*, 28(12), 2331–2336.
24. Rajaram N, Nguyen TH, Tunnell JW (2008). Lookup table-based inverse model for determining optical properties of turbid media. *J BiomedOptics*, 13(5), 050501.
25. Ramella-Roman J, Prahl S, Jacques S (2005). Three Monte Carlo programs of polarized light transport into scattering media: Part I. *Optics Express*, 13(12), 4420–4438.
26. Sandberg M, Zhang Q, Styf J, Gerdle B, Lindberg LG (2005). Non-invasive monitoring of muscle blood perfusion by photoplethysmography: Evaluation of a new application. *Acta Physiol Scand*, 183(4), 335–343.
27. Sassaroli A, Pierro M, Bergethon P, Fantini S (2012). Low-frequency spontaneous oscillations of cerebral hemodynamics investigated with near-infrared spectroscopy: A review. *IEEE J Sel Top Quantum Electron*, 18(4), 1478–1492.
28. Shafique M, Kyriacou PA, Pal SK (2012). Investigation of photoplethysmographic signals and blood oxygen saturation values on healthy volunteers during cuff-induced hypoperfusion using a multimode PPG/SpO(2) sensor. MedBiol EngComput, 50(6), 575–583.

29. Simpson CR, Kohl M, Essenpreis M, Cope M (1998). Near-infrared optical properties of ex vivo human skin and subcutaneous tissues measured using the Monte Carlo inversion technique. *Phys Med Biol*, 43(9), 2465–2478.
30. Wang L, Jacques SL, Zheng L (1995). MCML — Monte Carlo modeling of light transport in multi-layered tissues. *Comput Methods Programs Biomed*, 47(2), 131–146.
31. Xu M, Wang LV (2006). Photoacoustic imaging in biomedicine. *Review of Scientific Instruments*, 77(4), 041101–041101-22.
32. Zheng F, Sassaroli A, Fantini S (2010). Phasor representation of oxy- and deoxyhemoglobin concentrations: What is the meaning of out-of-phase oscillations as measured by near-infrared spectroscopy? *J Biomed Optics*, 15(4), 040512.

CHAPTER 6

MRI AND PET

JONATHAN P. DYKE
Assistant Research Professor, Physics in Radiology
Weill Cornell Medical College, New York, NY

6.1 History of 2D Radiologic Imaging in Bone

Adequate perfusion in bone is critical to maintain proper oxygenation, delivery of nutrients, and elimination of waste. The ability of radiologic imaging to detect changes in bone vasculature and intraosseous perfusion through the use of exogenous contrast agents has been examined for over 40 years. Two-dimensional (2D) planar techniques of x-ray and fluoroscopic imaging, along with gamma camera-based techniques, have been used to assess changes in skeletal circulation *in vivo*. Several examples of this technology applied to osteoarthritis (OA) are given as a foundation to these 2D radiologic techniques. A study was performed on normal and OA hips using x-ray techniques.[3] Measurement of intraosseous and intramedullary pressure, along with observation of contrast enhancement in the normal and OA femoral neck and head, was made. An increase in pressure and venous engorgement, seen as delayed drainage, was observed in OA bone using intraosseous phlebography and injection of iodinated contrast directly into the marrow cavity. Likewise, early gamma camera nuclear medicine studies were performed on OA and control hips to examine elimination of the radioisotope (^{131}NaI) in the femoral head and neck.[21] It was shown that the elimination rate in the femoral head of the OA-affected hip was reduced by 80% compared to that seen in control subjects. This showed the ability of radioisotopes to assess changes in skeletal circulation *in vivo*. Lastly, single photon emission computed tomography (SPECT) studies were performed on subjects with nodal OA using ^{99m}Tc-MDP.[11] This study showed a high degree of sensitivity in detecting abnormal tracer uptake in OA. However, there was decreased specificity associated with ^{99m}Tc-MDP uptake that requires additional study of the mechanism behind the uptake of the tracer *in vivo*. These studies and others pioneered the use of 2D radiologic imaging in assessing skeletal circulation.

6.2 3D Positron Emission Tomography (PET)/Computed Tomography (CT)

Several emerging imaging modalities began to gain ground in the 1970s. X-ray computed tomography (CT) was introduced, providing rapid three-dimensional (3D) density-based assessment of osseous structures. While CT attained excellent resolution of extraosseous vasculature using iodinated contrast agents, it has not achieved the same sensitivity in assessing intraosseous perfusion. During that same period, the nuclear medicine-based technology of positron emission tomography (PET) was developed. PET is a 3D functional and metabolic imaging technique that detects uptake of various radiolabeled pharmaceuticals or tracers *in vivo*.

The basic technique for PET scanning begins with a positron-emitting isotope that is typically created from a medical cyclotron but may also be eluted from an isotope generator. The cyclotron shown in Figure 6.1 accelerates protons that strike a target containing ^{18}O-enriched water, to produce a neutron and ^{18}F.

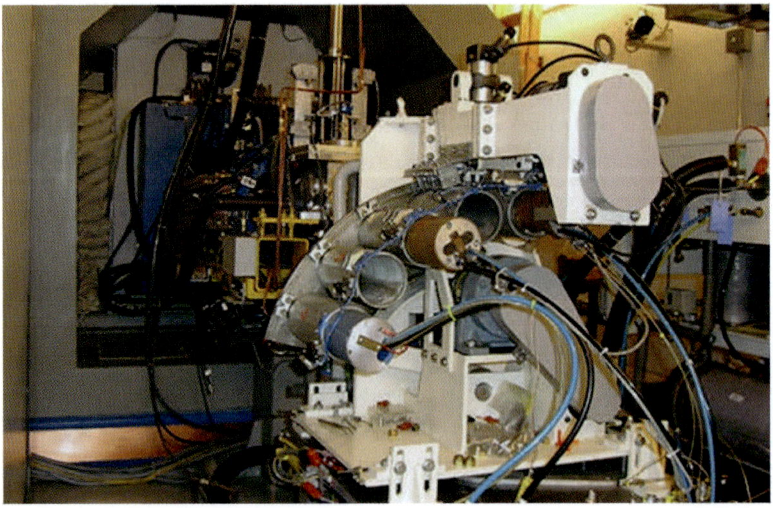

Fig. 6.1. A 19.2 MeV proton-producing cyclotron showing the automated target-changing mechanism.

Typically, the radioisotope is taken from the cyclotron area to a radiochemistry lab to bind the tracer with an amino acid or ligand specific to the disease or tissue to be studied. However, the ^{18}F ion produced directly from the product of the $^{18}O(p,n)^{18}F$ reaction requires no further processing to create ^{18}F-fluoride (sodium fluoride) which is the primary PET radioisotope used in imaging of skeletal circulation.[18] This tracer is injected intravenously and taken up by tissues at a rate defined by the metabolism in the target of interest. In the case of ^{18}F-fluoride, the tracer remains in the blood pool for approximately two minutes after which time it begins to bind with the hydroxyapatite in the bone matrix.[18] Pharmacokinetic modeling of dynamic uptake data then produces estimates of bone blood flow, blood volume, and net fluoride influx rate.

The tracer decays, emitting a positron (a positively charged electron) which decelerates in the tissue of interest and interacts with an electron. The annihilation of the e^+e^- pair produces two photons emitted almost back to back to each other. A ring of solid state scintillation detectors converts the photons into a burst of light on opposite sides of the ring. This results in a voltage in the photomultiplier tubes which is recorded as a coincidence event. In the clinic today, reconstruction algorithms employ a density-based attenuation correction provided by a simultaneously acquired CT scan. In practice, standalone PET scanners have been replaced by hybrid

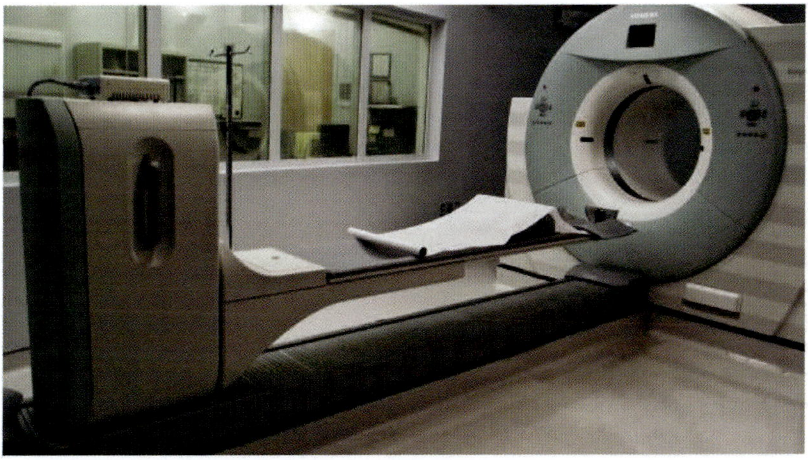

Fig. 6.2. A modern 64 slice PET/CT hybrid scanner allowing for rapid 3D imaging and dynamic acquisitions.

PET/CT scanners (Fig. 6.2). The PET scanner itself produces a metabolic image of the tracer uptake concentration that is fused to the CT scan.

6.3 3D Magnetic Resonance Imaging (MRI)

Following close behind, magnetic resonance imaging (MRI) became clinically available in the mid-1980's (Fig. 6.3). Using completely non-ionizing radiation in the spectrum of radio frequency (RF) waves, this modality produces the greatest soft tissue contrast available. However, as in PET, it also requires the use of exogenous contrast agents to assess perfusion in bone.

MRI is the imaging extension of nuclear magnetic resonance (NMR) that was developed in the 1940's for use in one-dimensional (1D) chemical spectroscopy. The main magnetic field in an MRI scanner contains a liquid helium-cooled super conducting magnet with a field strength of 3.0 tesla or 30,000 Gauss compared to the earth's magnetic field of 0.5 gauss. The hydrogen atoms in tissue act as individual bar magnets or nuclear magnetic moments that precess with a known frequency in the magnetic field. A number of the hydrogen atoms preferentially align with the main magnetic field and are flipped into the perpendicular plane by an RF pulse

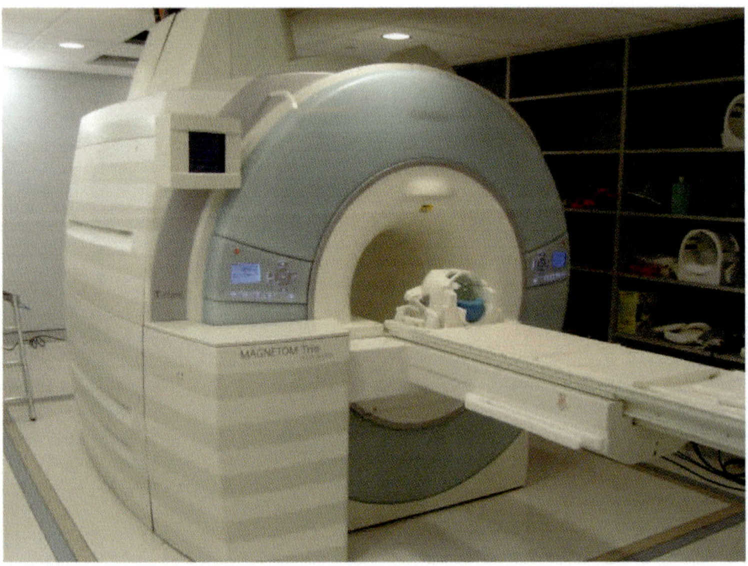

Fig. 6.3. A 3.0 Tesla MRI scanner for use in focal or whole body imaging.

at the Larmor frequency. Molecules then relax at different rates with the main magnetic field and with neighboring spins based on the structure and shielding of the compound. MRI relies on these differences in the relaxation times of molecules of the tissue of interest to produce image contrast. These differences in relaxation rates may be optimized by varying the timing of the MRI sequence parameters resulting in image weighting of specific contrast.

An RF coil or antenna is placed adjacent to the area of interest and detects a voltage as the nuclear magnetic moments or spins return to their fully relaxed state. Additional varying linear magnetic fields known as gradients assign a specific frequency to the signal recorded from each voxel in the image. Typically, an inverse Fourier transform is used to convert the spatial frequency data to an image. Injection of a gadolinium-based contrast agent shortens the relaxation times of adjacent water molecules to produce perfusion-related image contrast. Images of contrast uptake are acquired rapidly as a function of time allow for modeling of tracer kinetics in bone. Estimates of arterial inflow and venous outflow parameters are then possible. These techniques allow for quantitation of skeletal circulation using MRI contrast agents.

6.4 Multi-Modality Image Registration

Image co-registration algorithms are now available that allow for accurate fusion between modalities (MRI, PET/CT). This is of great value given that complementary information is obtained from both modalities providing a better and more complete understanding of the underlying mechanisms in skeletal circulation.

For example, current PET/CT platforms allow for simultaneous acquisition and fusion of PET and CT image sets during a single imaging session (Fig. 6.4). Co-registration of MRI with PET/CT images also provides useful information on uptake of various MRI contrast agents that may be correlated with metabolic PET maps of bone perfusion.

6.4.1 *Static vs. dynamic imaging techniques*

Historically, 2D radiologic techniques acquired planar images to assess tracer uptake in various phases of accumulation in bone. Recent advances in imaging hardware, computer processing, and memory capabilities now allow for rapid acquisition and reconstruction techniques that were not previously possible. This permits 3D dynamic uptake studies in both MRI

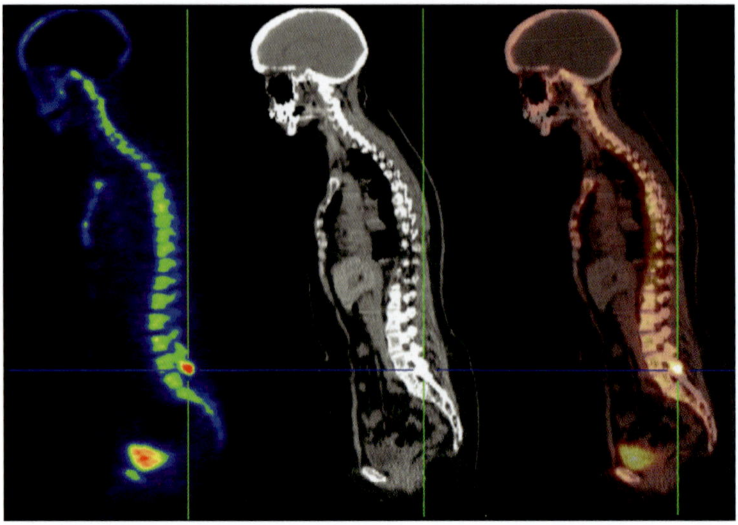

Fig. 6.4. A: ^{18}F-fluoride PET scan shows uptake in bone and tumor. B: corresponding CT scan. C: fused PET/CT scan showing metabolic uptake in relation to anatomy.

and PET on a per voxel basis with high temporal resolution. Each voxel contains a unique time intensity (activity) curve that displays uptake of the contrast agent or tracer as a function of time. These curves may be fitted with pharmacokinetic models to produce estimates of various perfusion parameters characterizing skeletal circulation that may be correlated with various clinical and histologic markers (Fig. 6.5). The resulting fit parameters may be used to create parametric perfusion maps describing the blood pool phase or binding of the specific agent to the bone matrix.

Dynamic acquisition allows more accurate characterization of bone perfusion than obtained at predefined static time points. Uptake characteristics of various tissues vary with their macroscopic vascular and microscopic angiogenic environments and may be monitored with 3D dynamic imaging techniques.

6.5 MRI Techniques

6.5.1 *Choice of MRI contrast agent*

The first clinically approved intravenous MRI contrast agent was Gd-DTPA (gadopentetatedimeglumine, Magnevist:Bayer-Schering Pharma) and was

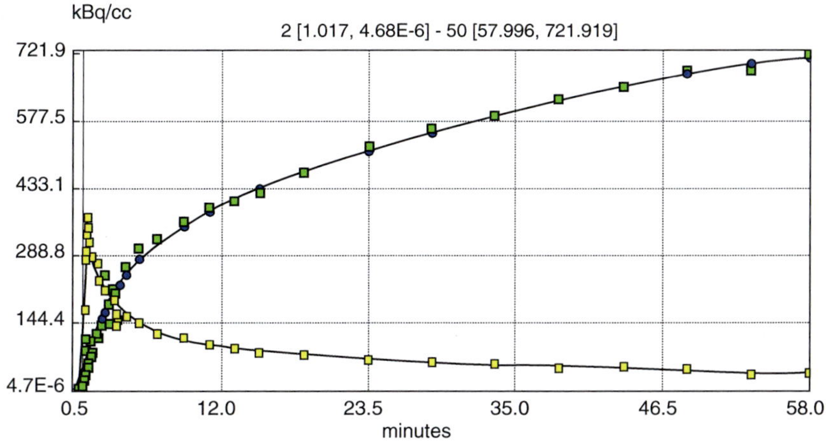

Fig. 6.5. Time activity curves showing ^{18}F-fluoride PET uptake in the medial tibial plateau (green) and femoral artery (yellow) of a preclinical pig model of OA. The three-compartment pharmacokinetic model fit is shown in blue.

introduced in 1987. This agent is known as a small molecular contrast medium (SMCM) having a molecular weight of 538 daltons with distribution and elimination half-lives of 12 and 100 minutes in plasma respectively. Approximately 20–30% of clinically indicated MRI scans utilize an injection of a paramagnetic gadolinium-based contrast agent. It is used in both T_1 and T_2^* weighted scans to increase visibility of tumors (primary and metastatic), vascularity (cardiac, large vessels), infection, inflammation, blood brain barrier disruption, and stroke. Gd-DTPA is taken up by normal and pathologic bone and may be used to assess the degree of perfusion *in vivo*.

A note should be included as to the current safety guidelines for use of gadolinium-based contrast agents in MRI. In 2006, it became known that gadolinium-based contrast agents (GBCAs) may be linked to the onset of a disease known as nephrogenic systemic fibrosis (NSF). Patients with compromised renal function or severe chronic kidney disease (CKD) may be at risk if proper clearance of the GBCA is not achieved. The risk occurs if the free gadolinium becomes unbound from the chelating agent. The American College of Radiology (ACR) and Food and Drug Administration (FDA) guidelines were immediately put into place to measure serum creatinine levels and to limit administration in patients with a glomerular filtration rate (GFR) $<30\,\text{mL/min/1.73m}^2$. A study was done at our combined university hospitals to assess the incidence of NSF over a ten-year period.[31]

There were no cases of NSF from a pool of 74,124 patients that received a standard dose of GBCA. In total, 15 patients receiving high doses of GBCA exhibited NSF, with all patients exhibiting an estimated GFR of less than 30 ml/min.

6.5.2 *Physiologic factors affecting contrast uptake in MRI*

Contrast uptake in bone as measured by dynamic contrast enhanced MRI (DCE-MRI) is dependent on many factors, including the degree of vascularity (angiogenesis), percentage of fatty and hematopoietic marrow, bone mineral density (BMD), and mechanical forces (pressure, stress, strain).[19] Fatty (yellow) marrow contains sparse vasculature in contrast to hematopoietic (red) marrow which has a richer, arborized vascular component.[5] Vascularity of both cortical and cancellous bone is also of great importance in designing and monitoring bone grafts.[16] Maximum revascularization and angiogenic activity are required to promote remodeling and incorporation of the graft into its environment.

6.5.3 *MRI acquisition techniques*

T_1-weighted DCE-MRI may be prescribed to quantitatively assess skeletal circulation in bone. Serum creatinine and GFR (>30 mL/min/1.73m^2) should be calculated for each subject prior to imaging. Online GFR calculators are available from the National Kidney Disease Education Program as part of the NIH NIDDK Institute.[2] Anatomic imaging and variable flip angle sequences should be run prior to injection for localization and T_1 measurement. A 2D or 3D fast spoiled gradient echo sequence should be prescribed that repeatedly covers the area of interest in a temporal resolution of less than 10 seconds.[1] The injection of a standard contrast dose (0.1 mmol/kg) into the right antecubital vein at a rate of 2–4 ml/sec should be performed after approximately 3–5 baseline images have been acquired. Fat suppression should be enabled in order to eliminate the signal from fatty marrow in normal bone that may conflict with the signal intensity of the contrast injection.

6.5.4 *DCE-MRI analysis techniques*

Qualitative estimates of perfusion may be readily performed by measuring the initial uptake slope (%/min), % enhancement ratio, or peak enhancement and initial area under the curve (IAUC) (%·min). Various pharmacokinetic models are available to provide semi-quantitative estimates of skeletal circulation. The Brix 2 compartment model gives estimates of amplitude (A), transfer rate (k_{ep}, min^{-1}), and elimination rate (k_{el}, min^{-1}) by fitting the time intensity curve (TIC) with a bi-exponential function.[8,35] Knowledge of the T_1 relaxation rate prior to injection and choice of an arterial input function allows estimation of the permeability surface area product (K_{trans}, min^{-1}), k_{ep}, and the extravascular extracellular space (v_e) via the Tofts-Kermode compartment model.[35,36]

6.5.5 *Normative DCE-MRI values in skeletal circulation*

Although MRI acquisition techniques and contrast agents vary across institutions, there are estimates of normal and regional bone perfusion in the literature. Chen *et al.* measured DCE-MRI perfusion parameters in normal vertebrae and demonstrated perfusion differences with age and gender.[9] The rate of peak enhancement with age was shown to decline faster in women than men. A study examined DCE-MRI uptake in the proximal femur in normal, osteopenic and osteoporotic subjects in conjunction with standard DEXA measurements of bone mineral density.[27] A significant correlation was seen in reduced patterns of perfusion in subjects that exhibited a reduction in bone mineral density over time. Our group also measured DCE uptake in the normal and injured femoral head using a quadrant-based analysis.[14]

Region	Agent	Parameters	Reference
Vertebrae	Gd-DTPA	Peak = 0.38/0.87(M/F), Slope = 1.53/2.31 (M/F), Age < 50 Peak = 0.25/0.18 (M/F), Slope = 1.30/0.82 (M/F), Age > 50	Chen, 2001
Vertebrae	Gd-DTPA	Plasma flow = 17, Plasma volume = 10, Extraction flow = 0.3	Biffar, 2010
Femoral head	Gd-DTPA	A = 0.53, k_{ep} = 1.76, k_{el} = 0.07, IAUC = 0.43, Peak = 0.39	Dyke, 2013

6.5.6 *Pathologic DCE-MRI values in skeletal circulation*

There are many disease-specific studies utilizing DCE-MRI to assess bone perfusion *in vivo*. A representative set of these results are given below.

Region	Agent	Parameters	Reference
Vertebral fracture	Gd-DTPA	Peak = 0.26/0.22 (M/F), Slope = 1.24/1.18(M/F), Age > 50 with compression fractures at other level	Chen, 2001
Vertebral fracture	Gd-DTPA	Plasma flow = 41, Plasma volume = 21, Extraction flow = 6, Interstitial volume = 19	Biffar, 2010
Femoral head w/FNF fracture	Gd-DTPA	A = 0.29, $k_{ep} = 1.19$, $k_{el} = 0.04$, IAUC = 0.17, Peak = 0.17	Dyke, 2013

6.5.7 *Clinical DCE-MRI applications*

6.5.7.1 *Osteogenic and Ewing's sarcomas*

Our group has used DCE-MRI to determine the percent necrosis in pediatric osteogenic and Ewing's sarcomas following induction chemotherapy.[15] DCE uptake parameters were significantly correlated with histologic necrosis grade, providing an *in vivo* estimate of treatment response. As seen in Fig. 6.6, the popliteal artery (region 2) yielded the fastest wash-in/wash-out characteristics as the feeding vessel for the region. An enhancing region at the tumor rim (region 4) also shows increased uptake compared to normal muscle (region 1). A final region (region 3) taken at the tumor center shows typical uptake in areas of necrosis following induction chemotherapy. Additionally, aggressive untreated tumors will often rapidly outgrow their blood supply, leaving a viable rim of enhancement and a necrotic center.

Receiver operator characteristics defined a predictive accuracy of 91% that was achieved using the inflow parameter (Ak_{ep}) in identifying the degree of tumor necrosis as >90% (grade III). Representative compartmental model fits of tumor regions of interest (ROI) for two patients

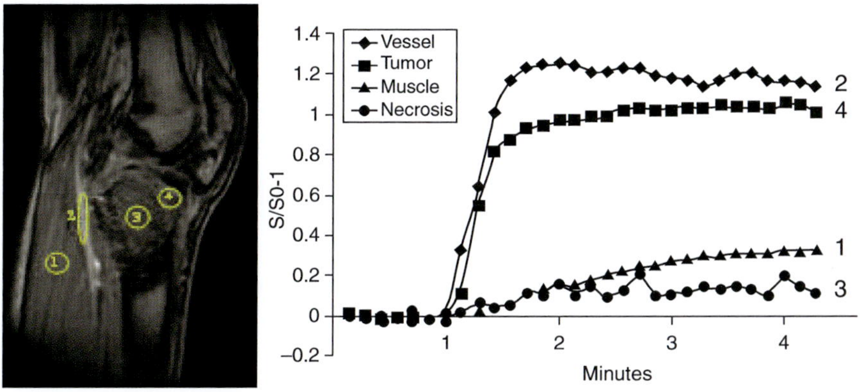

Fig. 6.6. Time intensity curves showing variable DCE-MRI enhancement patterns are given by tissue type following injection of Gd-DTPA in a pediatric osteogenic sarcoma.

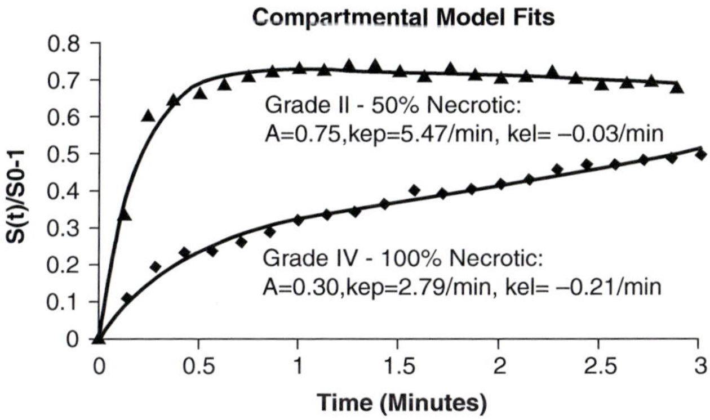

Fig. 6.7. Varying degrees of DCE-MRI enhancement may be seen with differing responses to treatment.

with differing chemotherapy responses are shown with their respective model parameters (Fig. 6.7).[15]

6.5.8 *Femoral neck fractures*

The ability of the orthopaedic trauma surgeon to know whether the blood supply feeding the femoral head has been compromised due to displaced fracture of the femoral neck is crucial. Proper healing requires an adequate blood supply to reduce the risk of avascular necrosis. Figure 6.8 shows

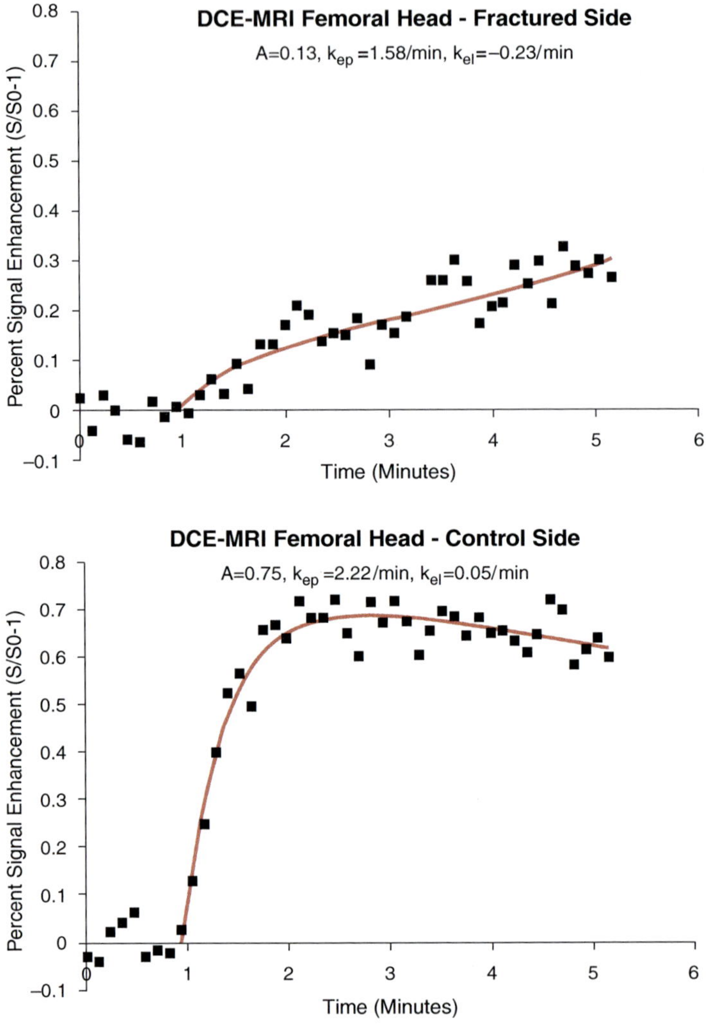

Fig. 6.8. DCE uptake in the femoral head on injured and contralateral sides is shown following fracture of the femoral neck.

reduced uptake in the entire femoral head on the fractured side compared to the control.

Additionally, our group has quantified perfusion differences in each quadrant of the femoral head in both control and injured sides.[14] The superomedial quadrant displayed decreased arterial and venous perfusion parameters in the femoral head. This confirms previous cadaveric studies that examined the distribution of blood vessels feeding the region.[7]

6.5.9 *Preclinical applications*

An application of DCE-MRI to skeletal circulation in OA has been shown by our group in the preclinical Dunkin-Hartley guinea pig model of osteoarthritis.[26] This animal model spontaneously and predictably develops OA on the medial side without surgical intervention and increases in severity with age.[4] DCE-MRI allows the assessment of arterial and venous perfusion parameters in the medial and lateral tibial plateau. The elimination rate or wash out (k_{el}) of the contrast was shown to decrease with increasing severity of OA as determined by histological Mankin score (Fig. 6.9). This change in perfusion in the subchondral bone, postulated to be a result of venous obstruction, spatially localized and temporally preceded Mankin score cartilage changes.

6.5.10 *Validation*

DCE-MRI techniques provide both qualitative and semi-quantitative estimates of skeletal circulation and bone perfusion by assessing uptake of the contrast agent as a function of time. Several studies have been performed to

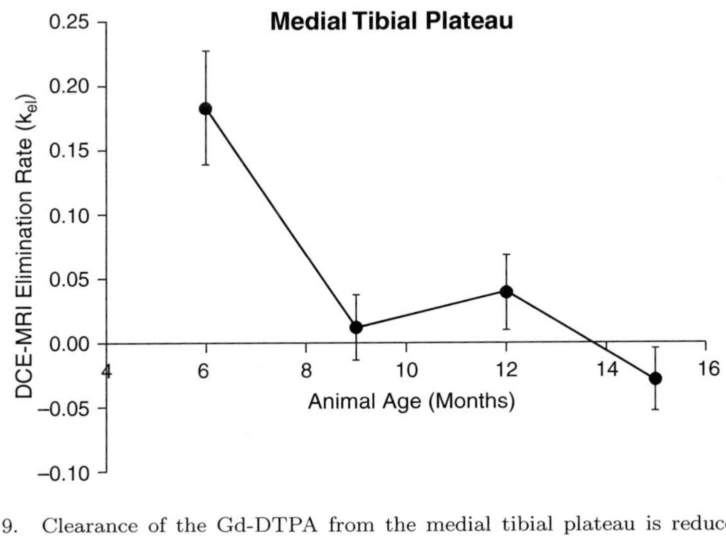

Fig. 6.9. Clearance of the Gd-DTPA from the medial tibial plateau is reduced at 9 months.

correlate various DCE-MRI parameters with external techniques. The gold standard of perfusion measurement has been radiolabeled microspheres. Cova *et al.* examined DCE-MRI uptake and radiolabeled microsphere deposition in the canine hip prior to and following femoral vessel occlusion.[10] A correlation was found between the DCE-MRI percent enhancement and absolute bone blood flow in units of ml/min/100g (average $r = 0.81$). Griffith *et al.* performed a DCE-MRI study in the hip of normal subjects as well as those with osteopenia and osteoporosis, correlating changes in perfusion indices with BMD and marrow fat content.[19] It was shown that an increase in bone marrow fat content had a greater role in decreasing perfusion indices in these populations than did decreased BMD. In addition, our previous study of osteogenic and Ewing's sarcomas contained a follow-up report in which we correlated the degree of MRI perfusion with histologic staining of vascular endothelial growth factor (VEGF) in the resected tumor.[23] A trend toward significance was seen between the arterial inflow (Ak_{ep}) parameter and the degree of VEGF positive staining ($p = 0.074$). Histochemical staining was performed in a rat model of head neck tumor xenografts.[33] This study confirmed a correlation between blood flow and volume as measured by DCE-MRI and CD31 (endothelial cells).

6.6 PET Techniques

6.6.1 *Choice of radiotracer*

The number of radiotracers available for use in PET imaging is limited only by the imagination and abilities of the radiochemist. Some of the more common PET isotopes are in order of increasing half-life: ^{15}O (~2 min), ^{13}N (~10 min), ^{11}C (~20 min), and ^{18}F (~110 min). The standard for blood flow measurement has always been ^{15}O-H_2O. Validation studies using this technique will be discussed later in this chapter. Production of this isotope requires imaging to be performed at the site of cyclotron production given the short half-life. However, the bone-seeking tracer, ^{18}F-fluoride (sodium fluoride), is readily available from many radioisotope vendors for use in both preclinical and clinical studies. While the SPECT tracer ^{99m}Tc-diphosphonate (MDP) has been widely used for bone scans, ^{18}F-fluoride has several advantages. ^{18}F-fluoride yields shorter scan times, higher bone-to-background ratio, and minimal serum protein binding. Studies have also shown it to have a higher diagnostic accuracy in detecting metastatic lesions.[22,32] PET technology provides 3D imaging and much higher spatial resolution than the 2D SPECT technique.

6.6.2 *PET acquisition techniques*

^{18}F-fluoride is injected using standard techniques with an activity of 185–370 MBq (5–10 mCi). (SNM guidelines) As a note, unlike ^{18}F-fluorodeoxyglucose (FDG) scans, subjects do not need to fast prior to imaging but should be well hydrated. The CT protocol should be acquired for attenuation correction of the PET images but may also be optimized to higher resolution should diagnostic information from the CT be required for the study. Static 3D image sets may be acquired 45 minutes after injection of the tracer. However, dynamic acquisition techniques must be acquired in order to yield estimates of bone blood flow and remodeling. Continuous acquisition mode allows rapid imaging ($\sim$3 sec/frame) during the blood pool phase in order to properly sample the arterial input function. The temporal sampling rate may be reduced to 1 min/frame thereafter out to 60 minutes. As in the DCE-MRI acquisition, the scanner should be started prior to injection to obtain several baseline image points.

6.6.3 *PET analysis techniques*

^{18}F-fluoride is a bone-seeking agent that was developed over 50 years ago and approved for clinical use in 1972.[6] After intravenous injection the ^{18}F-fluoride has a two-phase half-life of 24 minutes for the first phase and 2.6 hours for the second.[18] ^{18}F-fluoride estimates bone blood flow within the first two minutes after injection. After this time, the ^{18}F-ion binds to the hydroxyapatite at the bone surface and is incorporated into the bone matrix until remodeling occurs. Hawkins *et al.* proposed a three compartment model estimating skeletal blood flow (K_1) and a net fluoride influx rate (K_i) that estimates bone turnover.[20]

6.7 Normal ^{18}F-Fluoride PET Values in Skeletal Circulation

Several studies looked at normal and osteoporotic spine using PET perfusion parameters. Another group studied various bones [iliac ($n = 3$), scapula ($n = 1$), femur ($n = 4$), tibia ($n = 3$), vertebrae ($n = 1$) in both normal and Paget's disease subjects.[25]

Region	Parameters	Reference
Vertebrae	$K_1 = 0.091$, $K_i = 0.052$	Doot, 2010
Osteoporotic spine	$K_1 = 0.106$, $K_i = 0.035$, $k_3/(K_2+k_3) = 0.332$	Frost, 2010
Normal bones	$K_1 = 0.037$, $K_i = 0.016$	Installe, 2005

Units of K_1,K_i are ml/(cm^3 min)

6.8 Pathologic ^{18}F-fluoride PET Values in Skeletal Circulation

^{18}F-fluoride kinetics were shown to provide a statistically significant ($p < 0.001$) difference in uptake parameters between normal vertebrae and breast cancer metastasis.[12] Increases in PET perfusion parameters were also seen in the osteoporotic spine six months following treatment with Teriparatide.[17] Significant increases in K_1 and K_i were seen in the Paget's disease group compared to normal controls.[25]

Region	Parameters	Reference
Vertebral bone metastasis	$K_1 = 0.166$, $K_i = 0.103$	Doot, 2010
Osteoporotic spine 6 month post-Teriparatidetreatment	$K_1 = 0.108$, $K_i = 0.043$, $k_3/(K_2+k_3) = 0.403$	Frost, 2010
Paget's disease bones	$K_1 = 0.164$, $K_i = 0.114$	Installe, 2005

6.9 Clinical PET Applications

6.9.1 *Distal radius fracture healing*

Knowledge of clinical union after fracture is primarily assessed via x-ray imaging up to two months following initial injury. Different clinical scoring systems along with patient interaction are also useful in assessing healing. As shown in a rat model of femur fracture, ^{18}F-fluoride has the potential to detect non-union at an earlier time point than standard radiographic

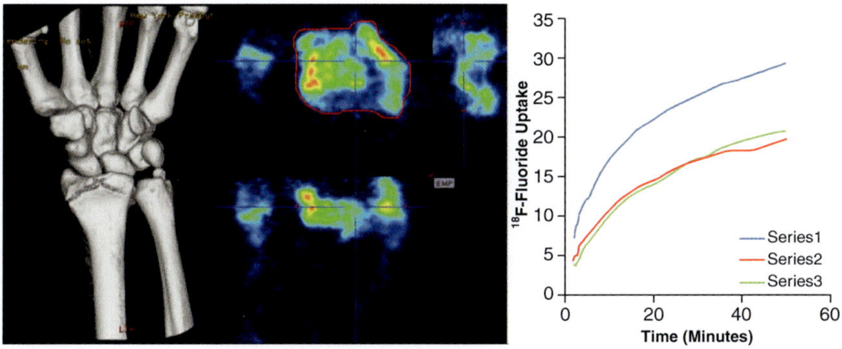

Fig. 6.10. Baseline CT and ^{18}F-fluoride PET images are shown of a distal radius fracture. Note the PET images also display uptake in the ulna due to a concurrent styloid fracture. This subject showed reduced PET uptake 1 and 2 months following initial insult.

techniques.[24] This knowledge would be useful in identifying candidates for use of bone morphogenic proteins, hormones, or other factors to stimulate healing. Our study examined subjects with non-displaced fractures of the distal radius using ^{18}F-fluoride PET (Fig. 6.10).[13]

6.9.2 *Oncologic ^{18}F-fluoride Imaging*

^{18}F-fluoride PET imaging plays a great role in the detection of osseous metastasis and bony infiltration.[29] Lesions that may show little or no uptake on standard ^{99m}Tc-MDP bone scintigraphy may show abnormally increased activity on ^{18}F-fluoride PET scans. Both techniques achieve high sensitivity in detecting sclerotic lesions in bone. ^{18}F-FDG does retain a slight advantage in detection of lytic and marrow-based lesions.[29] Figure 6.11 shows two patients utilizing whole body ^{18}F-fluoride PET imaging to determine the presence of osseous metastasis following treatment. Both patients show uptake determined to be due to degenerative or arthritic changes and not to the presence of abnormal osseous foci.

6.10 Preclinical PET Application

Our group has studied the preclinical Dunkin-Hartley model of guinea pig OA using ^{18}F-fluoride PET imaging (Fig. 6.12). Bone blood flow (K_1) and net fluoride influx rate (K_i) were shown to decrease along with

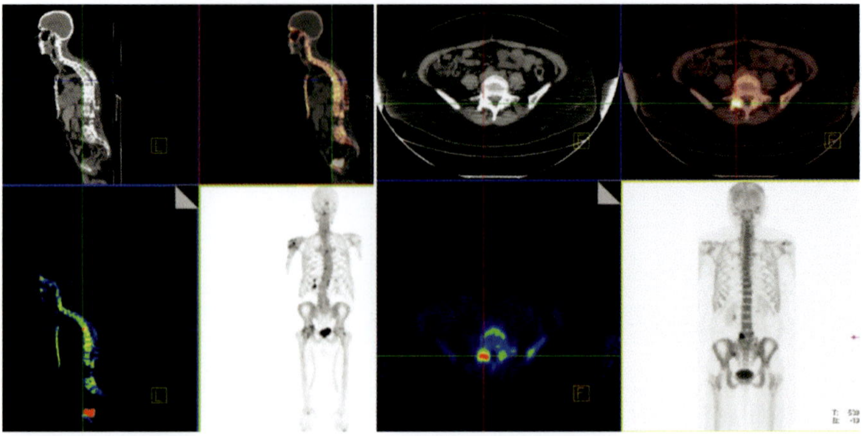

Fig. 6.11. A: Post-treatment follow-up evaluation of prostate carcinoma using 18.7 mCi of 18F-fluoride. B: Post-treatment follow-up evaluation of a neuroendocrine tumor using 15 mCi of 18F-fluoride. No evidence of abnormal osseous metastasis was found in either scan although degenerative changes due to arthritis were visible in both.

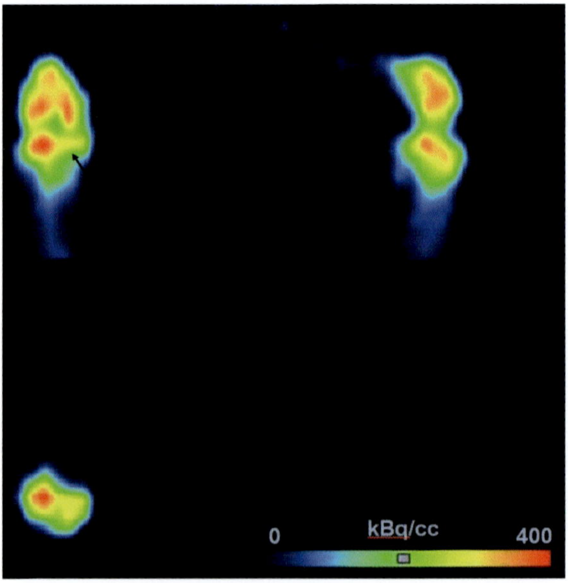

Fig. 6.12. Asymmetric ^{18}F-fluoride uptake may be seen in the guinea pig knee correlating with advanced OA on the medial side.

blood volume (V_b) with increasing histologic Mankin score. The technique shows promise to localize perfusion changes in subchondral bone due to OA.

6.10.1 *Validation*

A study was done in porcine bone using double tetracycline labeling to validate the mineral apposition rate (MAR) and correlate with ^{18}F-fluoride PET perfusion indices.[30] PET parameters of bone blood flow (K_1) and remodeling (K_i) were shown to significantly correlate with the measured MAR, confirming the utility of this imaging technique to assess bone formation. A second study correlated the gold standard of blood flow (^{15}O-H^2O) with ^{18}F-fluoride PET uptake in human subjects following total hip revision with impacted bone grafting.[34] A significant linear correlation ($r = 0.72$) was found with bone blood flow and K_i. These studies and others confirm the validity of ^{18}F-fluoride PET imaging to non-invasively assess perfusion parameters of skeletal circulation.[28]

6.11 Conclusions

The techniques of DCE-MRI and ^{18}F-fluoride PET continue to show promise as invaluable tools to assess skeletal circulation *in vivo*. Their use in localizing abnormalities in skeletal perfusion will play a major role in the management of many disease states. While oncologic imaging stands at the forefront of clinical utility for these techniques, their use is constantly being validated in many other fronts. Assessing underlying arterial and venous changes in subchondral bone perfusion may prove to unlock clues about the mechanism and etiology of osteoarthritis. Additional clinical utility for the orthopaedic trauma surgeon may be shown in assessing skeletal circulation using MRI and PET in various fracture states. Continued research in both modalities will provide normative perfusion indices that may be used as a reference for future applications of these techniques in evaluating skeletal circulation.

Acknowledgement

The author would like to thank the Citigroup Biomedical Imaging Center at Weill Cornell Medical College for Figures 6.1–6.3.

References

1. DCE-MRI Technical Committee. DCE-MRI Quantification Profile, Quantitative Imaging Biomarkers Alliance. QIBA, July 1, 2012; Version 1.0. Publicly Reviewed Version: Available from: RSNA.ORG/QIBA.
2. National Kidney Disease Education Program. National Istitute of Diabetes and Digestive and Kidney Diseases; [updated March 1, 2012; cited 2014]; Available from http://nkdep.nih.gov/lab-evaluation/gfr-calculators/adults-conventional-unit.asp.
3. Arnoldi CC, Linderholm H, Mussbichler H (1972). Venous engorgement and intraosseous hypertension in osteoarthritis of the hip. *J Bone Joint Surg Br*, 54(3), 409–421.
4. Bendele AM, Hulman JF (1988). Spontaneous cartilage degeneration in guinea pigs. *Arthritis Rheum*, 31, 561–565.
5. Biffar A, Dietrich O, Sourbron S, Duerr HR, Reiser MF, Baur-Melnyk A (2010). Diffusion and perfusion imaging of bone marrow. *Eur J Radiol*, 76(3), 323–328.
6. Blau M, Nagler W, Bender MA (1962). Fluorine-18: A new isotope for bone scanning. *J Nucl Med*, 3, 332–334.
7. Boraiah S, Dyke JP, Hettrich C, Parker RJ, Miller A, Helfet D, *et al.* (2009). Assessment of vascularity of the femoral head using gadolinium (Gd-DTPA)-enhanced magnetic resonance imaging: A cadaver study. *J Bone Joint Surg Br*, 91(1), 131–137.
8. Brix G, Semmler W, Port R, Schad LR, Layer G, Lorenz WJ (1991). Pharmacokinetic parameters in CNS Gd-DTPA enhanced MR imaging. *J Comput Assist Tomogr*, 15(4), 621–628.
9. Chen WT, Shih TT, Chen RC, Lo SY, Chou CT, Lee JM, *et al.* (2001). Vertebral bone marrow perfusion evaluated with dynamic contrast-enhanced MR imaging: Significance of aging and sex. *Radiology*, 220(1), 213–218.
10. Cova M, Kang YS, Tsukamoto H, Jones LC, McVeigh E, Neff BL, *et al.* (1991). Bone marrow perfusion evaluated with gadolinium-enhanced dynamic fast MR imaging in a dog model. *Radiology*, 179(2), 535–539.
11. Dieppe P, Cushnaghan J, Young P, Kirwan J (1993). Prediction of the progression of joint space narrowing in osteoarthritis of the knee by bone scintigraphy. *Ann Rheum Dis*, 52(8), 557–563.
12. Doot RK, Muzi M, Peterson LM, Schubert EK, Gralow JR, Specht JM, *et al.* (2010). Kinetic analysis of 18F-fluoride PET images of breast cancer bone metastases. *J Nucl Med*, 51(4), 521–527.
13. Dyke JP, Aaron RK (2010). Noninvasive methods of measuring bone blood perfusion. *Ann NY Acad Sci*, 1192, 95–102.
14. Dyke JP, Lazaro LE, Hettrich CM, Hentel KD, Helfet DL, Lorich DG (2015). Regional analysis of femoral head perfusion following displaced fractures of the femoral neck. *J Magn Reson Imaging*, 41(2), 550–554.

15. Dyke JP, Panicek DM, Healey JH, Meyers PA, Huvos AG, Schwartz LH, *et al.* (2003). Osteogenic and Ewing sarcomas: Estimation of necrotic fraction during induction chemotherapy with dynamic contrast-enhanced MR imaging. *Radiology*, 228(1), 271–278.
16. Finkemeier CG (2002). Bone-grafting and bone-graft substitutes. *J Bone Joint Surg Am*, 84-A(3), 454–464.
17. Frost ML, Siddique M, Blake GM, Moore AE, Schleyer PJ, Dunn JT, *et al.* (2011). Differential effects of teriparatide on regional bone formation using (18)F-fluoride positron emission tomography. *J Bone Miner Res*, 26(5), 1002–1011.
18. Grant FD, Fahey FH, Packard AB, Davis RT, Alavi A, Treves ST (2008). Skeletal PET with 18F-fluoride: Applying new technology to an old tracer. *J Nucl Med*, 49(1), 68–78.
19. Griffith JF, Yeung DK, Tsang PH, Choi KC, Kwok TC, Ahuja AT, *et al.* (2008). Compromised bone marrow perfusion in osteoporosis. *J Bone Miner Res*, 23(7), 1068–1075.
20. Hawkins RA, Choi Y, Huang SC, Hoh CK, Dahlbom M, Schiepers C, *et al.* (1992). Evaluation of the skeletal kinetics of fluorine-18-fluoride ion with PET. *J Nucl Med*, 33(5), 633–642.
21. Hernborg J (1969). Elimination of Na-131-I from the head and the neck of the femur in unaffected and osteoarthritic hip joints. *Arthritis Rheum*, 12(1), 30–33.
22. Hetzel M, Arslandemir C, Konig HH, Buck AK, Nussle K, Glatting G, *et al.* (2003). F-18 NaF PET for detection of bone metastases in lung cancer: Accuracy, cost-effectiveness, and impact on patient management. *J Bone Miner Res*, 18(12), 2206–2214.
23. Hoang BH, Dyke JP, Koutcher JA, Huvos AG, Mizobuchi H, Mazza BA, *et al.* (2004). VEGF expression in osteosarcoma correlates with vascular permeability by dynamic MRI. *Clin Orthop Relat Res*, 426, 32–38.
24. Hsu WK, Feeley BT, Krenek L, Stout DB, Chatziioannou AF, Lieberman JR (2007). The use of 18F-fluoride and 18F-FDG PET scans to assess fracture healing in a rat femur model. *Eur J Nucl Med Mol Imaging*, 34(8), 1291–1301.
25. Installé J, Nzeusseu A, Bol A, Depresseux G, Devogelaer JP, Lonneux M (2005). 18F-fluoride PET for monitoring therapeutic response in Paget's disease of bone. *J Nucl Med*, 46(10), 1650–1658.
26. Lee JH, Dyke JP, Ballon D, Ciombor DM, Rosenwasser MP, Aaron RK (2009). Subchondral fluid dynamics in a model of osteoarthritis: Use of dynamic contrast-enhanced magnetic resonance imaging. *Osteoarthritis and Cartilage*, 17(10), 1350–1355.
27. Ma HT, Griffith JF, Zhao X, Lv H, Yeung DK, Leung PC (2012). Relationship between marrow perfusion and bone mineral density: A pharmacokinetic study of DCE-MRI. *Conf Proc IEEE Eng Med Biol Soc*, 2012, 377–379.

28. Messa C, Goodman WG, Hoh CK, Choi Y, Nissenson AR, Salusky IB, *et al.* (1993). Bone metabolic activity measured with positron emission tomography and [18F]fluoride ion in renal osteodystrophy: Correlation with bone histomorphometry.*J Clin Endocr Metab*, 77(4), 949–955.
29. Mick CG, James T, Hill JD, Williams P, Perry M (2014). Molecular imaging in oncology: 18F-sodium fluoride PET imaging of osseous metastatic disease. *Am J Roentgenol*, 203(2), 263–271.
30. Piert M, Zittel TT, Becker GA, Jahn M, Stahlschmidt A, Maier G, *et al.* (2001). Assessment of porcine bone metabolism by dynamic. *J Nucl Med*, 42(7), 1091–1100.
31. Prince MR, Zhang H, Morris M, MacGregor JL, Grossman ME, Silberzweig J, *et al.* (2008). Incidence of nephrogenic systemic fibrosis at two large medical centers. *Radiology*, 248(3), 807–816.
32. Schirrmeister H, Guhlmann A, Kotzerke J, Santjohanser C, Kuhn T, Kreienberg R, *et al.* (1999). Early detection and accurate description of extent of metastatic bone disease in breast cancer with fluoride ion and positron emission tomography. *J Clin Oncol*, 17(8), 2381–2389.
33. Sterzik A, Paprottka PM, Zengel P, Hirner H, Rosspunt S, Eschbach R, *et al.* (2015). DCE-MRI biomarkers for monitoring an anti-angiogenic triple combination therapy in experimental hypopharynx carcinoma xenografts with immunohistochemical validation. *Acta Radiol*, 56(3), 294–303.
34. Temmerman OP, Raijmakers PG, Heyligers IC, Comans EF, Lubberink M, Teule GJ, *et al.* (2008). Bone metabolism after total hip revision surgery with impacted grafting: Evaluation using H2 15O and [18F]fluoride PET: A pilot study. *Mol Imaging Biol*, 10(5), 288–293.
35. Tofts PS (1997). Modeling tracer kinetics in dynamic Gd-DTPA MR imaging. *J Magn Reson Imaging*, 7(1), 91–101.
36. Tofts PS, Brix G, Buckley DL, Evelhoch JL, Henderson E, Knopp MV, *et al.* (1999). Estimating kinetic parameters from dynamic contrast-enhanced T(1)-weighted MRI of a diffusable tracer: Standardized quantities and symbols. *J Magn Reson Imaging*, 10(3), 223–232.

Part 3

Pathophysiology of Skeletal Circulation

CHAPTER 7

CIRCULATORY PATHOLOGY IN OSTEONECROSIS

LYNNE C. JONES

Associate Professor, Orthopaedic Surgery
Johns Hopkins University School of Medicine, Baltimore, MD

ROY K. AARON

Professor of Orthopaedic Surgery
The Warren Alpert Medical School of Brown University, Providence, RI

7.1 Introduction

The clinical features, etiology, and natural history of osteonecrosis (ON) have been well described.[1,19,60,66,98] This chapter focuses, and has a distinct emphasis, on circulatory pathologies and puts them in the context of the histopathology and pathomechanics of bone necrosis, subchondral resorption, subsequent subchondral fracture, collapse, and joint incongruity. ON has typically been classified by etiology and pathogenesis, and since most relevant studies of pathophysiology have been in late-stage human ON, combinations of pathologic observations and uncertainty as to their temporal sequences cloud the ability to finely parse out inciting primary and secondary events.[47,63,76] Various putative etiological conditions converge on a more or less stereotypical pathophysiology that reflects circulatory compromise. A unifying concept of the pathogenesis of ON emphasizes the role of circulatory occlusion leading to ischemia and osteocyte necrosis (Fig. 7.1). Many etiologies may contribute to the pathogenic mechanisms of vascular interruption, thrombotic occlusion, or extravascular compression, any of which may decrease perfusion and result in ischemia and necrosis.[1] It has been convenient to subdivide ON as traumatic and non-traumatic and to further subdivide non-traumatic ON as resulting from primarily intravascular pathology (e.g., hypercoagulation and thrombosis)

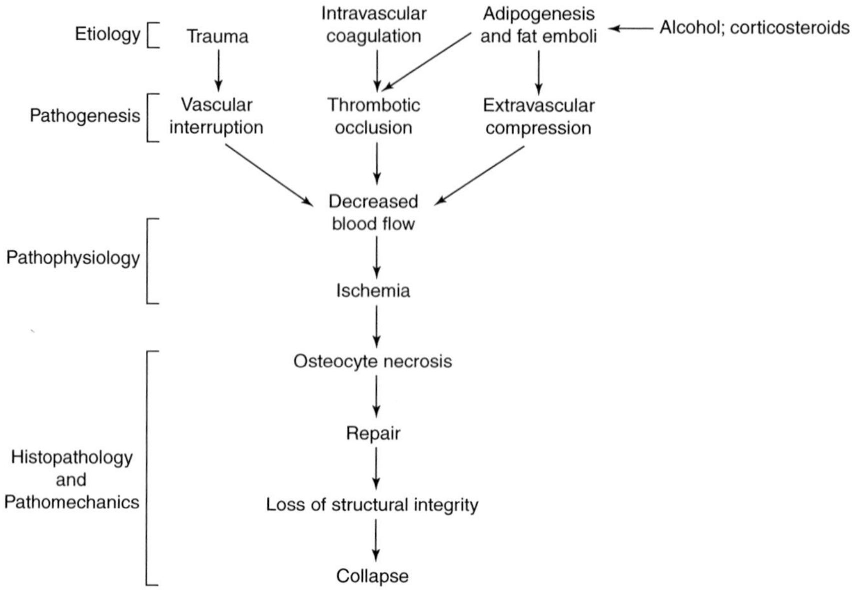

Fig. 7.1. A concept of pathogenesis of ON that unifies several etiologic and pathogenic hypotheses. *Source*: Aaron RK, Gray R. Osteonecrosis: Etiology, natural history, pathophysiology and diagnosis. In: Callaghan JJ, Rosenberg AG, Rubash HE, eds., *The Adult Hip*. Philadelphia, PA: Lippincott Williams, 463–476. Reprinted with permission from Wolters Kluwer Health.

or primarily extravascular pathology (e.g., adipocyte hypertrophy, Gaucher disease).

7.2 Histopathology and Pathomechanics

The pathologic features of ON focusing on vascularity are presented in this book in Chapter 8 and elsewhere.[1] In summary, the presence of necrotic bone induces a repair process in which bone resorption exceeds formation, leading to a loss of structural integrity in the subchondral trabeculae and, eventually, to subchondral collapse.[25–27] It is not the necrosis *per se* but rather the repair process dominated by bone resorption that leads to the loss of subchondral bone.[1] Finite element modeling has demonstrated that the resorption of subchondral trabeculae is the major contributor to the loss of structural integrity and eventual collapse and incongruity of the articular surface.[9]

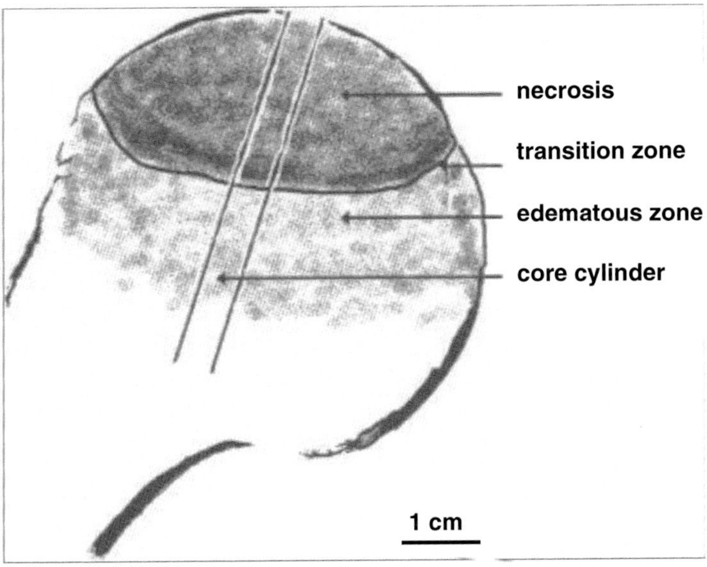

Fig. 7.2. Schematic view of ON femoral head showing necrotic, transitional, and edematous zones. *Source*: Radke, *et al.* (2006). Expression of the angiomatrix and angiogenic proteins CYR61, CTGF, and VEGF in osteonecrosis of the femoral head. *J Orthop Res*, 24(5): 945–952. Reprinted with permission.

The histopathology of ON has been well described.[8, 10, 16, 19, 43, 88] The necrotic area, usually encompassing the weight-bearing area of the femoral head, is characterized by absence of bone cells and necrotic marrow. It is described as containing granulation tissue reminiscent of caseating necrosis and containing saponified fat. Depending on the progression of the disease, it is often surrounded by a zone of repair with evidence of creeping substitution (new bone overlaying on dead bone) — sometimes called a rim of sclerosis. Beneath therepair zone is a hyperemic zone containing numerous blood vessels (Fig. 7.2). The histopathology of ON has been categorized by Ficat and Arlet as fourtypes:[19] type 1 (prenecrotic): plasmostasis, reticular proliferation, hemorrhage, accumulation of foam cells; type 2 (preradiologic): necrosis of fatty marrow; type 3: medullary necrosis with evidence of 50–100% of the trabecular lacunae empty; type 4: necrosis and fibrosis with foci of necrosis surrounded by new bone.[5, 36–38] Saito *et al.* described the histology of core biopsy specimens identifying four zones ranging from complete necrosis with ischemia (zone A) to transitional zones with necrosis containing evidence of old (zone B) or new hemorrhage (zone C) to intact bone (zone D) with living fatty or hematopoietic tissue.[82] A definitive diagnosis can be made when "creeping substitution" — new bone overlying necrotic bone — is detected.[8,41]

7.3 Vasculature and Vascular Pathology

The blood vessels that supply the femoral head include the medial and lateral circumflex, a vessel of the ligamentum teres, and the inguinal gluteal arteries. The medial circumflex and lateral circumflex arteries form a vascular ring around the femoral neck.[44,55,113] Two sets of retinacular vessels branch off from this ring including (1) metaphyseal branches which penetrate into the femoral neck and (2) epiphyseal branches which penetrate into the peripheral non-articular portion of the head to supply the epiphysis. Approximately 26 lateral epiphyseal arteries penetrate the femoral head posteriorly and superiorly supplying the lateral weight-bearing portion of the femoral head.[44] While it has also been shown that the inferior gluteal artery contributes significantly to the blood supply to the femoral head of developing fetuses, its role is less clear in adults.[113] The vessels of the ligamentum teres also carry a small supply to the femoral head, but its contribution to its blood supply is considered to be minimal.[44,113]

Veins are more difficult to visualize because venous valves may block retrograde extraosseous injections and veins are thinner walled and more collapsible than their arterial counterparts.[55] Epiphyseal and metaphyseal veins are more numerous than their corresponding arteries.[44] Veins within the medullary space, termed marrow sinusoids, drain through collecting ducts into the central venous sinus; a branch of the central venous sinus, the nutrient vein, passes through the nutrient foramen along with the nutrient artery.[44,55]

Several different pathologic mechanisms that may result in ischemia and subsequent lesions of ON include vascular disruption, intraosseous extravascular compression, extraosseous vascular constriction, and intravascular occlusion.[110]

7.3.1 *Vascular disruption*

The anatomy and location of the vessels to and from the femoral head make them especially vulnerable to trauma (Fig. 7.3). Trauma that compromises the femoral neck may compromise the vascular ring around the neck and the circulation to and from the femoral head. There is a notable incidence of ON with displaced and undisplaced femoral neck fractures, ranging from

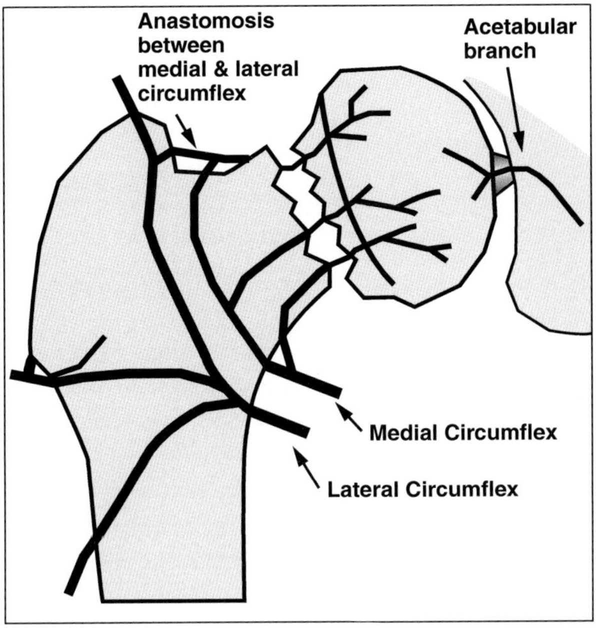

Fig. 7.3. Disruption of ascending vasculature and devascularization of the femoral head as a consequence of femoral neck fracture. *Source*: Johnson EO, Soultanis K, Soucacos PN (2004). Vascular anatomy and microcirculation of skeletal zones vulnerable to osteonecrosis: Vascularization of the femoral head. *Orthop Clin North Am*, 35(3), 285–291, viii. Reprinted with permission from Elsevier.

14.1 to 100%.[13] ON has also been reported to occur in association with hip dislocations (3% anterior; 13% posterior).[13]

Using superselective angiography, Atsumi and Kuroki identified five types of distributions of the superior retinacular arteries.[6] In normal cases, the superior retinacular arteries were characterized as arch type and extended to the center of the femoral head (type 1). The other types included(1) failure to visualize vessels due to extraosseous pathology (type 2) and(2) various degrees of small arterial penetration (types 3–5). The majority of the hips with early-stage necrosis demonstrated type 3 findings (the presence of small arteries penetrating where the superior retinacular arteries were normally located). The authors suggested that this represents revascularization. These findings were also noted in the contralateral "normal" hips and in normal hips with steroid administration. Further study is needed to determine whether these abnormalities existed before or after ON had been initiated. Serre and Simonfound normal femoral arteriograms with abnormal intraosseous phlebography in patients with ON of the femoral head.[86] Hungerford observed absent or incomplete filling of the main extraosseous veins, diaphyseal reflux, and stasis of contrast media on 5-min and subsequent films.[37]

7.3.2 *Intraosseous extravascular compression*

Prior to MRIs, core biopsies and intraosseous pressure measurements were often performed in order to confirm a diagnosis of ON. Examination of the core specimens indicated that there were increased numbers of adipocytes and adipocyte hypertrophy, frequently associated with high dose corticosteroid administration. Another finding was that patients with ON frequently exhibited elevated intraosseous pressures and abnormal stress tests.[19,37,45] A stress test involved the administration of a 5-ml bolus of saline into the head, creating a temporary increase in pressure. If normal, the pressure decreased rapidly following injection; if abnormal, the increase returned more slowly to pre-injection levels. Based upon these findings, it was suggested that ON developed as a consequence of compression of the thin-walled veins by encroaching adipocytes resulting in venous stasis.[39] This hypothesis was supported by observations of abnormal venograms.

The femoral head is a rigid compartment with marrow elements located within the spaces of trabecular bone. If there is an increase in intraosseous extravascular pressure, perfusion could be theoretically impaired. Intraosseous extravascular occlusion and intraosseous hypertension can conceivably occur if there is an increase in the adipocyte number and/or hypertrophy, or with increased numbers of Gaucher cells. Some experimental observations have reported the presence of intraosseous hypertension[70,101] but others have found that the measurement of intraosseous pressure lacks sufficient diagnostic precision, being neither sensitive nor specific.[1] Various observations have led to the conclusion that intraosseous hypertension, while often seen in ON, is a non-specific and secondary, perhaps contributory, but not causal, factor in ON.[49,50] Although the pathophysiology is not definitively known, intraosseous, space-occupying factors are clinically associated with ON.

7.3.2.1 *Lipid accumulation and lipocyte hypertrophy*

Lipid deposition and lipocyte hypertrophy have been observed in specimens of ON bone, often associated with corticosteroid or alcohol intake.[54,91,102]

It has been hypothesized that accumulating lipid and hypertrophic cells create extravascular pressure and decrease either arterial inflow or venous outflow, or both. Alcohol- or corticosteroid-associated adipogenesis may shift precursor cells from an osteocytic to an adipogenic lineage, thereby reducing the number of osteoprogenitor cells.[105]

7.3.2.2 *Gaucher disease*

Gaucher disease is associated with a high incidence of ON.[17] Gaucher cells are specialized cells that accumulate large amounts of glucocerebrosides, a type of glycosphingolipid. In Gaucher disease, there is substantial extravascular medullary infiltration by Gaucher cells resulting in an increase in intracortical pressure. It has been suggested that this increased pressure within the rigid compartment of the femoral head results in compression of the vascular sinusoids leading to bone ischemia.[85] This is explored further in Chapter 8.

7.3.3 *Extraosseous vascular constriction*

Impaired venous outflow (venous stasis) has been observed to increase intraosseous pressure, reduce perfusion, and result in hypoxia, and has been proposed as a cause of ON.[38, 104] Extraosseous venous obstruction has been implicated as a cause of venous stasis.[20] Hypoxia and reduced intraosseous fluid flow have been measured in the subchondral bone of hips with non-traumatic ON, suggesting a causal role in osteocyte necrosis.[20]

A number of laboratory studies have investigated the response of the endothelium and the effect on blood flow of ischemia following the clamping off of extraosseous blood vessels.[14, 97, 106] Ischemic skeletal muscle results in diminution of arterial diameters followed by active constriction, forcing blood elements distally and resulting in a reduced or even completely occluded lumens.[14] This study noted swelling of endothelia and leukocytes, erythrocyte rouleaux formation, and distortion of leukocytes and erythrocytes during ischemia. During reperfusion, alteration of flow patterns, vortex formation, regional stasis, focal hemorrhage, edema, vasospasm, platelet aggregation, erythrocyte sludging, adhesion and migration of leukocytes, and swelling of endothelia and leukocytes were observed. Winetet al. used intravital microscopy to study blood flow to bone.[36, 106] Using a model where they were able to clamp the right common iliac artery in rabbits, they were able to create ischemia to bone. Upon release of the clamp, they observed secondary ischemia/no-reflow and other evidence of reperfusion injury was observed.[36] This was associated with abnormally high leakage of FITC-D70 from the few vessels perfused during secondary ischemia, indicating that damage to the blood vessels had occurred. Further study is needed to investigate the possibility of reperfusion injury associated with ON; this has clinical ramifications regarding both an understanding of the pathogenesis and treatment of ON.

7.3.4 *Intravascular occlusion*

Intravascular occlusion may result from thrombosis, fat or gas embolism, or sickle cell aggregation. Fat emboli have been observed in cases of ON. Jones observed fat emboli in patients with dysbaric ON and following an allergic reaction to an insect bite, trauma, and alcohol.[46] He reported that "there were arterioles, capillaries, and sinusoids occluded by deformed fat emboli and fibrin thrombi".[46]

7.3.4.1 *Sickle cell anemia*

There is a strong association between sickle cell disease and ON.[69] The sickling of blood cells may lead to repeated ischemic events related to intravascular obstruction.[67,85] In adolescents with sickle cell disease, Hernigou and Bernaudin reported that the blood flow in the sinusoidal system was sluggish and the biochemical environment in this area facilitated the sickling process; blood containing sickled cells had high viscosity and produced a relative obstruction to blood flow in the sinusoidal system of the epiphysis.[33] This differs from other descriptions of ON in that the trabecular bone becomes necrotic while the marrow elements remain viable.[85,91] Furthermore, there is no blockage to revascularization and there is evidence of many cement lines indicating multiple attempts to heal the bone.[85] This is explored further in Chapter 8.

7.3.4.2 *Dysbarism*

In spite of our knowledge about the relationship between dysbarism (Caisson disease) and ON, ON continues to occur in as many as 34.5% of individuals exposed to compressed air in 2014.[62] With dysbarism, there is evidence of lipid dysregulation, coagulation abnormalities, and increased intracortical pressure.[76] Hutter *et al.* proposes that the ON is a consequence of intravascular obliteration by nitrogen bubbles or microthrombi or ofextraluminal obliteration by bone marrow gas or edema.[40] Another concept is that bubbles within the fatty marrow cause an increase in intramedullary pressure, occluding the intraosseous and extraosseous vessels, thereby leading to stasis of blood and subsequent ischemia of osteocytes.[87] J.P. Jones observed multiple gas bubbles within the large vessels and the fatty marrow of femoral and humeral heads associated with lipid and platelet aggregates on the surface of marrow bubbles. He also noted fibrin-platelet thrombi within dilated venous sinusoids adjacent to bubbles, and in veins, capillaries, and arterioles associated with intraosseous fat embolism and fibrin thrombi in the subchondral bone.[48] He proposed that injured marrow adipocytes can release liquid fat, thromboplastin, and other vasoactive substances that serve as procoagulants and trigger disseminated intravascular coagulation and ON. Unlike secondary and idiopathic ON of the femoral head, the regions affected by dysbarism may include the head, neck, and proximal shaft of the femur and humerus.[87]

7.3.4.3 *Hypercoagulation and thrombosis*

Intravascular occlusion resulting from thrombi within the microvascular circulation has been implicated in the development of ON of the femoral head. Thrombi may form in response to endothelial damage or dysfunction.[56] The consequences of thrombi range from a diminution of the blood flow through larger vessels to complete occlusion of smaller blood vessels. Evidence of endothelial damage and dysfunction in the bone of patients with ON include sinusoidal distension, thickening of the arteriolar walls, arteriolar thrombosis and fibrin thrombi in the subchondral Haversian capillaries, arterioles, and marrow sinusoids.[19,47] Thrombi have been detected in both intraosseous arterioles and venules.[84,92] Evidence of old and new intramedullary hemorrhage has also been observed.[47,82] Thrombi have been frequently observed when the inciting event for the ON is known (e.g., dysbaric ON).

In studies that are investigating a possible genetic predisposition in patients with ON, there has been a focus on the genes associated with hypofibrinolysis and thrombophilia.[28,31,51,111] Both disorders result in increased thrombi and blood flow impairment. Glueck *et al.* has observed that 4G/4G polymorphism for the gene for PAI-1 was associated with ON and that the gene product, PAI-Fx, was high in 31% of the ON patients as compared to the control subjects (3%).[29] With respect to thrombophilia, there is evidence of mutations of the genes for methylenetetrahydrofolate reductase (MTHFR), Factor V Leiden, and prothrombin. For example, Zalavras *et al.* reported that there was a significantly higher percentage of ON patients (18%) with the G1691A mutation of factor V Leiden as compared to controls (4.6%).[111]

Elevated coagulation factors can also be found in ON patients without evidence of genetic mutations. This acquired hypercoagulability may be related to other co-morbidities or to pharmaceutical treatment (for example, corticosteroids). Jones *et al.* found that 82.2% of ON patients had at least one abnormal coagulation factor compared to 30% of healthy controls.[52] Furthermore, almost 50% of the patients had two or more abnormalities as compared to 2.5% of the healthy controls. Regarding idiopathic ON (no identifiable risk factors), Jones *et al.* found at least one coagulation factor abnormality in the sera of all five patients in their study; high aCL IgG and PAI-1 were evident in four patients. Zalavras *et al.* reported low protein C, low protein S, high lipoprotein(a), and high von Willebrand factor levels present in a significantly higher proportion of patients with idiopathic ON (59%) and secondary ON (63%) compared with control subjects (8%).[109] In the same patient population, Cenni found higher plasminogen and D-dimer levels and lower protein C levels in patients with idiopathic ON than in healthy controls.[12]

7.4 Circulatory Pathophysiology and Vascular Pathology

Several investigators have studied the vasculature contained within and around ON lesions. In an examination of core biopsy specimens, Arlet *et al.* reported fewer thick- and thin-walled blood vessels as compared to samples from patients diagnosed with osteoarthritis or algodystrophy.[4] They observed fibrosis and thickening of the media with narrowing of the lumen. In a few of the cases, they found evidence of intravascular thrombosis. They also detected parietal ruptures and hemorrhages within the sinusoids. One limitation of this study is that there is no description of where within the affected tissue the vessels were located. Saito *et al.* reported that the number of blood vessels in the bone marrow was reduced in the necrotic core biopsies.[83] There was evidence of collapse and damaged wall structures, internal elastic membrane, tunica media of the arteriolar and arterial walls, and loss of elastin and collagen fibers, in vessels within the transitional zone. In a second study, this group expanded their study to include ON patients with abnormal MRI with normal scintigrams. As with the previous study, the most common pathological feature was evidence of both old and new hemorrhages. The study also demonstrated reduced blood vessel number and diameter, and structural damage to the vascular wall of arterioles. They did not observe structural damage within the veins and sinusoids. As the specimens were from patients with early-stage disease (pre-symptom; pre-radiologic), the investigators propose that arteriopathy is a specific and primary condition in early ON of the femoral head.

Using immunohistochemistry and the CD34 antibody, Radke *et al.* noted staining within the necrotic zone, indicating a high degree of vascularization.[79] This is in contradistinction to the findings of Li *et al.* who found no new vessels in the necrotic zone.[65] Vessels have been observed within the reparative, hyperemic/edematous zone where vessels might be expected to support the creeping substitution that occurs.

While it has been assumed that there is a decrease in blood flow with ON, this has been difficult to demonstrate since methods of measuring blood flow are invasive or destructive and not easily adapted for use clinically. Using laser Doppler flowmetry, Swiontkowski *et al.* found lower levels of blood cell flux in the region of the necrotic segment. In contrast, they noted higher values about the rim of the segment in four of five patients.[96] Fukioka *et al.* generated flow maps of the femoral head using the laser speckle method.[23] The blood flow level of the collapsed necrotic area was considerably lower (no overlap) than the intact area. With this method, they were able to clearly visualize the necrotic area in 92 of 100 cases.

7.4.1 *A special note on corticosteroids and ON*

Corticosteroids may exhibit several direct effects on the vasculature and blood flow.[56,57,76] They have been shown to alter vascular responsiveness to vasoactive substances and disturb the normal balance and regulation of vascular tone in endothelial tissues.[76] Corticosteroids can elevate peripheral resistance and arterial blood pressure.[57,76] Possible effects of corticosteroids, which may occur during the development of ON, are direct injury of endothelial cells, suppression of endothelial nitric oxide synthase activity, increased blood lipid levels, increase in coagulation factors, and inhibition of angiogenesis.[56,57,76,90] In an evaluation of femoral heads retrieved at autopsy with no history of hip problems, Hirano *et al.* observed no significant difference in the incidence of stenosis in the superior retinacular arteries between steroid- (intraosseous: 21.1–28.2%; extraosseous: 16.3–51.1%) and non-steroid-treated groups (intraosseous: 21.7–31.7%; extraosseous: 22.1–40.6%).[34] In contradistinction, the percentage of stenotic veins was significantly increased in the steroid-treated patients ($p < 0.0001$). The investigators suggest that their findings implicate stenotic changes in veins in the pathogenesis of ON.

Most impressions of the magnitude of the relationship between corticosteroid intake and ON have been formed from retrospective, uncontrolled, and cross-sectional studies that described the prevalence of corticosteroid use in patients with ON. However, only longitudinal, prospective studies of patients taking corticosteroids can determine the prevalence of ON in steroid-treated patients.[2] The few studies that have taken a prospective approach have determined that the prevalence of ON in patients taking corticosteroids varies between 4% and 7%.[18,99] In a prospective study of steroid-naïve patients, the prevalence of ON was determined to be 7% in patients with mixed etiologies and 16% in patients with renal transplantation.[2] Relative risks for duration, cumulative, and daily doses were determined.

7.5 The Failure of Neo-Angiogenesis

While the avascular lesion itself in ON is characterized by tissue often resembling caseating necrosis,[19] the tissue surrounding the bony lesion is often hypervascular with blood vessels beginning to penetrate the necrotic lesion. A few reports have shown that revascularization and repair is possible in cases of ON;[15,74] but most cases do not revascularize before subchondral collapse occurs and subsequent arthrosis occurs.[71] This may be related to the stage and size of the lesion.[93]

Since ON has long been considered a disease of the bone vasculature, the question arises whether angiogenesis is impaired as a pathogenic mechanism. Angiogenesis is defined as the growth of new capillary vessels and is characterized by soluble factors that are mitogenic for endothelial cells and is responsible for formation of new capillaries.[21] As previously discussed, there is evidence of angiogenesis in the reparative zone around necrotic lesions. The question can then be posed, why is this attempt at repair unsuccessful in most cases of femoral head necrosis? One hypothesis is that the mechanical integrity of the lesion is compromised before repair can be achieved. This may be a contributing factor, but probably does not explain why there are not significant in roads into the necrotic segment by newly formed vessels. The roles of angiogenic growth factors, especially those influenced by ischemia, are of interest in the regulation of angiogenesis in ON.

HIF-1α and vascular endothelial growth factor (VEGF) have been of particular interest. In a piglet model of ischemia, Kim *et al.* reported that, in the infarcted femoral heads, VEGF-IR and transcripts were not observed in the hypertrophic zone but could be identified in the proliferative zone above the necrotic hypertrophic zone.[59] In human tissue from patients with adult ON, Radke *et al.*[79] and Li *et al.*[65] reported increased VEGF expression in the reparative/edematous area surrounding the lesion. Li *et al.* reported an increase in HIF-1α in the fibrotic and transitional areas of the reparative zone.[65] Varoga observed VEGF expression in the transitional zone of ON femoral heads.[100] These findings have been corroborated by genetic studies demonstrating VEGF (A, B but not C or D) expression in the tissues and cells of ON patients.[72,107] HIF-1α is a transcription factor for VEGF and has been shown to increase significantly in response to hypoxia in diverse tissues.[78] VEGF has a number of biological activities including recruitment, promotion of growth, survival (anti-apoptotic factor), and activity of endothelial cells.[65,78] Increases in VEGF are also associated with increases in osteogenesis since angiogenesis and osteogenesis are coupled during bone repair.[65,94] Hong *et al.* found that a single polymorphism in the gene for VEGF-C was associated with an increased risk of ON.[35] The presence and potential role of other growth factors have also been explored. In a study of microRNAs, non-coding RNAs that are associated with the regulation of gene expression, Yamasaki identified miR-210 around the periphery of the necrotic area.[107] Radke *et al.* found the extracellular matrix proteins CYR61 and CTGF primarily in the edematous area although low levels were also detected in the areas of marrow fibrosis and the transitional zone.[79] Li *et al.* noted the presence of FGF-2 in the reparative zone.[65] In their study of gene polymorphisms, Hong *et al.* found that the highest risk for ON was noted for one single nucleotide polymorphism for the IGFBP3 gene, especially for patients with alcohol-associated or idiopathic ON.[35] IGFBP3 is insulin-like growth factor-binding protein 3 and also plays a role in hypoxia-induced angiogenesis. Despite the presence of various growth factors associated with angiogenesis in necrotic bone, new blood vessel invasion into the necrotic segment is not observed to any great degree.

There may be factors present in the necrotic bone that impair angiogenesis. These anti-angiogenic factors may include angiostatin, interferon-α, TGF-β, platelet factor IV, and prolactin.[90] Additionally, factors released from the dying cells and necrotic tissue may also inhibit angiogenesis. This has potential clinical ramifications for future treatments. There is considerable interest in the use of angiogenic VEGF as a treatment for ON. Evaluation of VEGF injected into ON femoral heads of animal models has suggested that it has the potential to stimulate angiogenesis and bony repair.[53,108] Questions concerning clinical applications include the size of the lesion, the presence of necrotic debris and saponified fat, and the lack of cells. Also there are concerns with adverse effects (e.g., tumorigenesis) that must be addressed before this technology can be translated into a viable treatment option.

The potential impact of damage to endothelial cells in the pathogenesis of ON is significant, and may play a role in early and late stages of the disease. Several investigators have observed damage to the endothelium and endothelial cells in ON.[4,65,83,89] Kerachian *et al.* proposed that damage to endothelial cells "may result in abnormal blood coagulation and thrombi formation".[56] This could then initiate a cascade of ischemia followed by apoptosis or necrosis of osteoblasts and osteocytes. One risk factor for ON, corticosteroid treatment, has the capacity to injure endothelial cells.[57] In an animal rabbit model of ON, He *et al.* observed decreased levels of 6-ketone prostaglandin $F_{1\alpha}$, a marker of endothelial cell injury.[32]

Using knockout mice, Fukumura *et al.* demonstrated that endothelial nitric oxide synthase (eNOS) plays a critical role in VEGF-induced angiogenesis and vascular permeability.[22] Koo *et al.* reported that the frequency of 4a allele for eNOS was significantly higher in patients (6.8% vs. 2.4%, $p < 0.0345$, OR 2.931, 95% CI 1.076–7.969) and in idiopathic ON subgroup (9.0% vs. 2.4%, $pc < 0.0297$, OR 3.976, 95% CI 1.356–11.631) than for controls.[61] The results of Gaglia *et al.* are in agreement with the findings of Koo *et al.*[24] Glueck *et al.* observed that the T-786C eNOS polymorphism was strongly associated with ON.[28] They suggest that the impairment of nitric oxide production by the T-786C eNOS polymorphism can result in vasoconstriction and platelet activation, recruitment, and aggregation in human subjects and diminish angiogenesis. Wang *et al.* investigated the possible role of inducible nitric oxide synthase (iNOS) in ON.[103] They found that the average percentage of iNOS positive osteocytes was higher in the ON, compared to normal or osteoarthritic, specimens.

7.6 Impact of Pathogenic Mechanisms on Treatment Approaches

There is considerable interest in identifying pharmaceutical interventions for the treatment of ON.[7,80] Approaches may be prophylactic or as treatment for early-stage disease prior to subchondral collapse and arthrosis. It must be realized that joint preservation depends upon early diagnosis and treatment before subchondral fracture. Pharmaceutical approaches that have been entertained have varied according to different underlying hypotheses for the pathogenesis of ON.

One study compared the diagnostic value of reactive examination by MRI of patients with hip pain to a prospective screening of patients newly exposed to corticosteroids and considered to be at high risk for ON.[2] Within two years, 9/80 (11%) of prospectively screened patients were diagnosed with ON, all at stage 0, I by the University of Pennsylvania staging system. All hips were successfully treated with bisphosphonates or core decompression. By contrast, of 100 patients diagnosed reactively with ON, 12 were stage I, 34 were stage II, 10 stage III, 29 stage IV, and 15 stage V. Within two years after diagnosis, 45% of these patients underwent hip replacement.

If intraosseous hypertension was proven to be a risk factor for ON, agents such as prostacyclin analogues, that increased venous outflow, might be effective as prophylactic agents. In a prospective study, treatment with Iloprost resulted in improvement in pain and Harris Hip scores in patients with early-stage ON.[42] This corresponded to a notable decrease in the extent of the bone marrow edema associated with the ON, as determined by MRI.

If increased adipocyte number and hypertrophy was shown to be a causal factor in ON, lipid lowering agents, including statins, might be effective in reducing this risk factor. Using a database of computerized prescription drug records, Prichett *et al.* identified 284 patients who were taking statin drugs concomitantly with high-dose steroids to determine whether ON had developed,[77] During a five-year period, only 1% (3 of 284) of patients developed ON. A more rigorous randomized, double-blinded study is needed to confirm these findings.

If hypercoagulability, due to thrombophilia or hypofibrinolysis, was shown to contribute to the development of ON, the use of anticoagulants or tranexamic acid may be effective treatments for ON. In a randomized study, Nagasawa *et al.* evaluated the effect of treating patients with warfarin while being treated with corticosteroids.[73] The patients treated with warfarin had a decreased incidence rate of ON (21%) as compared to control (33%) ($p > 0.05$). Glueck *et al.* also reported favorable results with treatment with enoxaparin, although they found that it was more effective in patients with primary ON than in those with secondary ON.[30]

Bisphophonates are in current widespread use for pre-collapse ON. Early reports are that they are highly effective in preventing clinical and radiographic progression.[3, 64, 75] The most likely mechanisms involve reduction in osteoclastic subchondral bone resorption and a "rebalancing" of the rates of resorption and formation in the repair process. Preventing the loss of subchondral bone integrity until bone formation can occur would theoretically reduce the risk of collapse and joint incongruity. This therapeutic strategy has the appeal of being potentially useful regardless of the etiologic mechanisms since it would be targeting the repair phase of ON. However, enthusiasm for bisphosphonates as a treatment for ON has been mitigated by a recent finding of no effect in a prospective, randomized controlled study[13] and potential complications.[58,81,95]

In addition to pharmaceutical interventions, physical treatments have been investigated that have vascular implications such as pulsed electromagnetic field therapy (PEMF), hyperbaric oxygen therapy, and extracorporeal shockwave therapy. In a study of patients treated with PEMF, Massari *et al.* reported that at two years, 94% of the stage 1 and 2 hips avoided surgery; this treatment was not effective in more advanced stages of ON.[68] To date, pulsed electromagnetic field therapy has not been approved for the treatment of ON. Hyperbaric oxygen might aid in providing increased oxygen early in ischemia by increasing the oxygen concentration of the extracellular fluid and by reducing edema by inducing vasoconstriction.[80] Camporesi *et al.*[11] evaluated the use of hyperbaric oxygen for the treatment of stage 2 ON lesions of the hip. Following treatment, significantly lower pain scores and lesion improvement were observed in the hyperbaric oxygen group as compared to the controls. As of the seven-year follow-up, no patients had undergone total hip arthroplasty. The results reported by Wang *et al.* with extracorporeal shockwave therapy (ESWT) were extremely favorable.[76] They found that in a comparison of ESWT to core decompression with fibular bone grafting for stage 1 to 3 ON of the hip, patients treated with ESWT had higher HSS hip scores (98 versus 77 points) and pain scores (0.4 versus 4.7) at two-year follow-up; fewer hips eventually required hip replacement (3 versus 9). Studies with physical techniques are relatively limited and further study is needed of each of these treatment alternatives.

7.7 Conclusions

For several decades there has been a search for a unifying concept for the pathogenesis of ON — especially for the femoral head. Controversy has surrounded whether the arterial supply or venous outflow plays a precipitating role, whether extravascular or intravascular events are primary, and whether there are direct effects on the blood vessels themselves. It may be that there are several different mechanisms involved at the onset of ON, based upon the variety of etiologic factors involved. These pathways may ultimately converge into a single pathway, as proposed by several investigators.[1,5,47,57,112] A better understanding of the etiologies and early pathophysiology is imperative to establishing effective prophylactic measures for ON. Until specific etiologies are identified at treatable stages, the most effective treatment strategy is surveillance of at-risk individuals and early intervention with medications that modify the bone remodeling response — trabecular resorption and subchondral fracture — common to all cases of ON.

References

1. Aaron RK, Gray RRL (2007). Osteonecrosis: Etiology, natural history, pathophysiology, and diagnosis. In: Callaghan JJ, Rosenberg AG, Rubash HE, eds., *The Adult Hip*. Philadelphia: Lippincott Williams and Wilkins, 463–476.
2. Aaron RK, Voisinet A, Racine J, Ali Y, Feller ER (2011). Corticosteroid-associated avascular necrosis: Dose relationships and early diagnosis. *Ann NY Acad Sci*, 1240, 38–46.
3. Agarwala S, Shah S, Joshi VR (2009). The use of alendronate in the treatment of avascular necrosis of the femoral head: Follow-up to eight years. *J Bone Joint Surg Br*, 91(8), 1013–1018.
4. Arlet J, Laroche M, Soler R, Thiechart M, Pieraggi MT, Mazieres B (1993). Histopathology of the vessels of the femoral heads in specimens of osteonecrosis, osteoarthritis and algodystrophy. *Clinical Rheumatology*, 12(2), 162–165.
5. Assouline-Dayan Y, Chang C, Greenspan A, Shoenfeld Y, Gershwin ME (2002). Pathogenesis and natural history of osteonecrosis. *Semin Arthritis Rheum*, 32(2), 94–124.
6. Atsumi T, Kuroki Y (1992). Role of impairment of blood supply of the femoral head in the pathogenesis of idiopathic osteonecrosis. *Clin Orthop Relat Res*, 277, 22–30.
7. Banerjee S, Issa K, Pivec R, Kapadia BH, Khanuja HS, Mont MA (2013). Osteonecrosis of the hip: Treatment options and outcomes. *Orthop Clin North Am*, 44(4), 463–476.
8. Bauer T, McCarthy JJ, Stulberg BN (1997). Osteonecrosis of the femoral head: Histologic diagnosis and findings after core biopsy. In: Urbaniak JR, Jones JP Jr, eds., *Osteonecrosis: Etiology, Diagnosis, and Treatment*. Rosemont, IL: AAOS, 73–79.
9. Brown TD, Baker KJ, Brand RA (1992). Structural consequences of subchondral bone involvement in segmental osteonecrosis of the femoral head. *J Orthop Res*, 10(1), 79–87.
10. Bullough PG (1997). The morbid analtomy of subchondral osteonecrosis. In: Urbaniak JR, Jones JP Jr, eds., *Osteonecrosis: Etiology, Diagnosis, and Treatment*. Rosemont, IL: AAOS, 69–72.

11. Camporesi EM, Vezzani G, Bosco G, Mangar D, Bernasek TL (2010). Hyperbaric oxygen therapy in femoral head necrosis. *J Arthroplasty*, 25(6 Suppl), 118–123.
12. Cenni E, Fotia C, Rustemi E, Yuasa K, Caltavuturo G, Giunti A, *et al.* (2011). Idiopathic and secondary osteonecrosis of the femoral head show different thrombophilic changes and normal or higher levels of platelet growth factors. *Acta Orthopaedica*, 82(1), 42–49.
13. Chen CH, Chang JK, Lai KA, Hou SM, Chang CH, Wang GJ (2012). Alendronate in the prevention of collapse of the femoral head in non-traumatic osteonecrosis: A two-year multicenter, prospective, randomized, double-blind, placebo-controlled study. *Arthritis Rheum*, 64(5), 1572–1578.
14. Chen LE, Seaber AV, Urbaniak JR (1997). Changes in microvasculature and flow dynamics in skeletal muscle during ischemia and perfusion. In: Urbaniak JR, Jones JP Jr, eds.,*Osteonecrosis: Etiology, Diagnosis and Treatment.* Rosemont, IL: AAOS.
15. Cheng EY, Thongtrangan I, Laorr A, Saleh KJ (2004). Spontaneous resolution of osteonecrosis of the femoral head. *J Bone Joint Surg Am*, 86-A(12), 2594–2599.
16. Chernetsky SG, Mont MA, LaPorte DM, Jones LC, Hungerford DS, McCarthy EF (1999). Pathologic features in steroid and nonsteroid associated osteonecrosis. *Clin Orthop Relat Res,* 368, 149–161.
17. Deegan PB, Pavlova E, Tindall J, Stein PE, Bearcroft P, Mehta A, *et al.* (2011). Osseous manifestations of adult Gaucher disease in the era of enzyme replacement therapy. *Medicine*, 90(1), 52–60.
18. Felson DT, Anderson JJ (1987). Across-study evaluation of association between steroid dose and bolus steroids and avascular necrosis of bone. *Lancet*, 1, 902–906.
19. Ficat RP, Arlet J (1980). *Ischemia and Necroses of Bone.* Baltimore, MD: Williams & Wilkins.
20. Findlay DM (2007). Vascular pathology and osteoarthritis. *Rheumatology*, 46(12), 1763–1768.
21. Folkman J, Merler E, Abernathy C, Williams G (1971). Isolation of a tumor factor responsible for angiogenesis. *J Exp Med*, 133(2), 275–288.
22. Fukumura D, Gohongi T, Kadambi A, Izumi Y, Ang J, Yun CO, *et al.* (2001). Predominant role of endothelial nitric oxide synthase in vascular endothelial growth factor-induced angiogenesis and vascular permeability. Proceedings of the National Academy of Sciences of the United States of America, 98(5), 2604–2609.
23. Fukuoka S, Hotokebuchi T, Jingushi S, Fujii H, Sugioka Y, Iwamoto Y (1999). Evaluation of blood flow within the subchondral bone of the femoral head: Use of the laser speckle method at surgery for osteonecrosis. *J Orthop Res*, 17(1), 80–87.
24. Gagala J, Buraczynska M, Mazurkiewicz T, Ksiazek A (2013). Endothelial nitric oxide synthase gene intron 4 polymorphism in non-traumatic osteonecrosis of the femoral head. *Int Orthop*, 37(7), 1381–1385.

25. Glimcher MJ, Kenzora JE (1979). The biology of osteonecrosis of the human femoral head and its clinical implications: I. Tissue biology. *Clin Orthop Relat Res*, 138, 284–309.
26. Glimcher MJ, Kenzora JE (1979). The biology of osteonecrosis of the human femoral head and its clinical implications: II. The pathological changes in the femoral head as an organ and in the hip joint. *Clin Orthop Relat Res*, 139, 283–312.
27. Glimcher MJ, Kenzora JE (1979). The biology of osteonecrosis of the human femoral head and its clinical implications: III. Discussion of the etiology and genesis of the pathological sequelae; comments on treatment. *Clin Orthop Relat Res*, 140, 273–312.
28. Glueck CJ, Freiberg RA, Boppana S, Wang P (2008). Thrombophilia, hypofibrinolysis, the eNOS T-786C polymorphism, and multifocal osteonecrosis. *J Bone Joint Surg Am*, 90(10), 2220–2229.
29. Glueck CJ, Freiberg RA, Fontaine RN, Tracy T, Wang P (2001). Hypofibrinolysis, thrombophilia, osteonecrosis. *Clin Orthop Relat Res*, (386), 19–33.
30. Glueck CJ, Freiberg RA, Sieve L, Wang P (2005). Enoxaparin prevents progression of stages I and II osteonecrosis of the hip. *Clin Orthop Relat Res*, 435, 164–170.
31. Hadjigeorgiou G, Dardiotis E, Dardioti M, Karantanas A, Dimitroulias A, Malizos K (2008). Genetic association studies in osteonecrosis of the femoral head: Mini review of the literature. *Skeletal Radiol*, 37(1), 1–7.
32. He W, Xu C, Fan Y, Fang B, Li X, Wang H, *et al.* (2004). Effects of the Chinese drugs for activating blood circulation on plasma TXB2 and 6-keto-PGF1alpha contents in rabbits with glucocorticoid-induced femoral head necrosis. *Journal of Traditional Chinese Medicine*, sponsored by All-China Association of Traditional Chinese Medicine, Academy of Traditional Chinese Medicine. 24(3), 233–237.
33. Hernigou P, Bernaudin F (1994). Course of bone tissue after bone marrow allograft in adolescents with sickle cell disease. *Revue de Chirurgie Orthopedique et Reparatrice de l'appareil Moteur*, 80(2), 138–143.
34. Hirano K, Tsutsui H, Sugioka Y, Sueishi K (1997). Histopathologic alterations of retinacular vessels and osteonecrosis. *Clin Orthop Relat Res*, 342, 192–204.
35. Hong JM, Kim TH, Kim HJ, Park EK, Yang EK, Kim SY (2010). Genetic association of angiogenesis- and hypoxia-related gene polymorphisms with osteonecrosis of the femoral head. *Exp Mol Med*, 42(5), 376–385.
36. Hsieh AS, Winet H, Bao JY, Stevanovic M (1999). Model for intravital microscopic evaluation of the effects of arterial occlusion-caused ischemia in bone. *Ann Biomed Eng*, 27(4), 508–516.
37. Hungerford DS (1975). Early diagnosis of ischemic necrosis of the femoral head. *The Johns Hopkins Medical Journal*, 137(6), 270–275.
38. Hungerford DS (1981). Pathogenetic considerations in ischemic necrosis of bone. *Can J Surg*, 24(6), 583–587.

39. Hungerford DS, Lennox DW (1985). The importance of increased intraosseous pressure in the development of osteonecrosis of the femoral head: Implications for treatment. *Orthop Clin North Am*, 16(4), 635–654.
40. Hutter CD (2000). Dysbaric osteonecrosis: a reassessment and hypothesis. *Medical Hypotheses*, 54(4), 585–590.
41. Inoue A, Ono K (1979). A histological study of idiopathic avascular necrosis of the head of the femur. *J Bone Joint Surg Br*, 61-B(2), 138–143.
42. Jager M, Zilkens C, Bittersohl B, Matheney T, Kozina G, Blondin D, *et al.* (2011). Efficiency of iloprost treatment for osseous malperfusion. *Int Orthop*, 35(5), 761–765.
43. Jergesen HE, Lang P, Moseley M, Genant HK (1990). Histologic correlation in magnetic resonance imaging of femoral head osteonecrosis. *Clin Orthop Relat Res*, 253, 150–163.
44. Johnson EO, Soultanis K, Soucacos PN (2004). Vascular anatomy and microcirculation of skeletal zones vulnerable to osteonecrosis: Vascularization of the femoral head. *Orthop Clin North Am*, 35(3), 285–291, viii.
45. Johnson L, ed. (1964). Histogenesis of avascular necrosis. Conference on Aseptic Necrosis of the Femoral Head, St Louis, MO.
46. Jones JP Jr (1993). Fat embolism, intravascular coagulation, and osteonecrosis. *Clin Orthop Relat Res*, 292, 294–308.
47. Jones JP Jr (1992). Intravascular coagulation and osteonecrosis. *Clin Orthop Relat Res*, 277, 41–53.
48. Jones JP Jr, Ramirez S, Doty SB (1993). The pathophysiologic role of fat in dysbaric osteonecrosis. *Clin Orthop Relat Res*, 296, 256–264.
49. Jones JP Jr (1994). Concepts of etiology and early pathogenesis of osteonecrosis. In: Schafer M, ed., AAOS Instructional Course Lectures. American Academy of Orthopaedic Surgeons, 499–512.
50. Jones JP Jr (1991). Etiology and pathogenesis of osteonecrosis. *Sem Arthroplasty*, 2, 160–168.
51. Jones LC, Ciombor DM (2014). Osteonecrosis and intravascular coagulation revisited. In: Koo KH, Mont MA, Jones LC, eds., *Osteonecrosis*. Seoul, Korea: Springer Verlag, 71–80.
52. Jones LC, Mont MA, Le TB, Petri M, Hungerford DS, Wang P, *et al.* (2003). Procoagulants and osteonecrosis. *JRheumatology*, 30(4), 783–791.
53. Katsube K, Bishop AT, Simari RD, Yla-Herttuala S, Friedrich PF (2005). Vascular endothelial growth factor (VEGF) gene transfer enhances surgical revascularization of necrotic bone. *J Orthop Res*, 23(2), 469–474.
54. Kawai K, Tamaki A, Hirohata K (1985). Steroid-induced accumulation of lipid in the osteocytes of the rabbit femoral head: A histochemical and electron microscopic study. *J Bone Joint Surg*, 67, 755–763.
55. Kelly PJ (1968). Anatomy, physiology, and pathology of the blood supply of bones. *J Bone Joint Surg Am*, 50(4), 766–783.
56. Kerachian MA, Harvey EJ, Cournoyer D, Chow TY, Seguin C (2006). Avascular necrosis of the femoral head: Vascular hypotheses: Endothelium. *J Endothelial Cell Research*, 13(4), 237–244.

57. Kerachian MA, Seguin C, Harvey EJ (2009). Glucocorticoids in osteonecrosis of the femoral head: A new understanding of the mechanisms of action. *J Steroid Biochem Mol Biol*, 114(3–5), 121–128.
58. Kharazmi M, Hallberg P, Michaelsson K (2014). Gender related difference in the risk of bisphosphonate associated a typical femoral fracture and osteonecrosis of the jaw. *Ann Rheum Dis,* 73(8), 1594.
59. Kim HK, Bian H, Randall T, Garces A, Gerstenfeld LC, Einhorn TA (2004). Increased VEGF expression in the epiphyseal cartilage after ischemic necrosis of the capital femoral epiphysis. *J Bone Miner Res*, 19(12), 2041–2048.
60. Koo KH, Mont MA, Jones LC (2014). *Osteonecrosis.* Berlin, Heidelberg: Springer Verlag.
61. Koo KH, Lee JS, Lee YJ, Kim KJ, Yoo JJ, Kim HJ (2006). Endothelial nitric oxide synthase gene polymorphisms in patients with nontraumatic femoral head osteonecrosis. *J Orthop Res*, 24(8), 1722–1728.
62. Kuang XY, Chen LJ, Li HL, Yao F, Xu JM, Huang F, *et al.* (2014). A study on dysbaric osteonecrosis in caisson workers. *Undersea and Hyperbaric Medicine*: Journal of the Undersea and Hyperbaric Medical Society, Inc. 41(3), 229–233.
63. Lafforgue P (2006). Pathophysiology and natural history of avascular necrosis of bone. *Joint Bone Spine*, 73(5), 500–507.
64. Lai KA, Shen WJ, Yang CY, Shao CJ, Hsu JT, Lin RM (2005). The use of alendronate to prevent early collapse of the femoral head in patients with nontraumatic osteonecrosis. A randomized clinical study. *J Bone Joint Surg Am*, 87(10), 2155–2159.
65. Li W, Sakai T, Nishii T, Nakamura N, Takao M, Yoshikawa H, *et al.* (2009). Distribution of TRAP-positive cells and expression of HIF-1alpha, VEGF, and FGF-2 in the reparative reaction in patients with osteonecrosis of the femoral head. *J Orthop Res*, 27(5), 694–700.
66. Lieberman JR, Berry DJ, Mont MA, Aaron RK, Callaghan JJ, Rajadhyaksha AD, *et al.* (2003). Osteonecrosis of the hip: Management in the 21st century. Instr Course Lectures, 52, 337–355.
67. Manwani D, Frenette PS (2013). Vaso-occlusion in sickle cell disease: Pathophysiology and novel targeted therapies. *Blood*, 122(24), 3892–3898.
68. Massari L, Fini M, Cadossi R, Setti S, Traina GC (2006). Biophysical stimulation with pulsed electromagnetic fields in osteonecrosis of the femoral head. *J Bone Joint Surg Am*, 88(Suppl 3), 56–60.
69. Matos MA, dos Santos Silva LL, Brito Fernandes R, Dias Malheiros C, Pinto da Silva BV (2012). Avascular necrosis of the femoral head in sickle cell disease patients. *Ortop Traumatol Rehabil*, 14, 155–160.
70. Miyanishi K, Yamamoto T, Irisa T, Yamashita A, Jingushi S, Noguchi Y, *et al.* (2002). Bone marrow fat cell enlargement and a rise in intraosseous pressure in steroid-treated rabbits with osteonecrosis. *Bone*, 30(1), 185–190.
71. Mont MA, Zywiel MG, Marker DR, McGrath MS, Delanois RE. The natural history of untreated asymptomatic osteonecrosis of the femoral head: Asystematic literature review. *J Bone Joint Surg Am*, 92(12), 2165–2170.

72. Mwale F, Wang H, Johnson AJ, Mont MA, Antoniou J (2011). Abnormal vascular endothelial growth factor expression in mesenchymal stem cells from both osteonecrotic and osteoarthritic hips. Bulletin of the NYU Hospital for Joint Diseases, 69(Suppl 1) S56–S61.
73. Nagasawa K, Tada Y, Koarada S, Tsukamoto H, Horiuchi T, Yoshizawa S, *et al.* (2006). Prevention of steroid-induced osteonecrosis of femoral head in systemic lupus erythematosus by anti-coagulant. *Lupus*, 15(6), 354–357.
74. Nakamura J, Harada Y, Oinuma K, Iida S, Kishida S, Takahashi K (2010). Spontaneous repair of asymptomatic osteonecrosis associated with corticosteroid therapy in systemic lupus erythematosus: 10-year minimum follow-up with MRI. *Lupus*, 19(11), 1307–1314.
75. Nishii T, Sugano N, Miki H, Hashimoto J, Yoshikawa H (2006). Does alendronate prevent collapse in osteonecrosis of the femoral head? *Clin Orthop Relat Res*, 443, 273–279.
76. Powell C, Chang C, Gershwin ME (2011). Current concepts on the pathogenesis and natural history of steroid-induced osteonecrosis. *Clin Rev Allergy Immunol*, 41(1), 102–113.
77. Pritchett JW (2001). Statin therapy decreases the risk of osteonecrosis in patients receiving steroids. *Clin Orthop Relat Res*, 386, 173–178.
78. Pugh CW, Ratcliffe PJ (2003). Regulation of angiogenesis by hypoxia: Role of the HIF system. *Nature Medicine*, 9(6), 677–684.
79. Radke S, Battmann A, Jatzke S, Eulert J, Jakob F, Schutze N (2006). Expression of the angiomatrix and angiogenic proteins CYR61, CTGF, and VEGF in osteonecrosis of the femoral head. *J Orthop Res*, 24(5), 945–952.
80. Rajpura A, Wright AC, Board TN (2011). Medical management of osteonecrosis of the hip: A review. *Hip International*, 21(4), 385–392.
81. Rasmusson L, Abtahi J (2014). Bisphosphonate associated osteonecrosis of the jaw: An update on pathophysiology, risk factors, and treatment. *International Journal of Dentistry*, 2014, 471035.
82. Saito S, Inoue A, Ono K (1987). Intramedullary haemorrhage as a possible cause of avascular necrosis of the femoral head. The histology of 16 femoral heads at the silent stage. *J Bone Joint Surg Br*, 69(3), 346–351.
83. Saito S, Ohzono K, Ono K (1992). Early arteriopathy and postulated pathogenesis of osteonecrosis of the femoral head: The intracapital arterioles. *Clin Orthop Relat Res*, 27, 98–110.
84. Saito S, Saito M, Nishina T, Ohzono K, Ono K (1989). Long-term results of total hip arthroplasty for osteonecrosis of the femoral head: A comparison with osteoarthritis. *Clin Orthop Relat Res*, 244, 198–207.
85. Schroer WC (1994). Current concepts on the pathogenesis of osteonecrosis of the femoral head. *Orthop Rev*, 23(6), 487–497.
86. Serre H, Simon L (1961). Primary osteonecrosis of the femoral head in adults. *Acta Rheumatologica Scandinavica*, 7, 265–286.
87. Sharareh B, Schwarzkopf R (2014). Dysbaric osteonecrosis: A literature review of pathophysiology, clinical presentation, and management. *Clinical Journal of Sport Medicine.*

88. Shi SH, Li ZR, Wang BL, Sun W, Cheng LM, Pan L, *et al.* (2010). Study on the relationship between sclerosis rim and bone morphogenetic proteins of osteonecrosis of the femoral head. *Zhonghua Wai Ke Za Zhi*, 48(17), 1305–1308.
89. Slichter SJ, Stegall P, Smith K, Huang TW, Harker LA (1981). Dysbaric osteonecrosis: A consequence of intravascular bubble formation, endothelial damage, and platelet thrombosis. *J Lab Clin Med*, 98(4), 568–590.
90. Smith DW (1997). Is avascular necrosis of the femoral head the result of inhibition of angiogenesis? *Medical Hypotheses*, 49(6), 497–500.
91. Solomon L (1981). Idiopathic necrosis of the femoral head: Pathogenesis and treatment. *Can J Surg,* 24(6), 573–578.
92. Starklint H, Lausten GS, Arnoldi CC (1995). Microvascular obstruction in avascular necrosis: Immunohistochemistry of 14 femoral heads. *Acta orthopaedica Scandinavica*, 66(1), 9–12.
93. Steinberg ME, Bands RE, Parry S, Hoffman E, Chan T, Hartman KM (1999). Does lesion size affect the outcome in avascular necrosis? *Clin Orthop Relat Res*, 367, 262–271.
94. Street J, Bao M, deGuzman L, Bunting S, Peale FV, Jr., Ferrara N, *et al.* (2002). Vascular endothelial growth factor stimulates bone repair by promoting angiogenesis and bone turnover. Proceedings of the National Academy of Sciences of the United States of America, 99(15), 9656–9661.
95. Suresh E, Pazianas M, Abrahamsen B (2014). Safety issues with bisphosphonate therapy for osteoporosis. *Rheumatology*, 53(1), 19–31.
96. Swiontkowski MF, Ganz R, Schlegel U, Perren SM (1987). Laser Doppler flowmetry for clinical evaluation of femoral head osteonecrosis: Preliminary experience. *Clin Orthop Relat Res*, 218, 181–185.
97. Swiontkowski MF, Senft D (1992). Cortical bone microperfusion: Response to ischemia and changes in major arterial blood flow. *J Orthop Res*, 10(3), 337–343.
98. Urbaniak JR, Jones JPJr (1997). *Osteonecrosis. Etiology, Diagnosis, and Treatment.* Rosemont, IL: AAOS.
99. Vakil N, Sparberg M (1989). Steroid related osteonecrosis in inflammatory bowel disease. *Gastroenterology*, 96, 62–67.
100. Varoga D, Drescher W, Pufe M, Groth G, Pufe T (2009). Differential expression of vascular endothelial growth factor in glucocorticoid-related osteonecrosis of the femoral head. *Clin Orthop Relat Res,* 467(12), 3273–3282.
101. Wang GJ, Lennox DW, Reger SI, Stamp WG, Hubbard SL (1981). Cortisone-induced intrafemoral head pressure change and its response to a drilling decompression method. *Clin Orthop Relat Res*, 159, 274–278.
102. Wang GJ, Sweet D, Reger SI, Thompson RC (1977). Fat-cell changes as a mechanism of avascular necrosis of the femoral head in cortisone-treated rabbits. *J Bone Joint Surg*, 59, 729–735.
103. Wang J, Kalhor A, Lu S, Crawford R, Ni JD, Xiao Y (2014). iNOS expression and osteocyte apoptosis in idiopathic, non-traumatic osteonecrosis. *Acta Orthopaedica*, 5, 1–8.

104. Wang L, Fritton SP, Weinbaum S, Cowin SC (2003). On bone adaptation due to venous stasis. *J Biomech*, 36(10), 1439–1451.
105. Wang Y, Li Y, Mao K, Li J, Cui Q, Wang GJ (2003). Alcohol-induced adipogenesis in bone and marrow: A possible mechanism for osteonecrosis. *Clin Orthop Relat Res*, 410, 213–224.
106. Winet H, Hsieh A, Bao JY (1998). Approaches to study of ischemia in bone. *J Biomed Mater Res*, 43(4), 410–421.
107. Yamasaki K, Nakasa T, Miyaki S, Yamasaki T, Yasunaga Y, Ochi M (2012). Angiogenic microRNA-210 is present in cells surrounding osteonecrosis. *J Orthop Res*, 30(8), 1263–1270.
108. Yang C, Yang S, Du J, Li J, Xu W, Xiong Y (2003). Experimental study of vascular endothelial growth factor gene therapy for avascular necrosis of the femoral head. *Journal of Huazhong University of Science and Technology Medical Sciences*, 23(3), 297–299, 316.
109. Zalavras C, Dailiana Z, Elisaf M, Bairaktari E, Vlachogiannopoulos P, Katsaraki A, *et al.* (2000). Potential aetiological factors concerning the development of osteonecrosis of the femoral head. *Eur J Clin Invest*, 30(3), 215–221.
110. Zalavras CG, Lieberman JR (2014). Osteonecrosis of the femoral head: Evaluation and treatment. *J Am AcadOrthop Surg*, 22(7), 455–464.
111. Zalavras CG, Vartholomatos G, Dokou E, Malizos KN (2004). Genetic background of osteonecrosis: Associated with thrombophilic mutations? *Clin Orthop Relat Res*, 422, 251–255.
112. Zizic TM, Lewis CG, Marcoux C, Hungerford DS (1989). The predictive value of hemodynamic studies in preclinical ischemic necrosis of bone. *Journal of Rheumatology*, 16(12), 1559–1564.
113. Zlotorowicz M, Czubak J, Caban A, Kozinski P, Boguslawska-Walecka R (2013). The blood supply to the femoral head after posterior fracture/dislocation of the hip, assessed by CT angiography. *Bone Joint J*, 95-B(11), 1453–1457.

CHAPTER 8

OSTEONECROSIS IN PATIENTS WITH SICKLE CELL ANEMIA AND OTHER HEMATOLOGIC DISORDERS

LUKE M. VAUGHAN

The Scripps Research Institute, La Jolla, CA

SARAH A. LONG, THOMAS SANTAMARÍA and MARC J. KAHN

Tulane University School of Medicine, New Orleans, LA

JOSEPHINA A. VOSSEN and MIRIAM A. BREDELLA

Department of Radiology
Massachusetts General Hospital, Boston, MA

ALAN L. SCHILLER

Department of Pathology
University of Hawaii, Honolulu, HI

HENRY J. MANKIN

Department of Orthopaedic Surgery
Massachusetts General Hospital, Boston, MA

The "Lazarus Dilemma": It's not the death that gets you. It's the resurrection!

Dr. Henry J. Mankin

8.1 Introduction

Bone infarction occurs when vascular flow is sufficiently impaired, or blocked, causing osteonecrosis. About 10,000–20,000 new cases are estimated each year; 21–37% of which are secondary to corticosteroid use.[19, 26] In the process of avascular necrosis, initially a variety of immunologic cells with repair capabilities from surrounding tissues, and vasoactive cytokines infiltrate the area, causing acute inflammation. Over the subsequent weeks and months, bone-resorbing osteoclasts in an acid-rich microenvironment, slowly bore into, or erode, the necrotic bone. These reparative replacement processes slowly begin at the interface between the viable and infarcted (non-viable) bone; however, these are often too slow to maintain the mechanical integrity of the periarticular bone, supporting the articular cartilage, leading to collapse of the subchondral supporting bony architecture, and ultimately, articular destruction.

Without the underlying structure or foundation of subchondral bone, the remaining tissue architecture collapses, as is observed with avascular necrosis in various disorders to be discussed, including sickle cell anemia and Gaucher disease. The actual process and cellular mechanism of corticosteroid-induced avascular necrosis is poorly understood. However, when present, it often produces significant morbidity and attendant disabilities, requiring various surgical management options, most typically joint replacement.[19]

The process in diaphyseal bone is similarly endosteal, affecting the cancellous or spongiosa bone marrow bearing areas, but typically manifests as an acute "bone crisis." The resorption or restoration process in the diaphysis typically is less critical, as cortical bone is relatively difficult to remove and naturally strong, as opposed to epiphyseal or metaphyseal, subchondral loci. Associated co-morbidities, such as osteomyelitis in sickle cell infarcts, are problematic, but can be effectively minimized with prophylactic antibiotic use, particular in infants and young children.[7,9] A similar issue arises in mandibular infarctions associated with osteoclast-inhibiting medications, such as bisphosphonates, as used in the treatment of osteoporosis, typically in locations juxtaposed to dental extraction sites.

8.2 Sickle Cell Disease and Osteonecrosis

Sickle cell disease (SCD) is caused by a selective genetic mutation in the beta chain of hemoglobin leading to the substitution of valine for glutamic acid at the sixth amino acid. This substitution results in an abnormal hemoglobin that polymerizes in physiologic states such as hypoxia or dehydration, leading to a distortion in the shape of red blood cells and giving them their characteristic sickled appearance.This gene is widely understood to have evolved and been preserved due to its protective effects against malaria when inherited as a single gene, and is observed in African, Middle

Eastern, Indian, and Mediterranean populations. The autosomal recessive sickle cell gene is present in 8% of the black African American population. While roughly 2 million people have sickle cell trait, one in every 500 black African Americans suffer from overt sickle cell disease, which currently affects approximately 70,000 people in the United States.[1] In addition to hemoglobin S, other hemoglobin variants can be co-inherited in a double heterozygote fashion and can also lead to human disease. Most notably, hemoglobin C in which glutamic acid at the sixth residue on the beta chain is replaced by lysine causes symptoms when co-inherited with hemoglobin S that are typically milder than those found in patients homozygous for hemoglobin S. An important exception is that patients with SC disease have more bone complications than patients with sickle cell disease.

Sickled hemoglobin leads to red cell hemolysis and a shortened red cell life span. Sickling also results in increased adhesion between cells, ultimately leading to vasoocclusive events in various organs including bone, brain, kidney, retina, liver and spleen.[5] Vasoocclusive crises can be precipitated by a low oxygen tension environment, which triggers hemoglobin precipitation leading to the sickling process. Sickling ultimately leads to thrombosis of the terminal vasculature.[6] Due to relatively low blood flow rates in bone; the osseous architecture creates a pathophysiologic niche for sickling to occur. In addition to *in situ* thrombosis, hemolysis leads to nitric oxide depletion due to scavenging by serum-free hemoglobin and leads to depletion of arginine, which is necessary for nitric acid production.[15] The combination of arterial constriction due to reduced nitric oxide and thrombosis leads to the clinical features seen during a vasoocclusive crisis. During a typical vasoocclusive crisis, patients experience pain in long bones, back, abdomen, and chest. Additionally, patients can have pulmonary complications of a sickle cell crisis and develop an acute chest syndrome characterized by fever, hypoxia, chest pain, and shortness of breath.

SCD often presents with characteristic osseous imaging features. Increased hemolysis results in persistence of the appendicular red marrow with widening of the medullary spaces and thinning of the cortical bone. In the spine, cortical thinning produces a biconcave deformity of the vertebral bodies (Fig. 8.1). Vasoocclusive events can lead to osseous infarction, typically occurring in the medullary cavity or epiphyses.[6] On MR imaging, chronic medullary infarcts have a thin low signal rim on all imaging sequences with a variable signal of the center. Osseous infarction in young children can occur in the small tubular bones of the hands and feet, termed dactylitis.[25] Radiographs demonstrate patchy

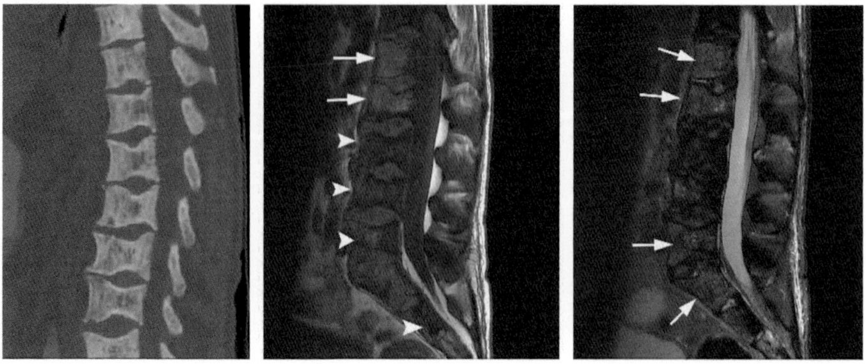

Fig. 8.1. Images of the lumbar spine in a patient with sickle cell anemia. (A *–left*): Sagittal CT image shows diffuse sclerosis and coarsening of the trabeculae and central endplate compression deformities resulting in characteristic H-shaped vertebral bodies. (B *–middle*): Sagittal T1-weighted MR image demonstrates diffuse low signal intensity of the vertebral bodies consistent with hyperplastic hematopoietic red marrow (arrowheads), which is replacing the normal bright fatty marrow (arrows). Concavity of the vertebral endplates at multiple levels is also seen. (C *–right*): Sagittal fat-suppressed T2-weighted image shows areas of high signal, consistent with active infarction (arrows).

areas of lucency with periosteal new bone formation and related growth abnormalities (Fig. 8.2).

Epiphyseal infarction (also commonly referred to as osteonecrosis, or avascular necrosis) often presents in the femoral and humeral head. On T2-weighted MR imaging, high signal intensity indicative of bone marrow edema and a serpiginous double line that consists of a hyperintense inner border and hypointense periphery can be seen (Fig. 8.3).[8] In later stages of avascular necrosis, radiographs typically demonstrate crescent-shaped subchondral lucencies and articular surface collapse (Fig. 8.4).[17]

In addition to osteonecrosis, osteomyelitis is seen in patients with sickle cell disease. Because patients homozygous for the sickle gene typically autoinfarct their spleens early in life, there is a high incidence of infection due to encapsulated organisms in patients with sickle cell anemia.[7,9] Interestingly, patients with sickle cell anemia are also prone to osteomyelitis with gram negative organisms such as salmonella. Distinguishing acute infection from infarction by imaging alone can be difficult but is important in light of correct and timely treatment. Radiographic features are often non-specific, showing periosteal inflammation, osteopenia, and sclerosis. Ultrasonography and radioisotope bone imaging may provide useful information in the

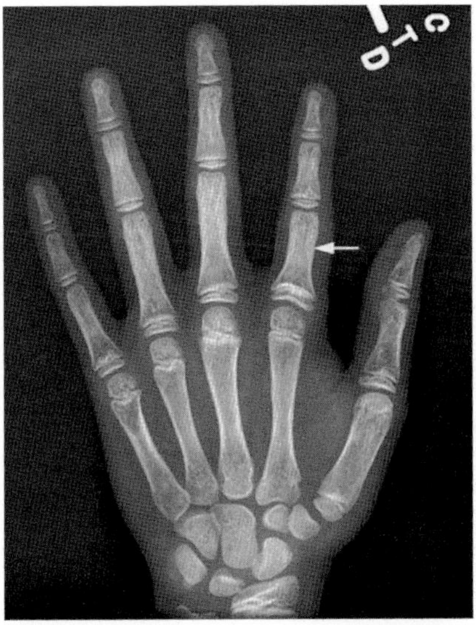

Fig. 8.2. Frontal radiograph of the left hand in a child with sickle cell anemia shows shortening of the second proximal phalanx (arrow). The restricted growth is secondary to childhood dactylitis and cartilage infarction during the growth period.

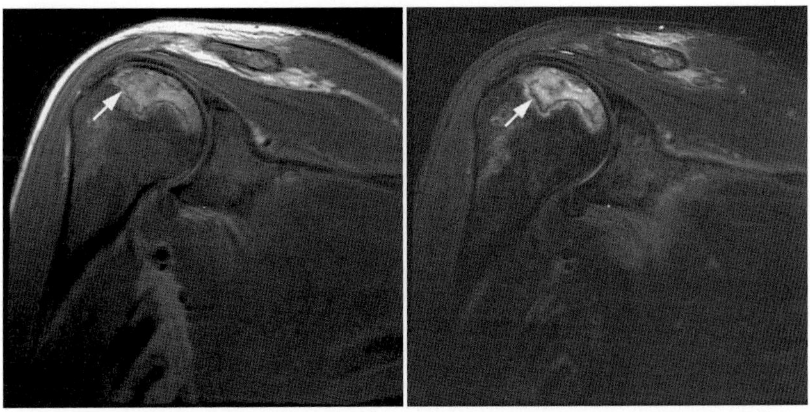

Fig. 8.3. MR images of the right shoulder in a patient with sickle cell anemia. Coronal oblique proton density-weighted (A –*left*) and fat-suppressed T2-weighted (B –*right*) images demonstrate abnormal bone marrow signal and edema within the epiphysis with serpiginous linear signal abnormality (arrows), consistent with avascular necrosis.

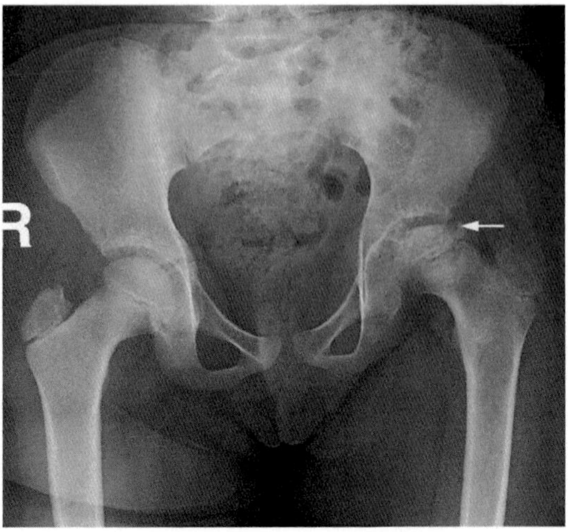

Fig. 8.4. Pelvic radiograph in a patient with sickle cell anemia shows sclerosis and crescent-shaped subchondral lucencies with articular surface collapse of the left femoral capital epiphysis (arrow), consistent with osteonecrosis.

early stages of acute osteomyelitis by showing features typical of inflammation.[11] MR imaging, in particular contrast enhanced T1-weighted imaging, is valuable by showing inflammatory osseous changes and associated soft tissue abnormalities in the setting of infection (Fig. 8.5).[13,27]

The most commonly seen bone complication in patients with sickle cell anemia is osteonecrosis of the humeral or femoral head, which is also called avascular necrosis (AVN). AVN likely results from infarction of the tenuous vascular supply to the femoral or humeral head but vitamin D deficiency has also been identified as a contributing factor.[2] Treatment for AVN is not standardized. Total hip arthroplasty can provide pain relief, and restoration of function in selected symptomatic patients with sickle cell disease and AVN.[14] Asymptomatic disease may not require therapy.[20] A recent Cochrane analysis was only able to identify one randomized trial involving hip AVN in patients with sickle cell disease. That study concluded that there was no advantage to adding hip core decompression to standard physical therapy with respect to major complications and pain.[18] Additionally, cementless prosthetic components may provide some advantage over those that are cemented.[12] For osteonecrosis of the humeral head, there is consensus that if left untreated, humeral head collapse will result, necessitating

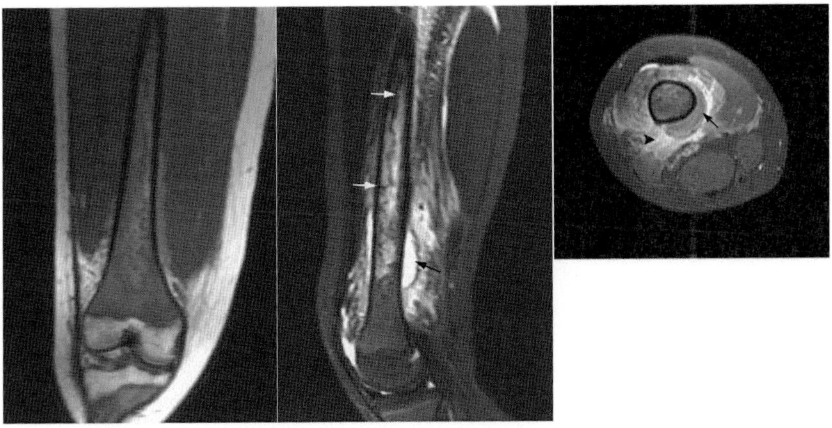

Fig. 8.5. MR images of the femur in a patient with sickle cell anemia and acute fever, lower extremity pain, and swelling. Coronal T1-weighted image (A –*left*) demonstrates diffuse low signal replacement of fatty marrow due to red marrow reconversion. Sagittal fat-suppressed T2-weighted image (B –*middle*) shows increased T2 signal involving the entire diaphysis with serpiginous areas of low signal intensity (white arrows), consistent with medullary bone infarcts. A T2 hyperintense collection around the lower aspect of the right femoral shaft (black arrow) is noted. Axial fat-suppressed T1-weighted image with intravenous gadolinium (C –*right*) demonstrates a non-enhancing collection (arrow) with surrounding enhancing inflammatory changes (arrowhead) which was found to represent an abscess likely related to underlying osteomyelitis.

surgical intervention.[22] As with hip arthroplasty, the optimal method of repair has not been determined.

8.2.1 *Pathology*

Osteonecrosis or AVN of bone, regardless of etiology, generally has common gross and histologic features. Osteonecrosis is the death of bone and marrow in the absence of infection. Cancellous necrotic bone heals by a process of "creeping substitution" where pluripotential mesenchymal cells and neovascular tissue form the granulation tissue. This tissue supplies osteoblasts for bone formation and vascular tissue, which will transport osteoclasts into the area for bone resorption. Often the residual necrotic trabeculae will be surface-coated with new lamellar or woven bone but some will be reabsorbed by osteoclasts as the invading or creeping neovascular tissue extends into and replaces the necrotic fatty marrow. Necrotic fat undergoes calcification to form fatty soaps. Since the necrotic trabeculae cannot

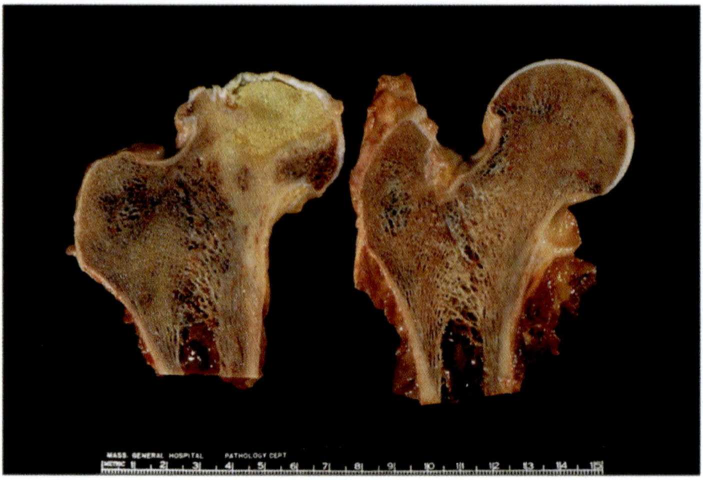

Fig. 8.6. The femoral heads of a 23-year-old black African college student who died of pulmonary emboli. Both femoral heads are shown and each has diffuse red marrow since anemia was severe. One femoral head has a classic appearance of osteonecrosis with a subchondral fracture, a wedge-shaped area of yellow-tan marrow, and dense collapsed trabecular bone. Courtesy of Dr. G. Petur Nielsen.

respond to continued stress, they often undergo microfracture producing collapse and compaction of the avascular area (Figs. 8.6–8.11).

Figure 8.6 illustrates the gross pathology of sickle cell disease involving both proximal femurs. The marrow is diffusely red since the patient was severely anemic. One femoral head has a wedge-shaped yellow subchondral area, which is the region of osteonecrosis caused by vascular insufficiency. There is a subchondral fracture with peeling away of the articular cartilage and the subchondral bone plate is separated from the marrow cavity by the fracture gap. This area is more radiodense with imaging studies because there is compaction of the necrotic cancellous bone, there is additional new bone formed by creeping substitution, and there is the presence of calcified fatty soaps secondary to necrosis of the fatty marrow. The opposite hip is intact.

In sickle cell disease, it is very difficult to see the deformed red blood cells clogging the vasculature adjacent to the ischemic areas. If the osteonecrotic areas are infected, inflammatory cells will predominate.

Necrotic cortical bone heals by tunneling into the dense compact lamellar bone, termed a "cortical cutting cone," where osteoclasts bore into the

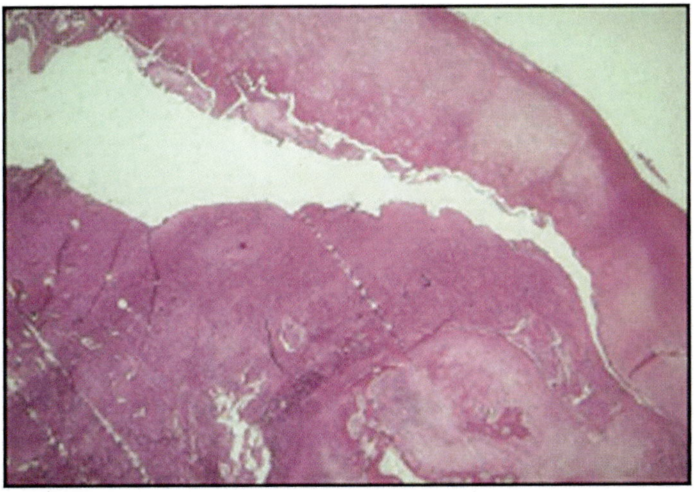

Fig. 8.7. A fracture at the subchondral bone plate which supports the normal-appearing articular cartilage. The necrotic marrow and trabecular bone are invaded by pluripotential mesenchymal cells and neovasculargranulation tissue.

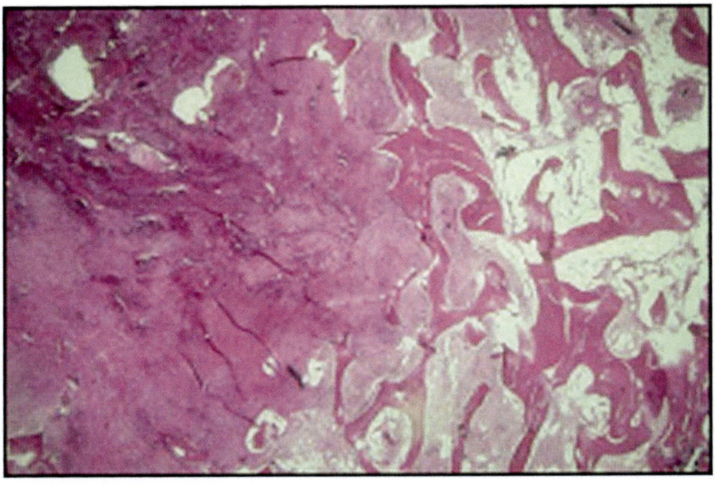

Fig. 8.8. The necrotic marrow and trabeculae are replaced by new woven bone and granulation tissue ("creeping substitution").

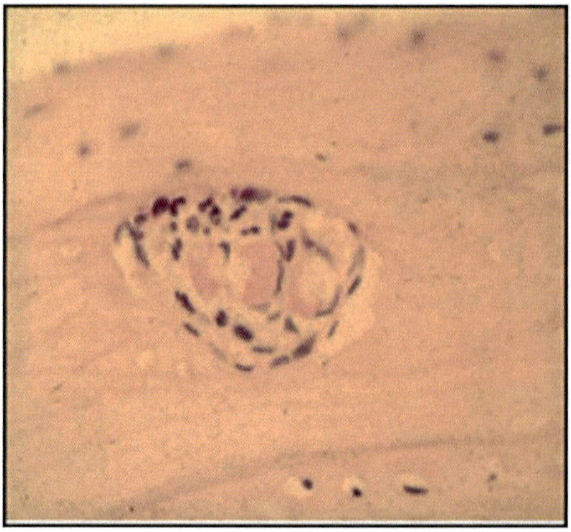

Fig. 8.9. A dead lamellar bone trabecula surface coated by live (osteocytes present) lamellar and woven bone with osteoclast resorption in the dead bone (creeping substitution).

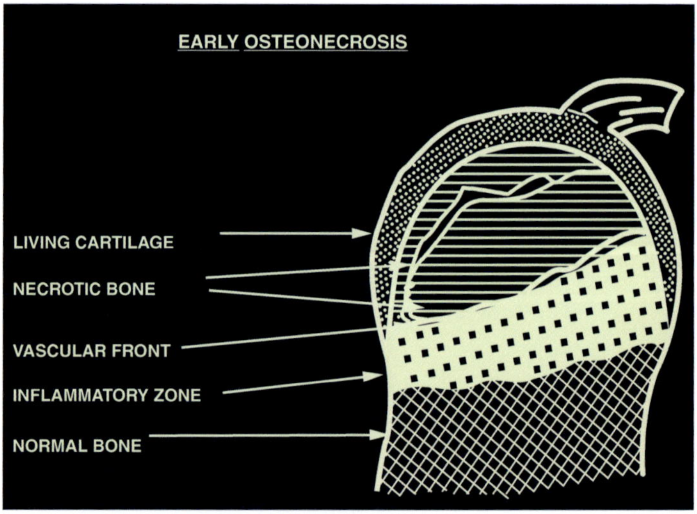

Fig. 8.10. A schematic drawing of osteonecrosis of the femoral head illustrating the regional areas of tissue findings.

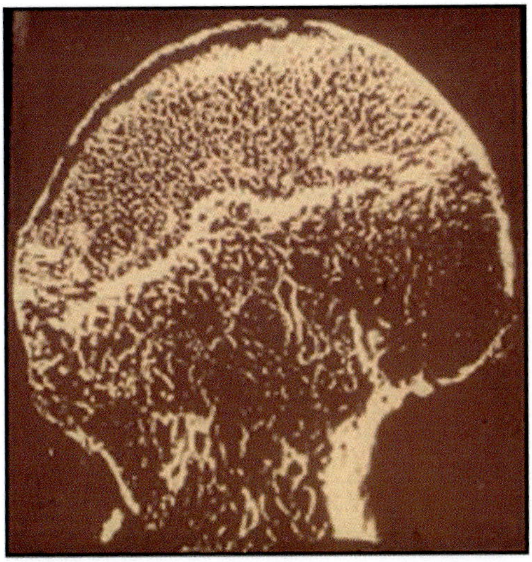

Fig. 8.11. A specimen radiograph of osteonecrosis illustrating the subchondral fracture and the necrotic area with trabecular thickening and collapse due to creeping substitution. There is a reactive zone of thickened bone with re-enforcement of trabeculae and neovascularization. Deep to this area, the remaining bone is osteoporotic due to clinical pain producing disuse atrophy.

cortex, usually from a vascular channel, with adjacent osteoblasts that add new woven or lamellar bone to the internal aspect of the defect (Fig. 8.12).

8.2.2 *Therapy*

Perhaps the best way to approach osteonecrosis in sickle cell patients is through prevention. One study suggested that optimal management of vasoocclusive crisis including pain control, hydration, rest, and crutches had a direct impact on the reduction of the incidence of AVN of the femoral head.[21] Despite a clear role for hydroxyurea in reducing vasoocclusive crisis in patients with sickle cell disease, hydroxyurea does not have a clear role in reducing the incidence of bone complications. Similarly, the role of bisphosphonate therapy has not been adequately studied in patients with sickle cell disease.

8.3 Gaucher Disease

Gaucher disease (GD) is a lysosomal storage disease caused by a deficiency in the enzyme, beta glucocerebrosidase, resulting in the accumulation

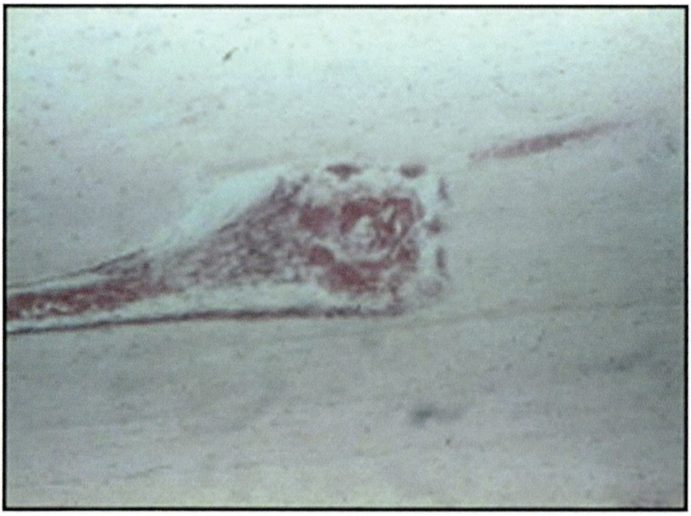

Fig. 8.12. A cortical cutting cone with the leading edge of the cone populated by osteoclasts tunneling into necrotic lamellar bone (no osteocytes), a central vascular supply, and trailing osteoblasts.

of the wax-like substance glucocerebroside in cells of the monocyte and macrophages lineage, typically in the liver, spleen, and bone marrow.[24] Gaucher disease patients typically develop anemia, hepatosplenomegaly, thrombocytopenia, osteoporosis, and juxta-articular infarctions, resulting in articular collapse with significant multifocal degenerative change often requiring joint replacement.[19] Long bone infarctions and acute crises, similar to those presenting in SCD, are debilitating. Currently, 20,000 people in the United States suffer from Gaucher disease, with an incidence of one in 75,000 people in the general population. However, the incidence is increased in the Ashkenazi Jewish population, where one in 12 individuals are carriers, and one in 850 manifest fulminant disease.While various forms can present, more than 90% of affected individuals exhibit Type 1 GD. This does not typically include neurological involvement, often termed non-neuropathic. Both Types 2 and 3 GD demonstrate extensive neurologic involvement, often severely limiting effective therapeutic intervention.

The availability of enzyme replacement therapies, first approved in the early 1990s, has dramatically improved the lives of those suffering with GD Type 1, accounting for 94% of all Gaucher disease cases.[3,19,24] While the 67-kDa enzyme glucocerebrosidase (alglucerase) was initially derived from large amounts of human placental tissue, the product was vastly improved with further purification and deglycosylation, with exposure of the glycoprotein's mannose residues further enhancing binding of macrophage mannose receptors.[24] The human recombinant cerebrosidase, imiglucerase, enzymatically equivalent to the native form, was approved for human use in the United States in 1994, and in Europe in 1997.[4] Two additional recombinant human enzyme variants are now available and another isoform is under clinical investigation.[24]

8.3.1 *Imaging*

The skeletal manifestations of Gaucher disease result in a variety of imaging features. Progressive accumulation of glucocerebrosides within the bone marrow cavity leads to a centrifugal expansion of red or hematopoietic bone marrow, mostly in the spine, pelvis, and diaphyseal region of the femur and humerus.[28] A pathological growth pattern with growth retardation and undertubulation with flaring of the distal metaphyses of the long bones is also seen, termed Erlenmeyer flask deformity (Fig. 8.13). Associated altered

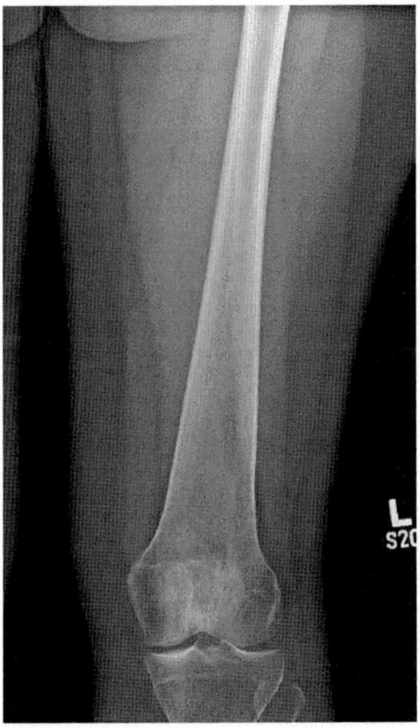

Fig. 8.13. Frontal radiograph of the left femur in a patient with Gaucher disease shows the abnormal growth (undertubulation) of the distal femoral metadiaphysis, termed Erlenmeyer flask deformity.

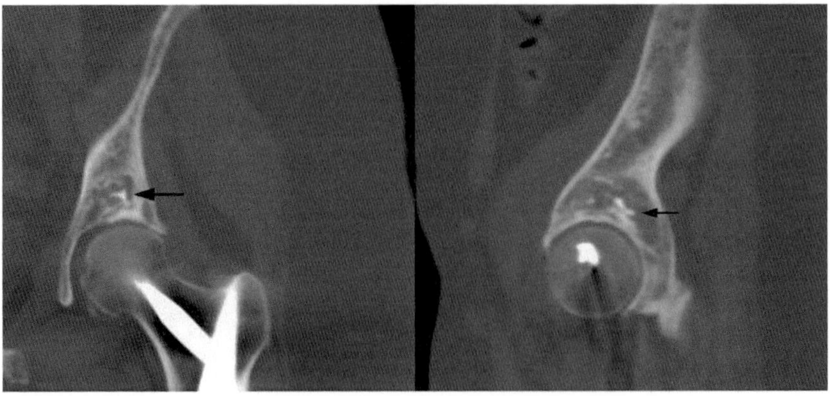

Fig. 8.14. Coronal (A –*left*) and sagittal (B –*right*) CT images of the left hip in a patient with Gaucher disease. There is subchondral lucency, sclerosis, and articular surface irregularity of the left acetabulum, consistent with avascular necrosis.

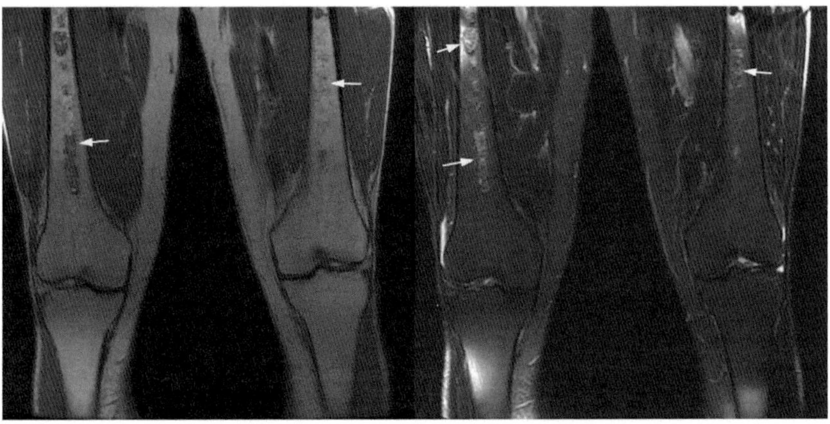

Fig. 8.15. MR images of bilateral femurs in a patient with Gaucher disease. Coronal T1-weighted (A –*left*) and fat-suppressed T2-weighted (B –*right*) images show serpiginous geographic signal abnormalities in the diaphysis, consistent with bone infarcts (arrows).

vascularity, changes in cytokine release, and increased local pressure lead to osteoporosis, cortical thinning, bone infarction, and avascular necrosis (Figs. 8.14 and 8.15).[16] MR imaging is the most sensitive imaging modality for the evaluation of bone manifestations in Gaucher disease. A number of semi-quantitative MRI methods have been developed to measure the amount of Gaucher cells infiltrate in the bone marrow.[23]

8.3.2 *Pathology*

The pathology of GD is caused by the presence of large histiocytes (Gaucher cells) stuffed with glucocerebroside that accumulates mainly in lysosomes (Fig. 8.16). These cells massively replace the marrow, presumably causing vascular compression leading to ischemia. The Gaucher cell is a macrophage (20–100 μm) with a small eccentric nucleus and clear cytoplasm with a fibrillar rather than a bubbly pattern. The cell is periodic acid-Schiff (PAS) stain positive.

The fibrillar pattern is the glucocerebroside stored in the lysosomes as parallel cylindrical structures (Fig. 8.17). The gross appearance of Gaucher osteonecrosis involving bone has bright yellow-orange marrow which replaces the normal fat with Gaucher cells. The osteonecrosis is typical but often with a brighter yellow-orange tissue in the marrow space (Fig. 8.18).

The histology is that of massive accumulation of Gaucher cells filling up the marrow space causing ischemia and crowding out and confining islets of hematopoietic elements (Fig. 8.19). In the necrotic areas, ghosts of dead Gaucher cells are present amongst the osteoporotic dead lamellar bone trabeculae (empty osteocyte lacunae) (Fig. 8.20).

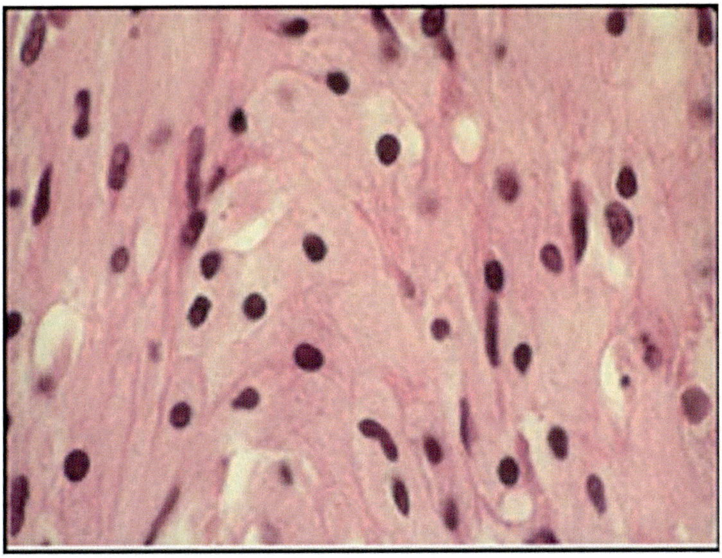

Fig. 8.16. The Gaucher cell is a large macrophage filled with glucocerebroside. Its nucleus is small and eccentric, and the cytoplasm has a linear or fibrillar pattern.

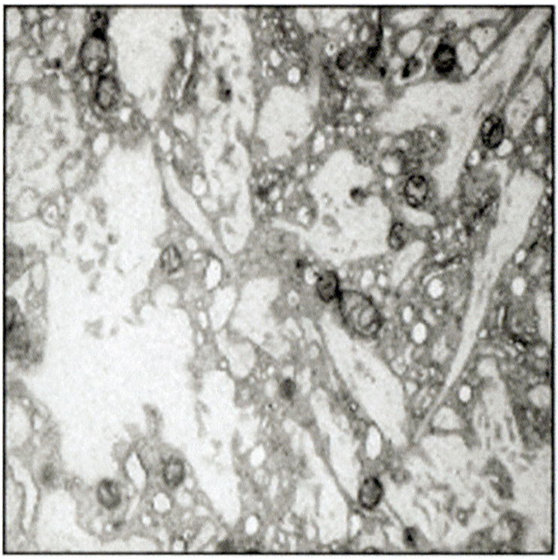

Fig. 8.17. An electron micrograph showing the glucocerebroside stored as cylinders or stacked tubes in the lysosomes, giving the cytoplasm a fibrillar appearance.

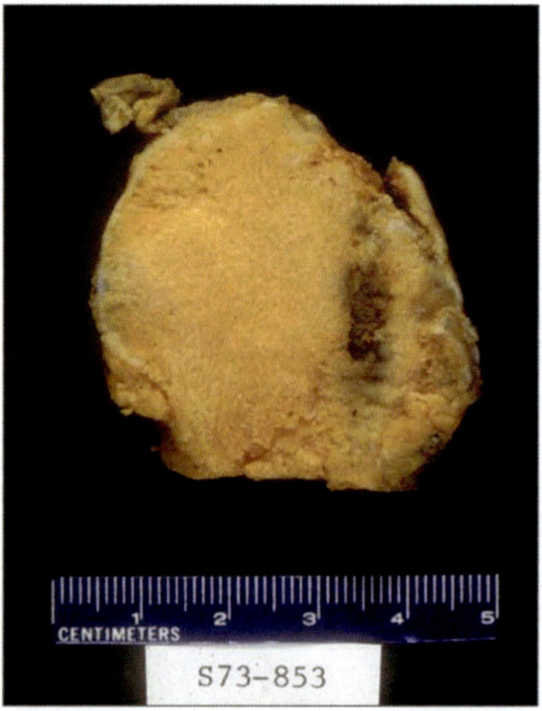

Fig. 8.18. Osteonecrosis of Gaucher disease has a classic appearance except that the marrow has a bright yellow-orange color produced by the accumulation of Gaucher cells.

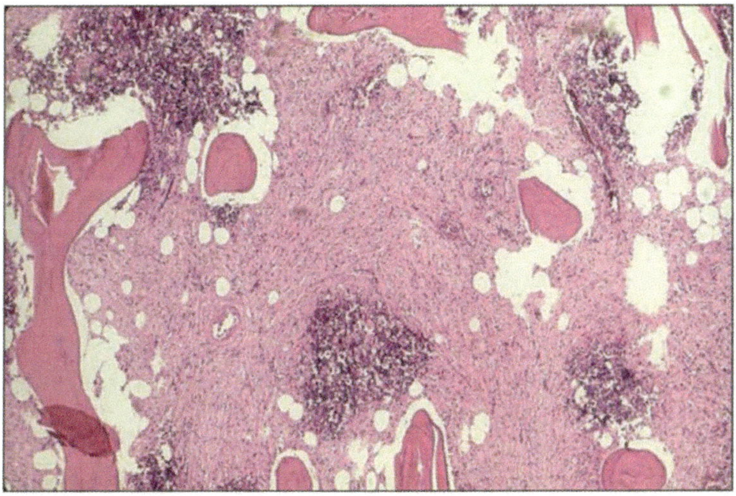

Fig. 8.19. Low power view with Gaucher cells replacing the fat and confining hematopoietic cells to islets. Osteoporosis observed.

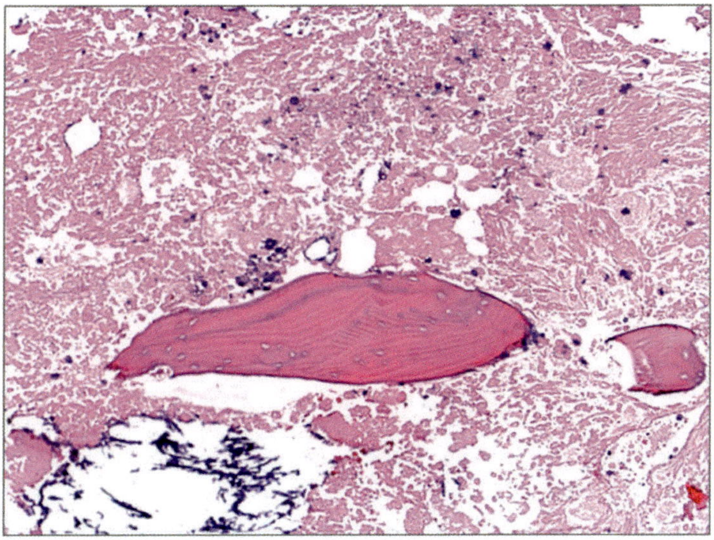

Fig. 8.20. A dead osteoporotic lamellar bone trabecula surrounded by necrotic Gaucher cells. Courtesy of Dr. G. Petur Nielsen.

If these areas are infected, inflammatory cells will be present, often with focal microabscesses.

8.4 Conclusion

Red cell adhesion mechanisms have been implicated in various disease entities, including sickle cell disease, Gaucher disease, and various thrombo-occlusive coagulopathies. Recent advances in our understanding of the pathophysiology of integrin-mediated, IgG- and laminin-related effects carry great clinical promise.[5,10] Current orthopedic management is restricted primarily to the late sequelae of bone infarction, particularly in a juxta-articular setting, as well as the associated increased risks of secondary bacterial seeding of osteonecrotic foci.[7,9]

Acknowledgements

The authors would like to acknowledge the extraordinary work of Dr. Henry J. Mankin on the occasion of his 86th birthday. A truly remarkable, super-productive career!

References

1. Anemia, Sickle Cell. Bethesda, MD: National Center for Biotechnology Available from: http://www.ncbi.nlm.nih.gov/books/NBK22238/.
2. Adams-Graves P, Daniels AB, Womack CR, Freire AX (2014). Bone mineral density patterns in vitamin D deficient African American men with sickle cell disease. *Am J Med Sci*, 347(4), 262–266.
3. Barton NW, Brady RO, Dambrosia JM, Di Bisceglie AM, Doppelt SH, Hill SC, *et al.* (1991). Replacement therapy for inherited enzyme deficiency: Macrophage-targeted glucocerebrosidase for Gaucher's disease. *N Engl J Med*, 324(21), 1464–1470.
4. Beutler E, Demina A, Laubscher K, Garver P, Gelbart T, Balicki D, *et al.* (1995). The clinical course of treated and untreated Gaucher disease: A study of 45 patients. *Blood Cells Mol Dis*, 21(2), 86–108.
5. Colin Y, Le Van Kim C, El Nemer W (2014). Red cell adhesion in human diseases. *Curr Opin Hematol*, 21(3), 186–192.
6. Ejindu VC, Hine AL, Mashayekhi M, Shorvon PJ, Misra RR (2007). Musculoskeletal manifestations of sickle cell disease. *Radiographics*, 27(4), 1005–1021.
7. Frenette PS, Atweh GF (2007). Sickle cell disease: Old discoveries, new concepts, and future promise. *J Clin Invest*, 117(4), 850–858.
8. Ganguly A, Boswell W, Aniq H (2011). Musculoskeletal manifestations of sickle cell anaemia: A pictorial review. *Anemia*, 2011, 794283.

9. Gaston MH, Verter JI, Woods G, Pegelow C, Kelleher J, Presbury G, *et al.* (1986). Prophylaxis with oral penicillin in children with sickle cell anemia: A randomized trial. *N Engl J Med*, 314(25), 1593–1599.
10. Gomez-Puerta JA, Peris P, Reverter JC, Espinosa G, Martinez-Ferrer A, Monegal A, *et al.* (2013). High prevalence of prothrombotic abnormalities in multifocal osteonecrosis: Description of a series and review of the literature. *Medicine*, 92(6), 295–304.
11. Inusa BP, Oyewo A, Brokke F, Santhikumaran G, Jogeesvaran KH (2013). Dilemma in differentiating between acute osteomyelitis and bone infarction in children with sickle cell disease: The role of ultrasound. *PloS One.* 8(6), e65001.
12. Issa K, Naziri Q, Maheshwari AV, Rasquinha VJ, Delanois RE, Mont MA (2013). Excellent results and minimal complications of total hip arthroplasty in sickle cell hemoglobinopathy at mid-term follow-up using cementless prosthetic components. *J Arthroplasty*, 28(9), 1693–1698.
13. Jain R, Sawhney S, Rizvi SG (2008). Acute bone crises in sickle cell disease: The T1 fat-saturated sequence in differentiation of acute bone infarcts from acute osteomyelitis. *Clin Radiol*, 63(1), 59–70.
14. Jeong GK, Ruchelsman DE, Jazrawi LM, Jaffe WL (2005). Total hip arthroplasty in sickle cell hemoglobinopathies. *J Am Acad Orthop Surg*, 13(3), 208–217.
15. Kahn MJ, Maley JH, Lasker GF, Kadowitz PJ (2013). Updated role of nitric oxide in disorders of erythrocyte function. *Cardiovascular and Hematological Disorders — Drug Targets*, 13(1), 83–87.
16. Katz R, Booth T, Hargunani R, Wylie P, Holloway B (2011). Radiological aspects of Gaucher disease: Skeletal radiology. 40(12), 1505–1513.
17. Madani G, Papadopoulou AM, Holloway B, Robins A, Davis J, Murray D (2007). The radiological manifestations of sickle cell disease. *Clin Radiol*, 62(6), 528–538.
18. Marti-Carvajal AJ, Sola I, Agreda-Perez LH (2014). Treatment for avascular necrosis of bone in people with sickle cell disease. The Cochrane Database of Systematic Reviews, 7, CD004344.
19. Mont MA, Hungerford DS (1995). Non-traumatic avascular necrosis of the femoral head. *J Bone Joint Surg Am*, 77(3), 459–474.
20. Mont MA, Zywiel MG, Marker DR, McGrath MS, Delanois RE (2010). The natural history of untreated asymptomatic osteonecrosis of the femoral head: Asystematic literature review. *J Bone Joint Surg Am*, 92(12), 2165–2170.
21. Mukisi-Mukaza M, Saint Martin C, Etienne-Julan M, Donkerwolcke M, Burny ME, Burny F (2011). Risk factors and impact of orthopaedic monitoring on the outcome of avascular necrosis of the femoral head in adults with sickle cell disease: 215 patients case study with control group. *Orthopaedics and Traumatology, Surgery and Research*, 97(8), 814–820.
22. Poignard A, Flouzat-Lachaniette CH, Amzallag J, Galacteros F, Hernigou P (2012). The natural progression of symptomatic humeral head osteonecrosis in adults with sickle cell disease. *J Bone Joint Surg Am*, 94(2), 156–162.

23. Robertson PL, Maas M, Goldblatt J (2007). Semiquantitative assessment of skeletal response to enzyme replacement therapy for Gaucher's disease using the bone marrow burden score. *Am J Roentgenol*, 188(6), 1521–1528.
24. Rosenbloom BE, Weinreb NJ (2013). Gaucher disease: A comprehensive review. *Crit RevOncog*, 18(3), 163–175.
25. Rosner F (1998). Hand-foot syndrome in sickle cell disease. *J Clin Oncol*, 16(2), 808–809.
26. Shigemura T, Nakamura J, Kishida S, Harada Y, Ohtori S, Kamikawa K, *et al.* (2011). Incidence of osteonecrosis associated with corticosteroid therapy among different underlying diseases: Prospective MRI study. *Rheumatology*, 50(11), 2023–2028.
27. Umans H, Haramati N, Flusser G (2000). The diagnostic role of gadolinium enhanced MRI in distinguishing between acute medullary bone infarct and osteomyelitis. *Magn Reson Imaging*, 18(3), 255–262.
28. Wenstrup RJ, Roca-Espiau M, Weinreb NJ, Bembi B (2002). Skeletal aspects of Gaucher disease: A review. *Br J Radiol*, 75(Suppl 1), A2–A12.

CHAPTER 9

FRACTURES AND BONE REPAIR

DEAN G. LORICH
Hospital for Special Surgery and Weill Cornell College of Medicine, New York, NY

LIONEL E. LAZARO
Orthopeadic Surgery Resident
Hospital for Special Surgery, New York, NY

9.1 Mature Long Bones Vascularity and Fractures

Bone perfusion derives from both the medullary and periosteal circulatory systems.[1–4] The medullary system is mainly comprised of the nutrient arteries which penetrate the diaphyseal cortex through vascular for aminas and supply both the medulla and inner $\frac{2}{3}$ of the cortex in a centrifugal fashion.[1–6] At the metaphysis and epiphysis, additional arterial systems penetrate the bone and join the medullary system supplying their respective segments of medulla and cortex. The periosteal system, mainly sustained by the surrounding muscles, provides a centripetal supply through small arterioles that pierce and supply the outer $\frac{1}{3}$ of the cortex, especially when the medullary blood supply has been interrupted.[7–9] These two microcirculations anastomose (medulloperiosteal anastomosis) within the cortex and allow for blood to flow through the cortex (Fig. 9.1).[2,10] Under normal conditions, the medullary system dominates the arterial supply.[1,2,10,11]

After fracture, an immediate decline of cortical blood flow of approximately 50% has been reported.[12] The mechanism of injury and the forces at the fracture site dictate the "personality of the fracture" and the associated soft-tissue injuries that affect the local blood supply. Additional factors also affect local blood supply and include the specific nature of patient management and fracture care — from initial transport and resuscitation to subsequent surgical intervention and implant placement.[13] The biologic responses during fracture healing depend on an intact blood supply,[10] and

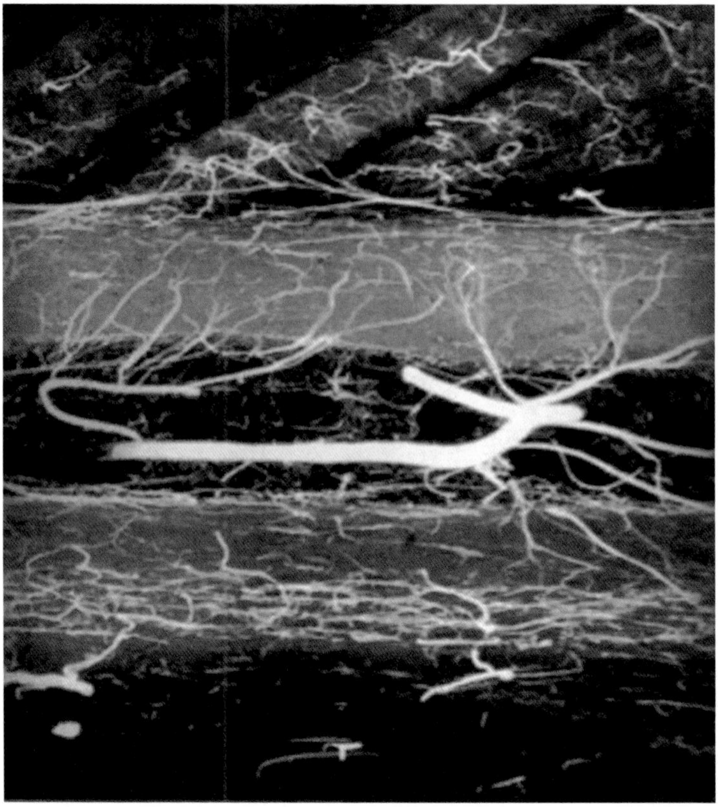

Fig. 9.1. Microangiogram depicts the intracortical anastomosis between the medullary circulation and periosteal circulation (medulloperiostealanastomosis). *Source*: Rhinelander FW (1968). The normal microcirculation of diaphyseal cortex and its response to fracture. *J Bone Joint Surg Am*, 50(4), 784–800. Reprinted with permission.

fracture management should focus on optimizing the fracture site environment for osseous healing.

With non-displaced fractures, an intact medullary circulatory system continues to dominate the blood supply throughout the entire healing process.[3] Displacement of fracture fragments interrupts the medullary system, the major contributor of blood flow to the cortical bone. The medulloperiosteal anastomoses are of significant importance, allowing the periosteal system to provide centripetal perfusion to the bone.[2,10] Fracture hematoma, which develops as the initial fracture healing response, interrupts communication of the medullary systems leaving the periosteal system as the sole connection of vascular supply between the fracture fragments through the external callus that initially forms.[10] Surrounding muscles are the immediate origin of the expanded periosteal circulation observed during displaced fractures.[2,4,10] Once endosteal osseous union and sufficient stabilization develops, the medullary capillaries can cross the fracture site and re-establish the normal predominant medullary circulation.[2,10]

The mechanical conditions created during fracture care determine the biologic response of fracture healing and associated angiogenesis.[13] When absolute fracture stability is achieved and the deformation, due to an applied given force (strain),[14] at the fracture site is <5%, primary bone/direct healing occurs without fracture callus.[15] This type of fracture healing is by osteonal bone remodeling, and consists of cutting cones that cross the fracture site.[13,16,17] With direct contact of the fracture edges, osteoclasts are followed by osteoblasts directly laying down lamellar bone. If there is a fracture gap of 200–500 microns, woven bone is laid down first which is then remodeled to lamellar bone, but at the expense of increased time.[13] Relative stability allows increased motion at the fracture site, but maintaining a mechanical strain between 5 and 15% creates secondary/indirect healing. This alternate form of fracture healing includes both intramembranous and endochondral bone formation. It is divided into fourstages: (1) inflammation, (2) soft callus formation, (3) hard callus formation, and (4) remodeling.[13] Ruptured blood vessels resulted in the initial fracture hematoma; granulation tissue follows that becomes soft callus, eliminating free motion, and subsequently becoming hard callus, finally remodeling to the native shape. The ideal fracture fixation provides the optimal stability to stimulate an adequate bone healing process and maintains the reduction until osseous union is achieved. Current fracture treatments fall within a spectrum of stability where each end of the spectrum can lead to a delay in fracture healing.[13]

9.2 Vascularity of Key Periarticular Bones

The composition of the metaphysis and epiphysis of both the proximal humerus and the proximal femur consists of mainly trabecular bone with a lesser component of cortical bone than the diaphysis and an excellent intraosseous anastomosis. When fractures occur through these bony segments, the arterial supply to the subchondral bone seems to be in great peril, and the development of osteonecrosis is of major concern. A careful surgical approach to achieve both an anatomic reduction and a stable fixation while maintaining the remaining blood supply is crucial to providing the ideal environment for fracture healing to occur. The arterial supply to these structures has received increased interest over the years. Much research has been focused on seeking a better understanding of the vascular injury during fracture and on new methods for optimizing surgical treatments of these injuries.

We performed cadaveric injection studies that provided qualitative and quantitative assessment of the vascularity of the humeral head, femoral head, patella, and talus.[18–23] This vascularity protocol utilizes gadolinium-enhanced magnetic resonance imaging (MRI) to quantify perfusion into a specific region of interest (ROI). Images were obtained using a 3.0 tesla GE MRI scanner (General Electric, Milwaukee, WI). High-resolution fat-suppressed three-dimensional gradient echo sequences were obtained both before and after administration of the contrast solution (gadolinium-diethylenetriaminepenta-acetic acid, Magnevist; Bayer Health Care Pharmaceuticals Inc., Wayne, NJ). Fat-suppressed images were used to eliminate bone marrow signal and provide improved detail of the contrast. Both pre- and post-contrast images produced weighted average of signal intensities and histograms, which were normalized using a baseline of non-enhancing muscle. A single reading of signal enhancement was obtained for each area on both the control and test specimens. Following the MRI protocol, a polyurethane compound, using an added color dye, is injected into the arterial system and subsequently, careful gross dissection of the arterial system is performed in order to confirm injection into the correct arterial system and to correlate MRI findings and the previously assessed anatomical findings.

9.2.1 *Humeral head vascularity*

The arterial supply to the humeral head arises from the axillary artery through the anterior and posterior humeral circumflex arteries.[24,25] The previous consensus in the literature was that the anterolateral branch of the anterior humeral circumflex artery provided the major blood supply to the humeral head.[24–27] Our study results demonstrated that the posterior humeral circumflex artery provides a greater percentage (64% versus 36%) of blood supply to the humeral head, than did the anterior humeral circumflex artery as previously thought (Fig. 9.2a,b). This study highlighted

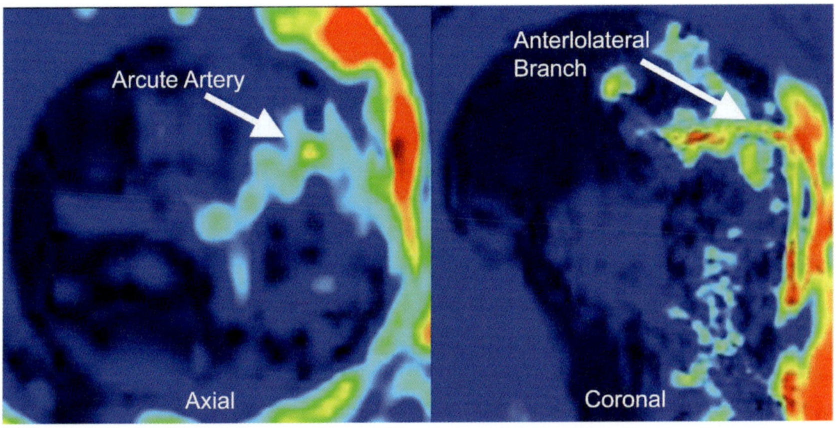

Fig. 9.2a. Contrast-enhanced MRI images that illustrate the anterior humeral circumflex artery perfusion through the arcuate artery (left axial image) and the anterolateral branch (right coronal image). *Source*: Hettrich CM, Boraiah S, Dyke JP, Neviaser A, Helfet DL, Lorich DG (2010). Quantitative assessment of the vascularity of the proximal part of the humerus. *J Bone Joint Surg Am*, 92(4), 943–948. Reprinted with permission.

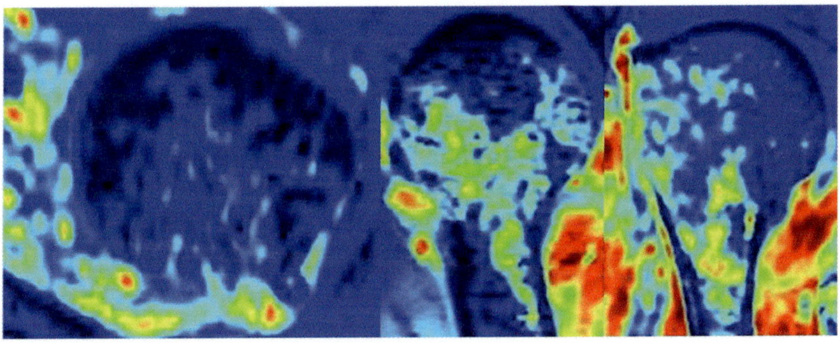

Fig. 9.2b. Contrast-enhanced MRI images that illustrate the posterior humeral circumflex artery perfusion to the entire humeral head (left – axial; middle — sagittal; right — coronal). *Source*: Hettrich CM, Boraiah S, Dyke JP, Neviaser A, Helfet DL, Lorich DG (2010). Quantitative assessment of the vascularity of the proximal part of the humerus. *J Bone Joint Surg Am*, 92(4). 943–948. Reprinted with permission.

the importance of avoiding dissection on the postero-medial aspect and to respect the posterior humeral circumflex artery during fracture manipulation and fixation. It provides a probable explanation for the relatively low rate of humeral head osteonecrosis following fixation of displaced three- and four-part proximal humerus fractures.[28]

9.2.2 *Femoral head vascularity*

Femoral head vascularity derives from three arterial systems: (1) retinacular, (2) foveolar, and (3) intraosseous.[29–34] The retinacular system is the dominant arterial supply to the femoral head,[29,32,34–38] and branches off from the medial (superior and inferior retinacular arteries) and lateral (anterior retinacular artery) femoral circumflex arteries. Once intracapsular, these terminal branches course within prolongations of the capsular wall, known as the retinacula of Weitbrecht,[29,31,39–42] and enter the femoral head-neck junction distal to the articular rim (Fig. 9.3).[30,32,37,43] With growth of the femoral neck during childhood, the anterior retinacular artery recedes to penetrate the anterior metaphyseal area, while the superior and inferior retinacular arteries advance and provide the predominant arterial supply to the femoral head.[32] Gross dissection of the terminal branches of the medial femoral circumflex artery (the superior and inferior retinacular arteries) demonstrated that these branches mainly penetrate the posterior-superior and posterior-inferior aspect of femoral head-neck junction (80% superiorly and 86% inferiorly),[44] with the superior retinacular artery being the primary blood supply to the femoral head.[1,3,6–10,12,15,23,24,26–28]

More recent studies have considered the inferior retinacular artery as a significant arterial supply to the femoral head, specifically when the superior retinacular system has been compromised. Our cadaveric studies, using quantitative contrast-enhanced MRI, demonstrated that 32–49% of femoral head perfusion is maintained when the inferior retinacular artery was preserved.[18,20] With fracture of the femoral neck, the inferior retinacular artery is protected by the inferior retinacula of Weitbrecht, which is separated and elevated from the femoral neck and can potentially avoid direct injury, contrary to the superior retinacular artery which courses in close proximity to the femoral neck and is at higher risk of injury in the event of a fracture (Fig. 9.4).[44–46] A clinical series of displaced femoral neck fractures reported intraoperative confirmation of an intact inferior retinacula of Weitbrecht in 98% ($^{108}/_{110}$) of cases.[47]

Our series of displaced femoral neck fractures, using dynamic contrast-enhanced MRI, demonstrated maintenance of some perfusion to the femoral head despite fracture displacement, presumably through the intact inferior retinacular artery (Fig. 9.5).[48] This study also demonstrated a decrease in venous outflow in the fractured side, probably secondary to the tamponade effect created by the contained intra-articular fracture hematoma.

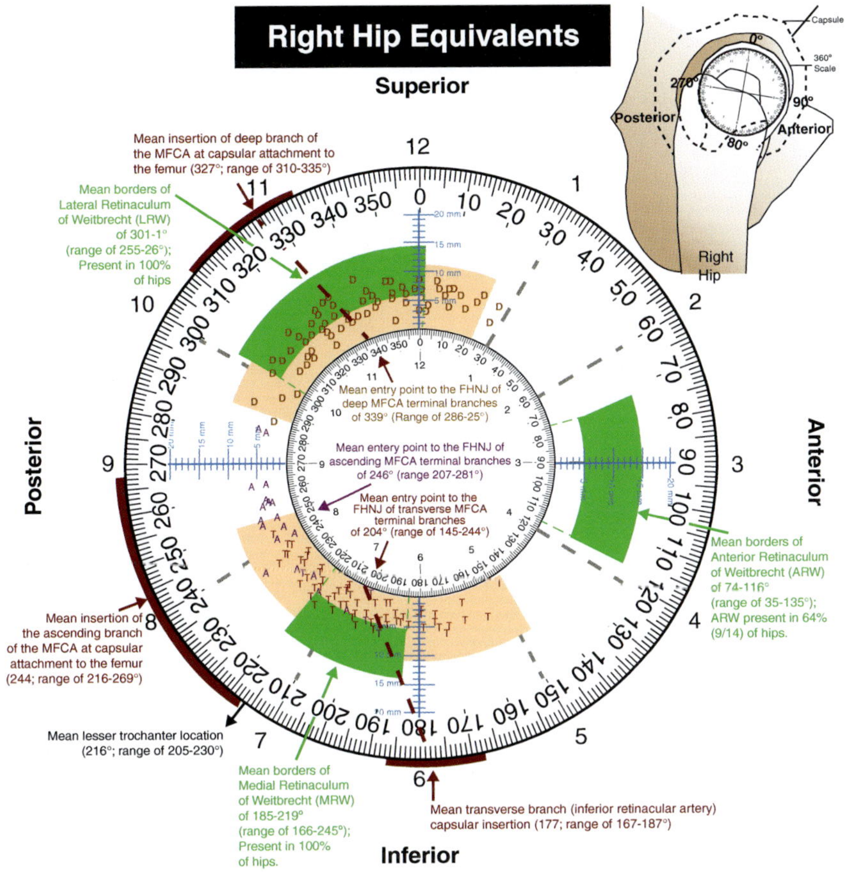

Fig. 9.3. The diagram depicts the combined results of 14 specimens. The outer circle represents the femoral capsular attachment; the inner circle represents the articular rim of the femoral head; and the millimeter scale represents the distance of the entry point of each terminal branch to the articular rim of the femoral head. MFCA = medial femoral circumflex artery; FHNJ = femoral head-neck junction. Entry point for the terminal branches: T = transverse MFCA; A = ascending MFCA; D = deep MFCA. *Source*: Lazaro LE, Klinger CE, Sculco PK, Helfet DL, Lorich DG (2015). Surgical Anatomy of the Medial Femoral Circumflex Artery Terminal Branches: Arterial Supply to the Femoral Head. (2015) *Bone and Joint Journal*, 97(9). Reprinted with permission.

9.2.3 *Patellar vascularity*

The arterial supply to the patella arises from the peripatellar anastomotic ring formed by the supreme genicular artery, superior/inferior

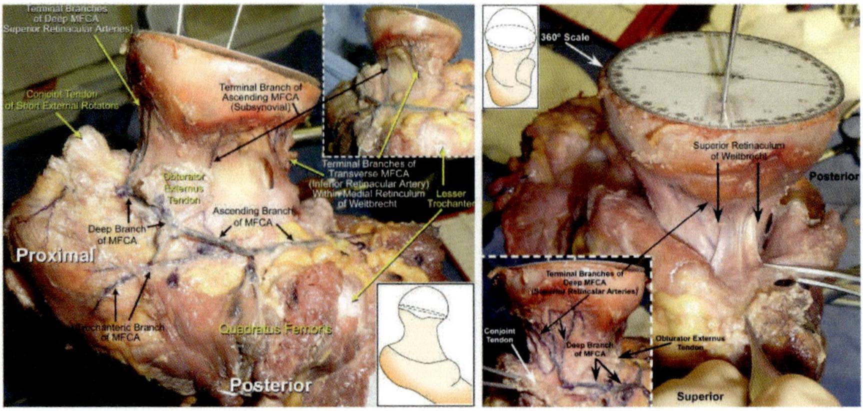

Fig. 9.4. The diagram demonstrates the intracapsular of the terminal braches arising from the medial femoral circumflex artery (MFCA). (Left) posterior aspect of one of the specimens demonstrates the posterior course of the MFCA, its relationship with the obturator externus muscle and conjoined tendon and the intracapsular course of the terminal braches. The inner square ilustrates the posterior inferior aspect of the femoral neck, illustrating the subsynovial course of the terminal branch of the ascending MFCA and intra-retinacular course of the inferior retinacular artery elevated off of the femoral neck. *Source*: Lazaro LE, Klinger CE, Sculco PK, Helfet DL, Lorich DG (2015). Surgical Anatomy of the Medial Femoral Circumflex Artery Terminal Branches: Arterial Supply to the Femoral Head. (2015) *Bone and Joint Journal*, 97(9). Reprinted with permission. (Right) superior aspect of a specimen that illustrates the superior retinaculum of Weitbrecht before and after (inner square) being incised, exposing the superior retinacular arteries (terminal branches of the deep MFCA) coursing closely against the femoral neck. *Source*: Lazaro LE, Klinger CE, Sculco PK, Helfet DL, Lorich DG (2015). Surgical Anatomy of the Medial Femoral Circumflex Artery Terminal Branches: Arterial Supply to the Femoral Head. (2015) *Bone and Joint Journal*, 97(9). Reprinted with permission.

medial genicular arteries, superior/inferior lateral genicular artery, and the anterior tibial recurrent artery (Fig. 9.6);[21, 49] Quantitative and qualitative MRI data demonstrated that the dominant arterial system penetrates the patella at the distal pole mainly inferomedially (80%), supporting the recommendation of preserving the distal pole and the infrapatellar fatpad and the associated anastomotic network (Fig. 9.7).[21] Transverse fractures of the patella jeopardize the blood supply to the proximal fragment with an average reduction of 36% (Fig. 9.8), probably contributing to the frequent reports of residual persistent pain following patellar fractures despite osseous union and articular congruency.[21, 49]

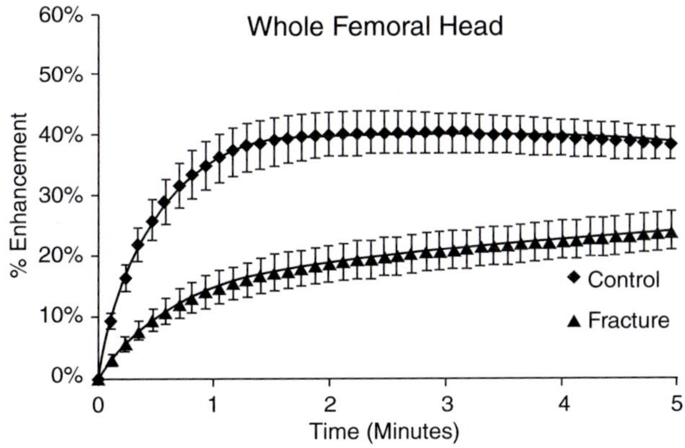

Fig. 9.5. Average time intensity curves of the dynamic contrast enhanced MRI ($n = 27$) demonstrating the perfusion to the entire femoral head on both the injured and contralateral (uninjured) hips. *Source*: Dyke JP, Lazaro LE, Hettrich CM, Hentel KD, Helfet DL, Lorich DG (2013). Regional analysis of femoral head perfusion following displaced fractures of the femoral neck. *J Magn Reson Imaging*. Reprinted with permission.

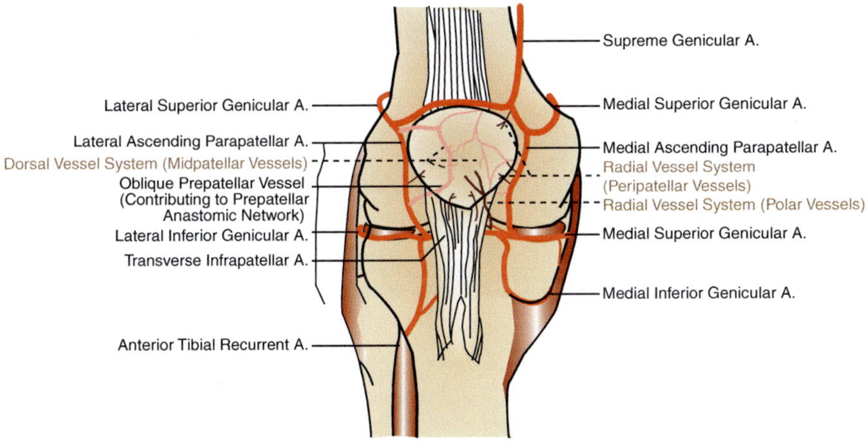

Fig. 9.6. The drawing depicts the extraosseous and intraosseous vasculature of the patella. The terminal branches supplying the patella penetrate the patella at the anterior cortex from the dorsal vessel system (mid-patellar vessels, shown in orange color), and the radial vessel system supplies the terminal branches entering at the border of the patella (peripatellar and polar vessels, shown in brown color). *Source*: Lazaro LE, Wellman DS, Klinger CE, Dyke JP, Pardee NC, Sculco PK, Helfet DL, Lorich DG (2013). Quantitative and qualitative assessment of bone perfusion and arterial contributions in a patellar fracture model using gadolinium-enhanced magnetic resonance imaging: A cadaveric study. *J Bone Joint Surg Am*, 95(19), e1401–e1407. Reprinted with permission.

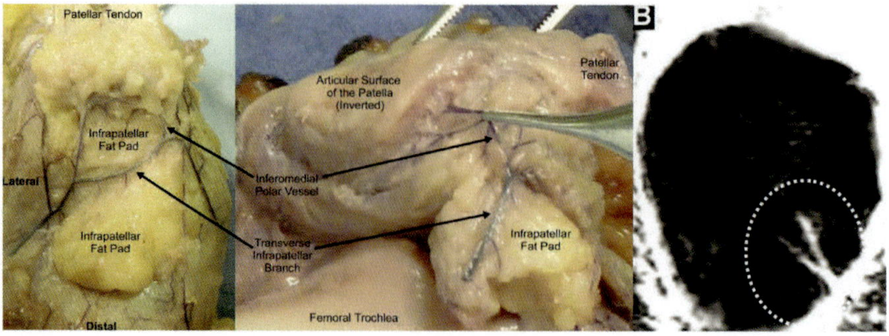

Fig. 9.7. Gross dissection of the infrapatellar fat pad area illustrates the transverse infrapatellar branch giving off the polar vessels and connecting the medial and lateral vessels of the peripatellar anastomotic ring. (Left) the patellar tendon was detached and elevated proximally to illustrate the infrapatellar area posterior to the patellar tendon. (Middle) A lateral arthrotomy was performed and the patella was inverted to illustrate the polar vessels penetrating the patella on the inferiomedial aspect of the distal pole, posterior to the patellar tendon and anterior to the articular cartilage. (Right) the coronal MRI image revealed the dominant vessel entering at the inferior pole at the inferomedial aspect. *Source*: Lazaro LE, Wellman DS, Klinger CE, Dyke JP, Pardee NC, Sculco PK, Helfet DL, Lorich DG (2013). Quantitative and qualitative assessment of bone perfusion and arterial contributions in a patellar fracture model using gadolinium-enhanced magnetic resonance imaging: Acadaveric study. *J Bone Joint Surg Am*, 95(19), e1401–e1407. Reprinted with permission.

9.2.4 *Talar vascularity*

Arterial supply to the talus derives from an anastomotic network of three arterial branches that supply the distal part of the leg (anterior tibial, posterior tibial, and perforating peroneal arteries).[22, 23, 50–53] A large surface area of the talus is covered by articular cartilage, and the arterial perforating sites are limited. Consensus on the main blood supply to the talus has shifted from the anterior tibial artery through the superior surface of the body and neck,[53, 54] to the posterior tibial artery.[50–52] Based on the latter view, the arterial supply to the body of the talus is mainly by retrograde flow and is in danger with displaced fractures of the talar neck predisposing the talar body to osteonecrosis. Our quantitative MRI results demonstrated that the arterial supply comes mainly from the posterior tibial (47%) and anterior tibial arteries (36%), with lesser contributions coming from the peroneal penetrating arteries (17%) (Fig. 9.9a, b).[22] The main contribution of the posterior tibial artery coupled with the rich intra- and extraosseous anastomosis may help explain the low incidence of talar body osteonecrosis following talar neck fractures.[22]

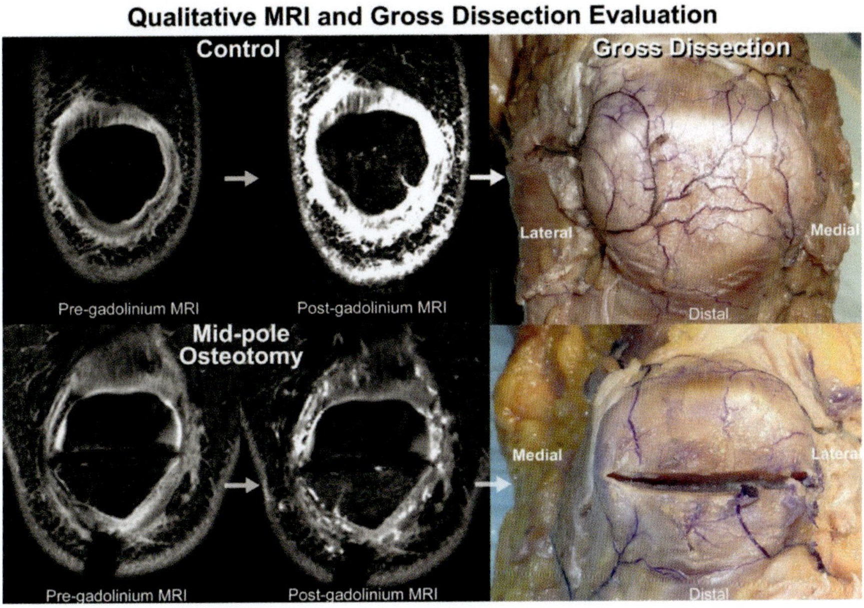

Fig. 9.8. Demonstration of MRI and gross dissection on a matched pair of the mid-pole osteotomy group. *Source*: Lazaro LE, Wellman DS, Klinger CE, Dyke JP, Pardee NC, Sculco PK, Helfet DL, Lorich DG (2013). Quantitative and qualitative assessment of bone perfusion and arterial contributions in a patellar fracture model using gadolinium-enhanced magnetic resonance imaging: a cadaveric study. *J Bone Joint Surg Am*, 95(19), e1401–e1407. Reprinted with permission.

9.3 Femoral Neck Fracture: A Challenging Periarticular Fracture

Surgical preservation of the native femoral head following femoral neck fractures remains a difficult challenge,[46,55] and continues to be associated with high re-operation rates (20–64%).[56–61] The leading complications are fracture non-union (30%),[61] femoral head osteonecrosis (25–45%).[62] These reported complications and re-operation rates often prompt surgeons to replace the femoral head instead of opting for fracture fixation.[56,63] The biological limitations for fracture healing coupled with the instability often created by suboptimal reduction and/or poor biomechanical constructs, seem to be the crux of the problem in femoral neck fractures.[46,64]

The femoral neck is an intracapsular structure, and the periosteum lacks the cambium layer and the ability to form periosteal callus.[65–67] Fracture

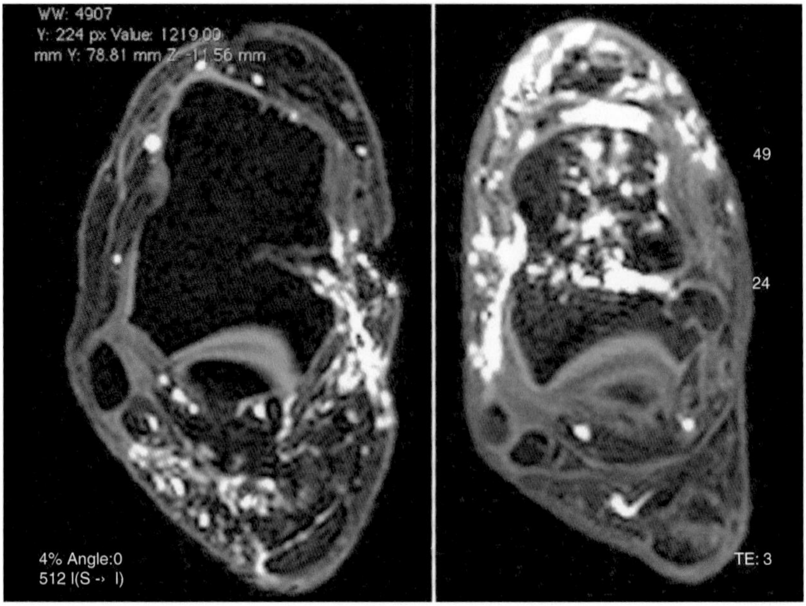

Fig. 9.9a. Post-contrast gadolinium-enhanced MRI of a matched pair with one side with posterior tibial artery ligated (left) and without the posterior tibial artery ligated (right). *Source*: Miller AN, Prasarn ML, Dyke JP, Helfet DL, Lorich DG (2011). Quantitative assessment of the vascularity of the talus with gadolinium-enhanced magnetic resonance imaging. *J Bone Joint Surg Am*, 93(12), 1116–1121. Reprinted with permission.

healing at the femoral neck requires a stable fixation construct that controls the deforming forces and strain at the fracture site to allow for primary/direct bone healing. The femoral metaphysis and femoral neck are comprised of mainly a dense arrangement of cancellous bone, which constitutes the internal weight-bearing system, and is covered by a thin cortex.[68] With fracture of the femoral neck, the compression side is often comminuted[46, 69] and anatomical re-apposition of the fracture fragments is difficult to obtain, especially when attempting closed reduction.[46, 70] The usual constructs for femoral neck fractures allow sliding and dynamic compression at the fracture site during physiological loading to increase chances for fracture healing. But this type of fixation permits motion and increased strain at the fracture site, potentially hindering revascularization crossing the fracture and direct bone healing. These constructs invariably lead to femoral neck shortening (<5 mm in 30–66%).[71–73] The resulting malunion negatively affects hip joint biomechanics and patients' ultimate functional

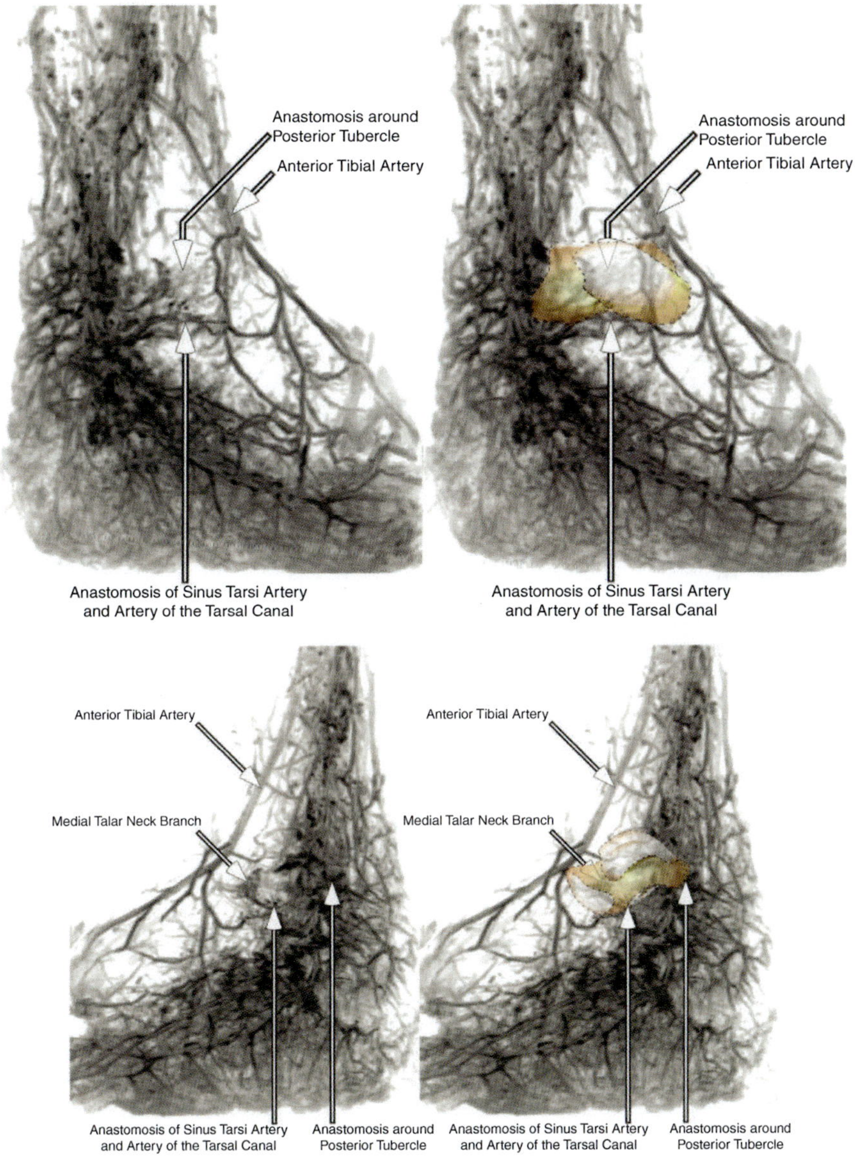

Fig. 9.9b. (Top) the 3D reconstruction images depict the extensive anastomosis about the talus at the sinus tarsi. (Bottom) the lower images demonstratethe anastomosis around the posterior tubercle. *Source*: Prasarn ML, Miller AN, Dyke JP, Helfet DL, Lorich DG (2010). Arterial anatomy of the talus: A cadaver and gadolinium-enhanced MRI study. *Foot Ankle Int.* 31(11), 987–993. Reprinted with permission.

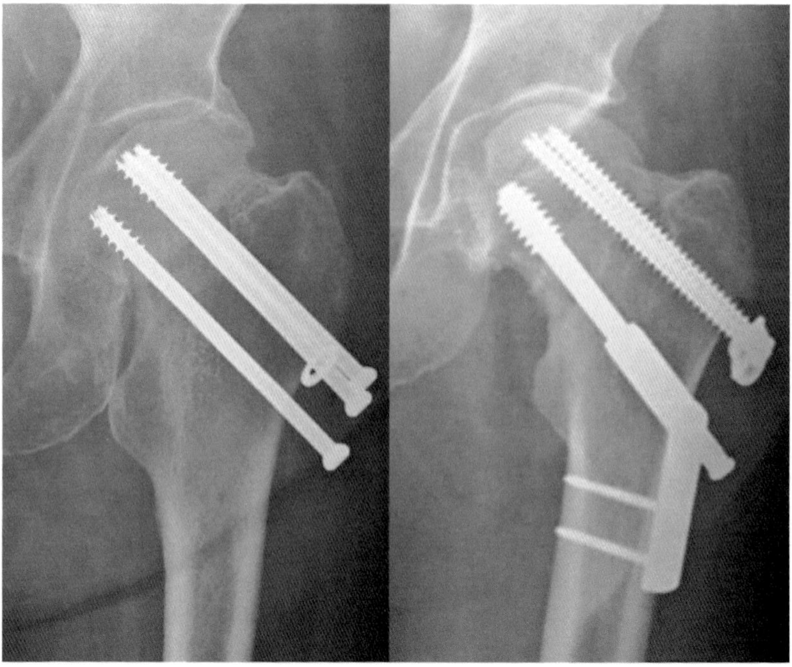

Fig. 9.10. Radiographs demonstrating two constructs that allowed for compression at the fracture side with physiological loading. It demonstrates the shortening of the femoral neck. *Source*: Lorich D, Lazaro L, Boraiah S (2013). *Master Technique in Orthopaedic Surgery: Femoral Neck Fracture Open Reduction and Internal Fixation*, thirded., Wiss D, ed. Philadelphia, PA: Lippincott Williams & Wilkins. Reprinted with permission.

ability (Fig. 9.10).[71, 72, 74–76] To improve stability, surgeons often depend upon valgus malreduction "valgus impacted" and accept rotatory malposition, which further alters the hip joint biomechanics and the already tenuous blood supply.[77, 78]

In 1961, Garden[46] stated that the solution for fixation of femoral neck fractures relies on both anatomical reduction of the internal weight-bearing system and adequate stability of the construct. Several randomized studies comparing different sliding constructs have failed to demonstrate a difference in osseous union, osteonecrosis, and re-operation rates.[56, 79–84] Globally, orthopaedic surgeons agree that the ideal construct would allow intraoperative compression and minimize femoral neck shortening.[85] Open, near-anatomic reductions coupled with non-sliding constructs, using fully threaded screws, resulted in high union rates with minimal femoral neck shortening.[86] In one study, a posterolateral proximal femoral locking plate, with multiple non-parallel converging/diverging screws was used in an attempt to better prevent neck shortening; however, this fixation resulted in poor outcomes and high rates of catastrophic failure (37%).[87] The increased stiffness of this design prevented motion and dynamization of the fracture, putting all the mechanical stress on the implant and resulting in bone-screw interface failure or fatigue failure of the implant. It became clear that some motion and fracture dynamization is necessary to avoid the catastrophic implant failure seen in a rigid fixed-angle plate construct.

With increased consideration of the functional anatomy of the hip joint, it is hypothesized that the optimal construct should provide angle and length stability, withstanding the deforming forces crossing the fracture and allowing controlled microdynamization. To achieve these requirements, we augmented a fully threaded screw construct with an endosteal fibular allograft serving as a biologic dowel. This structural graft is placed at the compression side of the fracture to rebuild the comminuted femoral neck and increase the stability of the construct (Fig. 9.11a,b,c). Immediately after fixation, the smooth edges of the allograft can permit some motion, but the fully threaded screws provide length stability. Over time the bone-screw interface weakens;[88–90] however, the allograft undergoes osseous incorporation,[90–92] increasing the strength of the host bone-allograft interface and the overall stability of the construct. Clinical and radiographic results of this novel length- and angle-stable construct using a biologic dowel demonstrated high union rates (85%), minimal femoral neck shortening (< 5 mm; 0%), low re-operation rate (15%), and excellent clinical outcomes (Hip Harris Score: 91 ± 13.2) and radiographic outcomes (osteonecrosis and segmental collapse rates of 0%).[92]

Compromise of the femoral head vascularity with subsequent development of osteonecrosis and late segmental collapse is of significant concern following displaced femoral neck fractures. A presumed etiologic cause of this condition is a decrease in arterial in-flow caused either directly by disruption of the terminal vessels and/or indirectly by tamponade secondary to development of an intra-articular fracture hematoma. In displaced femoral neck fractures, vascular disruption of the intraosseous nutrient artery and the superior retinacular artery are presumed to occur due to the close proximity of those arteries to the femoral neck. The vascular supply from the inferior retinacular artery and foveal artery may be preserved since these arteries are protected by the inferior retinaculum of Weitbrecht and the ligamentumteres, respectively. Dynamic contrast-enhanced MRI of acute

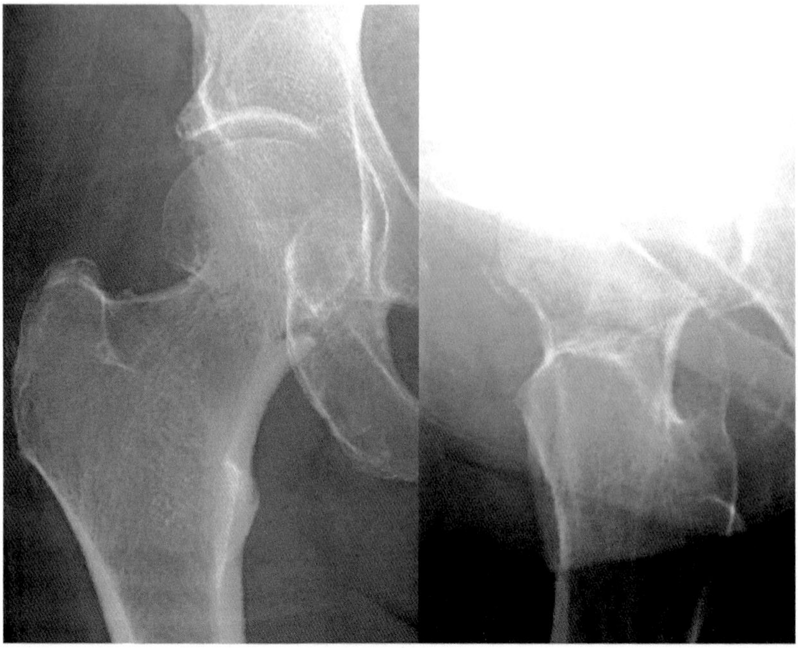

Fig. 9.11a. AP and lateral radiograph of a displaced femoral neck fracture. *Source*: Lorich D, Lazaro L, Boraiah S (2013). *Master Technique in Orthopaedic Surgery: Femoral Neck Fracture Open Reduction and Internal Fixation*, thirded., Wiss D, ed. Philadelphia, PA: Lippincott Williams & Wilkins. Reprinted with permission.

displaced femoral neck fractures demonstrated impairment of both arterial inflow and venous outflow of the entire femoral head, especially at the supero-medial segments.[48] These segments subsequently demonstrated a high incidence (76%) of localized osteonecrosis on follow-up MRI, but radiographically there was neither any sign of osteonecrosis nor segmental collapse at the latest follow-up (average 17.6 ± 6.6 months).[92,93] A longer follow-up is needed to fully assess FH viability given that segmental collapse usually developed two to three years after the injury. In 1971, Garden[94] challenged the conventional wisdom that impaired vascularity of the femoral head is the main cause for failure and complication following fixation of femoral neck fracture. He suggested that late segmental collapse of the femoral head is a remodeling process that develops in response to hip joint incongruity.[94] Despite the high incidence of osteonecrosis of the

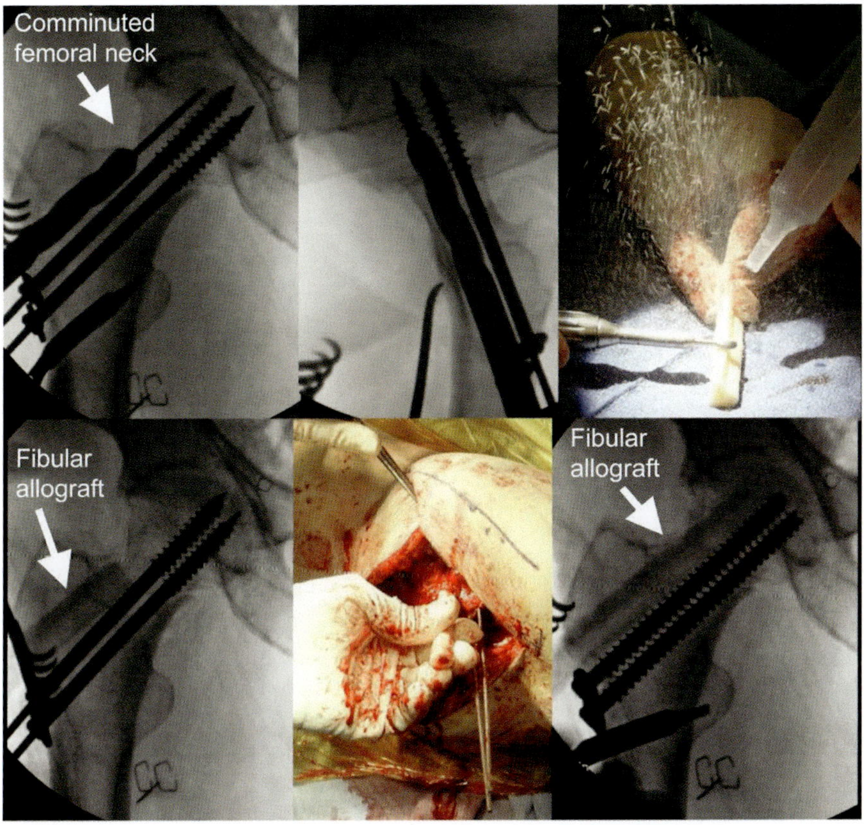

Fig. 9.11b. Intraoperative fluoroscopic images demonstrating correction of coronal plane deformity (valgus). Terminally threaded guide wires are used as a joystick to control fragments and achieve anatomical reduction. The bull stick pusher is used to control deforming forces in the sagittal plane. *Source*: Lorich D, Lazaro L, Boraiah S (2013). *Master Technique in Orthopaedic Surgery: Femoral Neck Fracture Open Reduction and Internal Fixation*, thirded., Wiss D, ed. Philadelphia, PA: Lippincott Williams & Wilkins. Reprinted with permission.

femoral head based on MRI, excellent radiographic and functional outcomes were obtained by maintaining anatomical reduction with a length- and angle-stable construct.[92] Fracture reduction and stable fixation are crucial to avoiding complications and re-operations following internal fixation of femoral neck fractures. Preserving the remaining blood supply to the femoral head and maintaining the congruity of the hip joint, by means of an

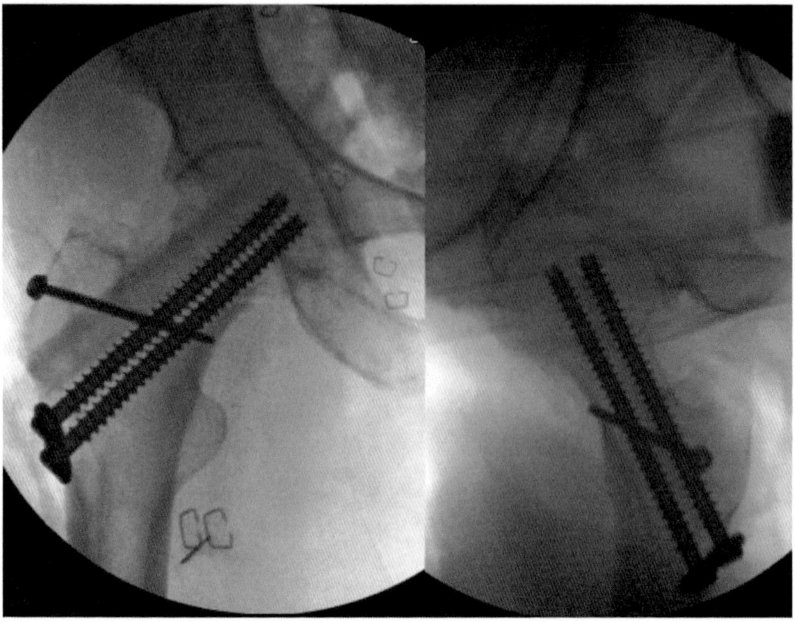

Fig. 9.11c. Fluoroscopic view demonstrating the cannulated drill used to form the track for the fibula allograft. A burr is used to contour the biologic implant to a core diameter of 10–11 mm. The implant is tapped gently into the subchondral bone. The partially threaded screws are then replaced with fully threaded screws. *Source*: Lorich D, Lazaro L, Boraiah S (2013). *Master Technique in Orthopaedic Surgery: Femoral Neck Fracture Open Reduction and Internal Fixation*, third ed., Wiss D, ed. Philadelphia, PA: Lippincott Williams & Wilkins. Reprinted with permission.

angle and length stable fixation construct, seems to provide the ideal environment for fracture healing and revascularization of the injured femoral head.

References

1. Der schenkelhalsbruch: Ein mechanisches Problem. By Dr. Friedrich Pauwels (Aachen, 1936). Royal 8vo. pp. 157, with 186 illustrations. Ferdinand Enke (Stuttgart, 1935). Paper covers, RM. 13.60; bound, RM. 15.00. *Br J Surg.* 23(92), 874.
2. Banks HH. Factors influencing the result in fractures of the femoral neck (1962). *J Bone Joint Surg,* 44(5), 931–964.
3. Banks HH (1968). Tissue response at the fracture site in femoral neck fractures. *Clin Orthop Relat Res,* 61, 116–128.

4. Benterud JG, Husby T, Nordsletten L, Alho A (1997). Fixation of displaced femoral neck fractures with a sliding screw plate and a cancellous screw or two Olmed screws: A prospective, randomized study of 225 elderly patients with a three-year follow-up. *Annales chirurgiae et gynaecologiae*, 86(4), 338–342.
5. Berkes MB, Little MT, Lazaro LE, Cymerman RM, Helfet DL, Lorich DG (2012). Catastrophic failure after open reduction internal fixation of femoral neck fractures with a novel locking plate implant. *J Orthop Trauma.*
6. Boraiah S, Dyke JP, Hettrich C, Parker RJ, Miller A, Helfet D, Lorich D (2009). Assessment of vascularity of the femoral head using gadolinium (Gd-DTPA)-enhanced magnetic resonance imaging: Acadaver study. *J Bone Joint Surg Br*, 91, 131–137.
7. Boraiah S, Paul O, Hammoud S, Gardner MJ, Helfet DL, Lorich DG (2010). Predictable healing of femoral neck fractures treated with intraoperative compression and length-stable implants. *J Trauma*, 69(1), 142–147.
8. Brookes M (1958). The vascular architecture of tubular bone in the rat. *The Anatomical Record.* 132(1), 25–47.
9. Brookes M (1958). The vascularization of long bones in the human foetus. *J Anat*, 92(2), 261–267.
10. Brooks CH, Revell WJ, Heatley FW (1993). Vascularity of the humeral head after proximal humeral fractures. An anatomical cadaver study. *J Bone Joint Surg Br,* 75(1), 132–136.
11. Claes LE, Heigele CA (1999). Magnitudes of local stress and strain along bony surfaces predict the course and type of fracture healing. *J Biomech*, 32(3), 255–266.
12. Cleveland M, Fielding JW (1954). A continuing end-result study of intracapsular fracture of the neck of the femur. *J Bone Joint Surg Am,* 36-a(5), 1020–1030.
13. Depreux R, Hollingshausen (1963). Arterial vascularization of the astragalus. *Lille chirurgical*, 18, 188–194.
14. Dyke JP, Lazaro LE, Hettrich CM, Hentel KD, Helfet DL, Lorich DG (2013). Regional analysis of femoral head perfusion following displaced fractures of the femoral neck. *J Magn Reson Imaging.*
15. Frangenheim P (1906). Studien uber Schenkelhalsgrakturen und die Vorgange bei ihrer Heilung. *Dsch Z Chir*, 401–455.
16. Garden RS (1961). Low-angle fixation in fractures of the femoral neck. *J Bone Joint Surg Br*, 43, 647–663.
17. Garden RS (1971). Malreduction and avascular necrosis in subcapital fractures of the femur. *J Bone Joint Surg Br*, 53(2), 183–197.
18. Garden RS (1964). Stability and union in subcapital fractures of the femur. *J Bone Joint Surg Br*, 46, 630–647.
19. Garden RS (1961). The structure and function of the proximal end of the femur. *J Bone Joint Surg Br*, 43-B(3), 576–589.
20. Gautier E, Ganz K, Krugel N, Gill T, Ganz R (2000). Anatomy of the medial femoral circumflex artery and its surgical implications. *J Bone Joint Surg Br*, 82(5), 679–683.

21. Gelberman RH, Mortensen WW (1983). The arterial anatomy of the talus. *Foot and Ankle*, 4(2), 64–72.
22. Gerber C, Schneeberger AG, Vinh TS (1990). The arterial vascularization of the humeral head: An anatomical study. *J Bone Joint Surg Am*, 72(10), 1486–1494.
23. Gojda J, Bartonicek J (2012). The retinacula of Weitbrecht in the adult hip. *Surg Radiol Anat*, 34(1), 31–38.
24. Grundnes O, Reikeras O (1992). Blood flow and mechanical properties of healing bone: Femoral osteotomies studied in rats. *Acta Orthop Scand*, 63(5), 487–491.
25. Gurney B, Mermier C, Robergs R, Gibson A, Rivero D (2001). Effects of limb-length discrepancy on gait economy and lower-extremity muscle activity in older adults. *J Bone Joint Surg Am*, 83-A(6), 907–915.
26. Haliburton RA, Sullivan CR, Kelly PJ, Peterson LF (1958). The extra-osseous and intra-osseous blood supply of the talus. *J Bone Joint Surg Am*, 40-a(5), 1115–1120.
27. Harrison MH, Schajowicz F, Trueta J (1953). Osteoarthritis of the hip: A study of the nature and evolution of the disease. *J Bone Joint Surg Br*, 35-B(4), 598–626.
28. Harty M (1953). Blood supply of the femoral head. *Br Med J*, 2(4848), 1236–1237.
29. Hettrich CM, Boraiah S, Dyke JP, Neviaser A, Helfet DL, Lorich DG (2010). Quantitative assessment of the vascularity of the proximal part of the humerus. *J Bone Joint Surg Am*, 92, 943–948.
30. Howe WW, Jr., Lacey T, Schwartz RP (1950). A study of the gross anatomy of the arteries supplying the proximal portion of the femur and the acetabulum. *J Bone Joint Surg Am*, 32(A:4), 856–866.
31. Ito K, Perren S (2007). Biology and biomechanics in bone healing. In: Ruedi T, Buckley R, Moran C, eds., *AO Principles of Fracture Management*, second expanded edition. Stuttgart, New York: Georg Thieme Verlag, 9–31.
32. Johnson RW Jr (1968). A physiological study of the blood supply of the diaphysis. *Clin Orthop Relat Res*, 56, 5–11.
33. Judet J, Judet R, Lagrange J, Dunoyer J (1955). A study of the arterial vascularization of the femoral neck in the adult. *J Bone Joint Surg Am*, 37-a(4), 663–680.
34. Kalhor M, Beck M, Huff TW, Ganz R (2009). Capsular and pericapsular contributions to acetabular and femoral head perfusion. *J Bone Joint Surg Am*, 91(2), 409–418.
35. Kalhor M, Horowitz K, Gharehdaghi J, Beck M, Ganz R. Anatomic variations in femoral head circulation (2012). *Hip Int (Journal of Clinical and Experimental Research on Hip Pathology and Therapy)*, 22(3), 307–312.
36. Kelly PJ (1968). Anatomy, physiology, and pathology of the blood supply of bones. *J Bone Joint Surg Am*, 50(4), 766–783.
37. Kuokkanen H, Korkala O, Antti-Poika I, Tolonen J, Lehtimaki MY, Silvennoinen T (1991). Three cancellous bone screws versus a screw-angle plate

in the treatment of Garden I and II fractures of the femoral neck. *Acta Orthopaedica Belgica*, 57(1), 53–57.

38. Laing PG (1956). The arterial supply of the adult humerus. *J Bone Joint Surg Am*, 38-a(5), 1105–1116.
39. Lavigne M, Kalhor M, Beck M, Ganz R, Leunig M (2005). Distribution of vascular for amina around the femoral head and neck junction: Relevance for conservative intracapsular procedures of the hip. *Orthop Clin North Am*, 36(2), 171–176, viii.
40. Lazaro L, Dyke J, Farshad-Amacker N, Helfet D, Potter H, Lorich D (2014). Femoral head osteonecrosis following anatomic stable fixation of femoral neck fractures: An in-vivo MRI study. *Am Acad Orthop Surg*, LA2014.
41. Lazaro L, Farshad-Amacker N, Dyke J, Birnbaum J, Helfet D, Potter H, Lorich D (2013). Osseous incorporation of fibular allograft used to augment construct for femoral neck freactures: An in-vivo MRI study. Orthopaedic Trauma Association 29th Annual Meeting, Phoenix, AZ, October 2013.
42. Lazaro L, Klinger C, Sculco P, Helfet D, Lorich D (2014). Terminal branches of the medial femoral circumflex artery: Arterial supply to the femoral head. *Bone Joint J*. In submission.
43. Lazaro LE, Birnbaum J, Farshad-Amacker N, Helfet DL, Potter HG, Lorich DG (2014). Endosteal biologic augmentation reduces complications associated with fixation of displaced femoral neck fractures. *The Journal of Orthopaedic Trauma*. In submission.
44. Lazaro LE, Sculco PK, Pardee NC, Klinger CE, Dyke JP, Helfet DL, Lorich DG (2013). Assessment of femoral head and head-neck junction perfusion following surgical hip dislocation using gadolinium-enhanced magnetic resonance imaging: a cadaveric study. *J Bone Joint Surg Am*, 95(23), e1821–e1828.
45. Lazaro LE, Wellman DS, Klinger CE, Dyke JP, Pardee NC, Sculco PK, Helfet DL, Lorich DG (2013). Quantitative and qualitative assessment of bone perfusion and arterial contributions in a patellar fracture model using gadolinium-enhanced magnetic resonance imaging: Acadaveric study. *J Bone Joint Surg Am*, 95(19), e1401–e1407.
46. Lopez-Curto JA, Bassingthwaighte JB, Kelly PJ (1980). Anatomy of the microvasculature of the tibial diaphysis of the adult dog. *J Bone Joint Surg Am*, 62(8), 1362–1369.
47. Lorich D, Lazaro L, Boraiah S (2013). *Master Technique in Orthopaedic Surgery: Femoral Neck Fracture Open Reduction and Internal Fixation*, thirded. Wiss D, ed. Philadelphia, PA: Lippincott Williams & Wilkins.
48. Lu-Yao GL, Keller RB, Littenberg B, Wennberg JE (1994). Outcomes after displaced fractures of the femoral neck: A meta-analysis of one hundred and six published reports. *J Bone Joint Surg Am*, 6(1), 15–25.
49. Macaulay W, Pagnotto MR, Iorio R, Mont MA, Saleh KJ (2006). Displaced femoral neck fractures in the elderly: Hemiarthroplasty versus total hip arthroplasty. *J Am Acad Orthop Surg*, 14(5), 287–293.
50. Madsen F, Linde F, Andersen E, Birke H, Hvass I, Poulsen TD (1987). Fixation of displaced femoral neck fractures: A comparison between sliding

screw plate and four cancellous bone screws. *Acta Orthop Scand,* 58(3), 212–216.

51. Masson M, Parker MJ, Fleischer S (2003). Internal fixation versus arthroplasty for intracapsular proximal femoral fractures in adults. The Cochrane Database of Systematic Reviews, (2), Cd001708.
52. Meyer C, Alt V, Hassanin H, Heiss C, Stahl JP, Giebel G, *et al.* (2005). The arteries of the humeral head and their relevance in fracture treatment. *Surg Radiol Anat,* 27(3), 232–237.
53. Miller AN, Prasarn ML, Dyke JP, Helfet DL, Lorich DG (2011). Quantitative assessment of the vascularity of the talus with gadolinium-enhanced magnetic resonance imaging. *J Bone Joint Surg Am*, 93(12), 1116–1121.
54. Miyamoto RG, Kaplan KM, Levine BR, Egol KA, Zuckerman JD (2008). Surgical management of hip fractures: An evidence-based review of the literature. I: femoral neck fractures. *J Am Acad Orthop Surg,* 16(10), 596–607.
55. Mulfinger GL, Trueta J (1970). The blood supply of the talus. *J Bone Joint Surg Br*, 52(1), 160–167.
56. Nagi ON, Dhillon MS, Aggarwal S (2004). The long term fate of the fibula when used as an intraosseous graft. *Acta Orthopaedica Belgica*, 70(4), 322–326.
57. Nagi ON, Gautam VK, Marya SK (1986). Treatment of femoral neck fractures with a cancellous screw and fibular graft. *J Bone Joint Surg Br*, 68(3), 387–391.
58. Neviaser AS, Hettrich CM, Dines JS, Lorich DG (2011). Rate of avascular necrosis following proximal humerus fractures treated with a lateral locking plate and endosteal implant. *Arch Orthop Trauma Surg*, 131(12), 1617–1622.
59. Nikolopoulos KE, Papadakis SA, Kateros KT, Themistocleous GS, Vlamis JA, Papagelopoulos PJ, *et al.* (2003). Long-term outcome of patients with avascular necrosis, after internal fixation of femoral neck fractures. *Injury*, 34, 525–528.
60. Ogden JA (1974). Changing patterns of proximal femoral vascularity. *J Bone Joint Surg Am*, 56(5), 941–950.
61. Pajenda G, Vecsei V, Reddy B, Heinz T (2000). Treatment of talar neck fractures: Clinical results of 50 patients. *J Foot Ankle Surg*, 39(6), 365–375.
62. Papadakis SA, Segos D, Kouvaras I, Dagas S, Malakasis M, Grivas TB (2009). Integrity of posterior retinaculum after displaced femoral neck fractures. *Injury*, 40(3), 277–279.
63. Parker MJ, Blundell C (1998). Choice of implant for internal fixation of femoral neck fractures: Meta-analysis of 25 randomised trials including 4,925 patients. *Acta Orthop Scan*, 69(2), 138–143.
64. Parker MJ, Khan RJ, Crawford J, Pryor GA (2002). Hemiarthroplasty versus internal fixation for displaced intracapsular hip fractures in the elderly: A randomised trial of 455 patients. *J Bone Joint Surg Br*, 84(8), 1150–1155.
65. Parker MJ, Stockton G (2001). Internal fixation implants for intracapsular proximal femoral fractures in adults. The Cochrane Database of Systematic Reviews, (4), Cd001467.

66. Patrick J (1949). Intracapsular fractures of the femur treated with a combined Smith-Petersen nail and fibular graft. *J Bone Joint Surg Am*, 31a(1), 67–80.
67. Paus A, Gjengedal E, Hareide A, Jorgensen JJ (1986). Dislocated fractures of the femoral neck treated with von Bahr screws or hip compression screw: Results of a prospective, randomized study. *Journal of the Oslo City Hospitals*, 36(5–6), 55–61.
68. Perren S, Cordey J (1980). The concept of interfragmentary strain. Berlin, Heidelberg, New York: Spinger Verlag.
69. Prasarn ML, Miller AN, Dyke JP, Helfet DL, Lorich DG (2010). Arterial anatomy of the talus: Acadaver and gadolinium-enhanced MRI study. *Foot Ankle Int*, 31, 987–993.
70. Puolakka TJ, Laine HJ, Tarvainen T, Aho H (2001). Thompson hemiarthroplasty is superior to Ullevaal screws in treating displaced femoral neck fractures in patients over 75 years. A prospective randomized study with two-year follow-up. *Annales Chirurgiae et Gynaecologiae*, 90(3), 225–228.
71. Rahn BA, Gallinaro P, Baltensperger A, Perren SM (1971). Primary bone healing: An experimental study in the rabbit. *J Bone Joint Surg Am,* 53(4), 783–786.
72. Rhinelander FW (1968). The normal microcirculation of diaphyseal cortex and its response to fracture. *J Bone Joint Surg Am,* 50(4), 784–800.
73. Rhinelander FW (1974). Tibial blood supply in relation to fracture healing. *Clin Orthop Relat Res,* (105), 34–81.
74. Rhinelander FW, Baragry R (1962). Microangiography in bone healing: I. Undisplaced closed fractures. *J Bone Joint Surg Am,* 44-a, 1273–1298.
75. Rhinelander FW, Phillips RS, Steel WM, Beer JC (1968). Microangiography in bone healing: II. Displaced closed fractures. *J Bone Joint Surg Am*, 50(4), 643–662 passim.
76. Roden M, Schon M, Fredin H (2003). Treatment of displaced femoral neck fractures: Arandomized minimum 5-year follow-up study of screws and bipolar hemiprostheses in 100 patients. *ActaOrthop Scand*, 74(1), 42–44.
77. Scapinelli R (1967). Blood supply of the human patella: Its relation to ischaemic necrosis after fracture. *J Bone Joint Surg Br*, 49(3), 563–570.
78. Schenk R, Willenegger H (1963). On the histological picture of so-called primary healing of pressure osteosynthesis in experimental osteotomies in the dog. *Experientia*, 19, 593–595.
79. Schmorl G (1924). *Die Pathologische Anatomie der Schenkelhalsbrakturen.* Munchen: MedWschr.
80. Sevitt S, Thompson RG (1965). The distribution and anastomoses of arteries supplying the head and neckof the femur. *J Bone Joint Surg Br*, 47, 560–573.
81. Smith FB (1959). Effects of rotatory and valgus malpositions on blood supply to the femoral head observations at arthroplasty. *J Bone Joint Surg*, 41(5), 800–815.
82. Smith LD (1953). Hip fractures: the role of muscle contraction or intrinsic forces in the causation of fractures of the femoral neck. *J Bone Joint Surg Am*, 35-a(2), 367–383.

83. Tidermark J, Ponzer S, Svensson O, Soderqvist A, Tornkvist H (2003). Internal fixation compared with total hip replacement for displaced femoral neck fractures in the elderly: A randomised, controlled trial. *J Bone Joint Surg Br*, 85(3), 380–388.
84. Trueta J (1957). The normal vascular anatomy of the human femoral head during growth. *J Bone Joint Surg Br*, 39-b(2), 358–394.
85. Trueta J, Caladias AX (1964). A study of the blood supply of the long bones. *Surg Gynecol Obstet*, 118, 485–498.
86. Trueta J, Cavadias AX (1955). Vascular changes caused by the Kuntscher type of nailing: An experimental study in the rabbit. *J Bone Joint Surg Br*, 37-b(3), 492–505.
87. Tucker FR (1949). Arterial supply to the femoral head and its clinical importance. *J Bone Joint Surg Br*, 31B(1), 82–93.
88. Walmsley T (1916). A note on the retinacula of Weitbrecht. *J Anat*, 51(Pt 1), 61–64.
89. Weil YA, Khoury A, Zuaiter I, Safran O, Liebergall M, Mosheiff R (2012). Femoral neck shortening and varus collapse after navigated fixation of intracapsular femoral neck fractures. *J Orthop Trauma*, 26(1), 19–23.
90. Wendt M, Cass J, Trousdale R (2013). Incidence of radiographic cam-type impingement in young patients (<50) after femoral neck fracture treated with reduction and internal fixation. *HSS J*, 9(2), 113–117.
91. Wolcott WE (1943). The evolution of the circulation in the developing femoral head and neck. *Surg Gynecol Obstet*, 77, 185.
92. Zlowodzki M, Ayieni O, Petrisor BA, Bhandari M (2008). Femoral neck shortening after fracture fixation with multiple cancellous screws: Incidence and effect on function. *J Trauma*, 64(1), 163–169.
93. Zlowodzki M, Brink O, Switzer J, Wingerter S, Woodall J, Jr., Petrisor BA, *et al.* (2008). The effect of shortening and varus collapse of the femoral neck on function after fixation of intracapsular fracture of the hip: A multi-centre cohort study. *J Bone Joint Surg Br*, 90(11), 1487–1494.
94. Zlowodzki M, Jonsson A, Paulke R, Kregor PJ, Bhandari M (2007). Shortening after femoral neck fracture fixation: Is there a solution? *Clin Orthop Relat Res*, 461, 213–218.

CHAPTER 10

JOINT INFLAMMATION AND SYNOVITIS

ALISSA J. BURGE
Assistant Attending Radiologist
Department of Radiology and Imaging
Hospital for Special Surgery, New York, NY
Assistant Professor of Radiology
Weill Medical College of Cornell University, New York, NY

10.1 Introduction to Joint Inflammation and Synovitis

10.1.1 *Joint tissues: Synovial*

Synovial joints contain a variety of different tissues, each type having varying degrees of vascularization. While some tissues are highly vascular, others, such as articular cartilage, are avascular, receiving nutrients via diffusion from synovial fluid or from the subchondral bone. The synovium consists of a lining (the layer closest to the synovial fluid) and a sublining, which is thicker and situated subjacent to the lining. Normal synovium is highly vascular, with a dense highly fenestrated capillary network, and the majority of the vessels being located within the portions of the sublining layer closest to the lining and capsule. In normal joints, vascular anatomy is typically highly organized; however, in the setting of arthritis and inflammation, vascular plasticity, the ability of the vascular system to remodel in response to stimuli, leads to abnormal redistribution of blood vessels, which may compromise both regulation of blood flow to the joint, as well as the functional capacity of the altered tissues.[12]

10.1.2 *Joint tissues: Non-synovial*

Non-synovial tissues comprising a typical synovial joint may include ligaments, articular cartilage, menisci, tendons, muscles, bursae, and bone.

Ligamentous vascular density varies based on the ligament in question. For example, while the cruciate ligaments possess both deep and superficial vessels, they also appear to be dependent on synovial fluid for their nutrient supply, and have been shown experimentally to be sustained by the synovial fluid in the absence of normal vascular supply for a limited time with relatively normal function.

Tendons have been shown to have a variable vascular supply, with both vascular and avascular segments, as well as highly vascularized tendon sheaths which function similarly to the synovial lining, providing nutritional support to the superficial portions of the tendons.

The fibrocartilaginous menisci are partially vascularized, with blood supply entering the meniscus peripherally, and diminishing toward the central and inner portions, such that the free edge of the meniscus is avascular. Devascularization progresses with age; vessels are only present in the portion of the meniscus closest to the joint capsule in adults over 50 years of age.

The periarticular portions of bones are generally highly vascular, while the supporting joint capsule is typically avascular. Articular cartilage, as previously mentioned, is avascular and receives nutrient supply from the synovial fluid and subchondral bone.[12]

10.1.3 *Vascular changes in joint inflammation*

Vascular plasticity is a necessary adaptive mechanism to altered stresses and tissue damage incurred over the lifespan of a joint. While certain changes in the vascular anatomy may be considered a normal part of the aging process, vascular plasticity may also result in architectural changes that hinder normal tissue function.

In patients with inflammatory arthritides, such as rheumatoid arthritis, as the synovial lining becomes inflamed and hyperplastic, the depth of blood vessels from the synovial surface increases, resulting in an increase in the distance over which nutrients must travel and therefore decreased efficacy with regard to nourishing the articular cartilage. Localized hypoxia may stimulate angiogenesis and a resultant immature vascular architecture. As this process progresses, the growing synovial pannus may invade nonsynovial structures such as adjacent bone and articular cartilage, resulting in local tissue damage. Additionally, vascularization of the normally avascular articular cartilage may result in functional compromise, leading to further joint damage.[12]

10.2 Joint Inflammation and Synovitis in Clinical Practice

10.2.1 *Inflammatory arthropathies*

Inflammatory arthritis is an umbrella term encompassing a variety of arthritides, largely considered autoimmune, the hallmark of which is synovial inflammation, as opposed to osteoarthritis, which is considered primarily a degenerative process, though a component of inflammation may be present.

Rheumatoid arthritis is a common and classic example of inflammatory arthropathy, and is classically described as a symmetric inflammatory peripheral polyarthropathy. Diagnostic criteria include polyarthritis involving three or more joints, positive serologic markers (these include rheumatoid factor, anti-cyclic citrullinated peptides, C reactive protein, and erythrocyte sedimentation rate), with duration of symptoms for more than six weeks, and exclusion of similar diseases, though not all of the diagnostic criteria are met in certain patients with rheumatoid arthritis. The arthropathy typically involves the hands and wrists, as well as a component of soft tissue swelling. Additional clinical features include morning stiffness and rheumatoid nodules. Early recognition and treatment of the disease is crucial in minimizing joint damage and resultant disability.[35]

A variety of other inflammatory arthropathies exist, and may be difficult to differentiate from rheumatoid arthritis, particularly early in the clinical course. More commonly encountered examples of these conditions include psoriatic arthritis, reactive arthritis (including Reiter's syndrome), and arthritis of inflammatory bowel disease.

Psoriatic arthritis is an inflammatory arthropathy encountered in patients with psoriasis, affecting approximately 4–30% of this patient population. Typically, joint involvement is polyarticular or oligoarticular, with various patterns of involvement described:

- Distal, as characterized by involvement of the DIP joints
- Asymmetric oligoarthritis, as characterized by asymmetric involvement of <5 small and/or large joints
- Symmetric polyarthritis, which is often indistinguishable from rheumatoid arthritis
- Arthritis mutilans, characterized by a destructive arthritis
- Spondyloarthritis, characterized by sacroiliitis and/or spondylitis

Additional clinical manifestations may include enthesitis, tenosynovitis, dactylitis, and nail lesions. Laboratory findings are non-specific, and may include elevated acute phase reactants and HLA-B27; rheumatoid factor is positive in a minority of patients.[8,14]

Reactive arthritis is an uncommon disease affecting young adults, typically defined as a seronegative spondyloarthropathy resulting in arthritis following an infection; this term includes but is not limited to patients who fulfill the clinical criteria for Reiter's syndrome. Organisms implicated in reactive arthritis include Chlamydia trachomatis, Yersinia, Salmonella, Shigella, Campylobacter, Escherichia coli, Clostridium difficile, and Chlamydophilapneumoniae. Clinical features include mono- or oligoarticular arthritis, often involving the lower extremities. The development of this arthritis often follows the initial infectious episode by several days to weeks. Additional signs and symptoms include enthesitis; dactylitis; conjunctivitis; oral, skin, and genital lesions; nail changes; and constitutional symptoms such as fever and malaise. Laboratory findings include evidence of preceding infection, elevated acute phase reactants, HLA-B27, and evidence of inflammatory synovitis. Treatment involves therapy directed at both the initial infection as well as the subsequent arthritis, which commonly involves non-steroidal anti-inflammatory drugs (NSAIDs) and/or glucocorticoids. The development of chronic refractory arthritis may require the use of disease modifying anti-rheumatic agents (DMARDs).[17,39]

Arthritis associated with inflammatory bowel disease may occur in approximately 9–53% of this patient population, and appears to be more common in patients with ulcerative colitis and those Crohn's patients with colonic involvement. Peripheral arthritis has been divided into type 1 (acute, pauciarticular, and remitting) and type II (chronic, polyarticular, and relapsing) subtypes. While type I most commonly involves the knees, type 2 most commonly involves the MCP joints. Additionally, sacroiliitis and spondylitis may occur. Laboratory findings are again somewhat nonspecific, and may include elevated acute phase reactants, HLA-B27, and evidence of inflammatory synovitis.[32]

10.2.2 *Crystalline arthropathies*

Crystalline arthropathies result from the deposition of various crystals within the joints and periarticular soft tissues. Gout is the most common of these conditions, with an estimated prevalence of 3–8 million individuals in the United States, and involves the accumulation of monosodium urate crystals secondary to longstanding hyperuricemia. Clinical manifestations include recurrent attacks of inflammatory arthritis, chronic arthropathy, tophaceous deposits of urate crystals, nephrolithiasis, and chronic nephropathy. An acute attack of gout is characterized by severe pain, redness, and swelling typically involving the lower extremities, most commonly the great toe or knee. Inflammation, however, typically extends beyond the affected joint. Locations more commonly affected in recurrent gout include the ankle, wrist, fingers, and olecranon bursa. Definitive diagnosis of gout typically requires identification of characteristic urate crystals with the synovial fluid aspirated from an affected joint. In the absence of this finding, gout may be diagnosed tentatively based on a combination of classic clinical signs and symptoms in the setting of hyperuricemia and typical imaging findings.[2,5,7]

Various clinical syndromes have been associated with the deposition of calcium pyrophosphate (CPPD) within the tissues; these include:

- Pseudogout: attacks of crystal-induced synovitis clinically similar to gout, but precipitated by CPPD.
- Chondrocalcinosis: deposition of CPPD crystals within hyaline and fibrocartilage, resulting in mineralization.
- Pyrophosphate arthropathy: joint disease related to CPPD.

The majority of joints affected by CPPD deposition are asymptomatic. In patients with acute pseudogout, the clinical manifestations closely resemble those of gout, with acute onset of pain and swelling, though most commonly involve the knee rather than the great toe. Differences in joint involvement, however, are insufficient to differentiate the two conditions — this is optimally accomplished by identification of characteristic crystals on microscopy of synovial fluid obtained from an affected joint. Longstanding joint disease related to CPPD may have a joint distribution resembling that of gout, rheumatoid arthritis, osteoarthritis, and/or neuropathic arthroses, complicating diagnosis.[3,30]

10.2.3 *Hemophilia*

Hemophilia is a term referring to bleeding disorders linked to deficiency of certain clotting factors, with hemophilia A (factor XIII deficiency) being more common than hemophilia B (factor IX deficiency). Most often, these patients tend to bleed into muscles, and, more commonly, joints, resulting in a characteristic arthrosis. Recurrent spontaneous hemarthroses in patients with severe disease commonly affect the ankles, knees, and elbows, contributing to synovitis and joint destruction related to iron deposition and fibrosis. Prophylactic treatment with factor replacement therapy has been shown to result in a decreased risk of spontaneous hemarthrosis and subsequently reduced risk of hemophiliac arthropathy.[13]

10.2.4 *Synovial proliferative disease*

Pigmented villonodular synovitis (PVNS) is a rare condition of unclear etiology resulting in proliferation of synovial tissue within joints, tendon sheaths, and bursae. Diffuse and nodular forms are classically described, with the diffuse form being more common, and frequently affecting the larger joints. Clinical manifestations may include pain and swelling. Joint involvement is typically monoarticular. Extra-articular PVNS commonly involves the tendon sheath, resulting in a localized soft tissue mass, referred to as giant cell tumor of the tendon sheath.[26,36]

Synovial chondromatosis is another rare proliferative disorder of the joints in which there is cartilaginous metaplasia of the synovium, which produces nodules of cartilage that subsequently break off and form numerous loose intra-articular bodies. These bodies, nourished by the synovial fluid, may grow, calcify, or ossify, ultimately resulting in mechanical damage to the articular cartilage. Clinical symptoms include pain, swelling, mechanical symptoms such as catching and locking, and limited range of motion. Joint involvement is typically monoarticular, most commonly involving the knee, followed by the hip, elbow, and shoulder.

10.2.5 *Post-surgical*

Patients with surgical implants may develop synovitis on the basis of a reaction to various types of wear debris. This most commonly occurs in the setting of joint arthroplasty, in which these implants are subject to load bearing and repetitive motion, predisposing the components to stresses leading to implant wear.

Joint arthroplasties incorporating polyethylene components are extremely common; therefore, wear-induced synovitis related to polymeric debris is commonly encountered in patients with these implants. Particulate polymeric wear debris incite a histiocytic foreign body reaction in which tissue macrophages attempt to phagocytize particulate debris. For bodies too large to be phagocytized, macrophages fuse to form foreign body giant cells, secrete degradative agents, and encapsulate the body in a collagenous shell to isolate it from surrounding host tissues. Polymeric wear typically results in a synovitis and, if longstanding, can result in osteolysis about the implant.[10, 11]

Joint arthroplasties incorporating metal-on-metal bearings and junctions have been implicated in the development of a more aggressive type of wear-related reaction termed adverse local tissue reaction (ALTR). In this type of reaction, analogous to a type IV hypersensitivity reaction, wear debris acting as haptens complex with local proteins, are presented by surface complexes of local cells, and recognized by sensitized CD8 cytotoxic T cells, which destroy the "infected" presenting cell. CD4 helper T cells activate macrophages and produce interleukins which activate eosinophils. This process may result in a severe synovitis with aggressive and rapidly progressive tissue damage.[10, 11]

Hemarthrosis has been described as a complication of arthroplasty, and less commonly of arthroscopy. Recurrent bleeding into the joint space may lead to synovitis and joint destruction, in a similar fashion to hemophiliac arthropathy. Clinical manifestations include pain and swelling. Diagnosis commonly involves joint aspirate and/or imaging, in the setting of a history of preceding surgery.[10, 23]

While infection may occur in non-surgical settings, it is encountered with increased frequency in post-operative patients, in both acute/subacute and more chronic settings. In the more acute setting, post-operative edema and fluid may be present, complicating the diagnosis of infection.[9, 10]

10.3 Imaging of Joint Inflammation and Synovitis

A variety of imaging modalities have been employed in the diagnosis, monitoring, and post-treatment follow-up of pathologic conditions involving joint inflammation and synovitis. These modalities each have their particular strengths and weaknesses, and should be considered complimentary to a certain extent, though some modalities, such as magnetic resonance imaging (MRI), do offer a superior combination of sensitivity and specificity for diagnosis and monitoring of joint inflammation and synovitis. In a clinical context, diagnostic imaging continues to gain importance, not only in establishing an initial diagnosis, but also in terms of determining treatment strategy and efficacy.

10.3.1 *Standard clinical imaging*

10.3.1.1 *Radiographs*

Conventional radiographs provide a general assessment of the osseous structures, with less sensitive evaluation of the soft tissues. While the synovium is not directly imaged utilizing radiography, this is often the first modality employed in the clinical assessment of suspected inflammatory conditions involving the joints. Imaging findings are therefore typically limited to the late effects of synovial expansion upon the osseous structures, such as erosions and areas of soft tissue mineralization (Fig. 10.1), though areas of soft tissue swelling and other soft tissue changes, such as tophaceous deposits in the setting of gout (Fig. 10.2), may also be evident. Ultimately, radiographs are relatively insensitive for detection

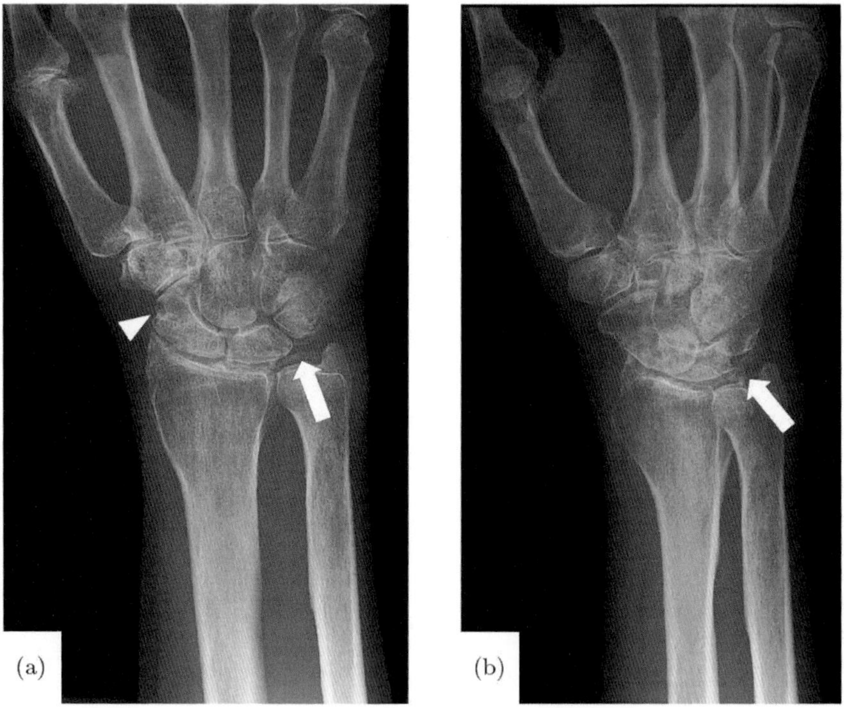

Fig. 10.1. Radiographs in a 70-year-old man with a history of hemochromatosis and CPPD arthropathy demonstrate indolent osseous erosions (white arrowhead) as well as mineralization of the articular disc of the triangular fibrocartilage complex (white arrow) related to CPPD deposition.

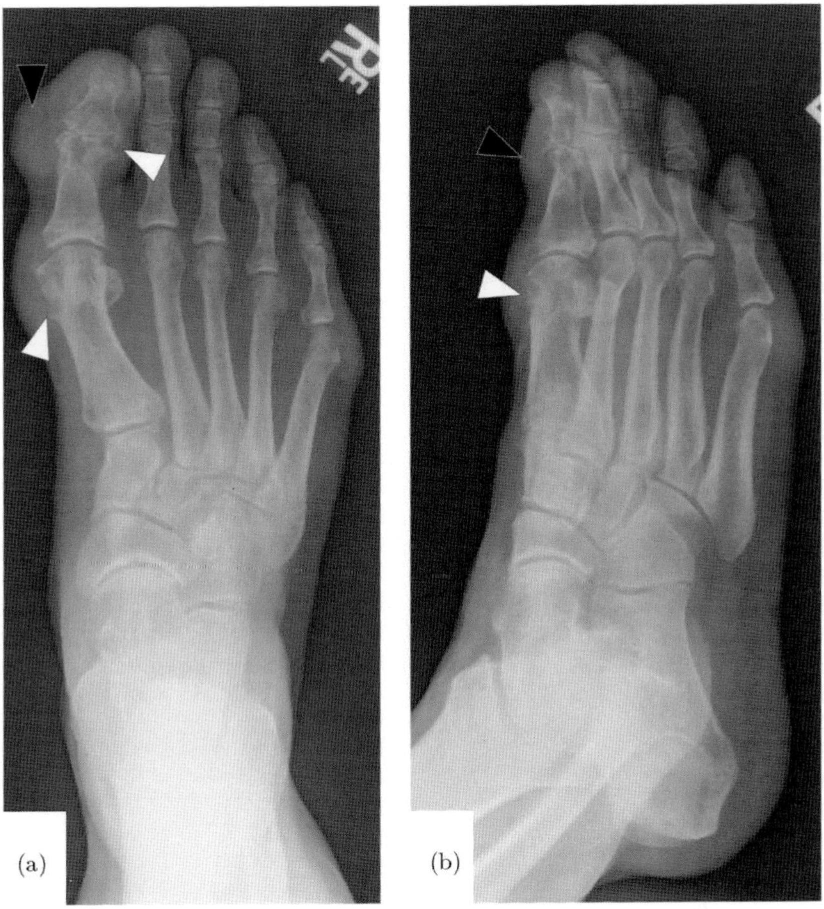

Fig. 10.2. Radiographs in a 68-year-old man with a history of longstanding gout demonstrate osseous erosions (white arrowheads) and soft tissue swelling related to tophaceous deposits (black arrowheads).

of early disease, typically depicting only later manifestations of joint inflammation.[19] However, radiographs, due to their ease of acquisition and ability to cover multiple joints, remain an effective modality for monitoring progression and/or treatment of known disease.[19]

10.3.1.2 *Arthrography*

Like radiographs, conventional arthrography does not allow direct visualization of the synovium; however, instillation of intra-articular contrast

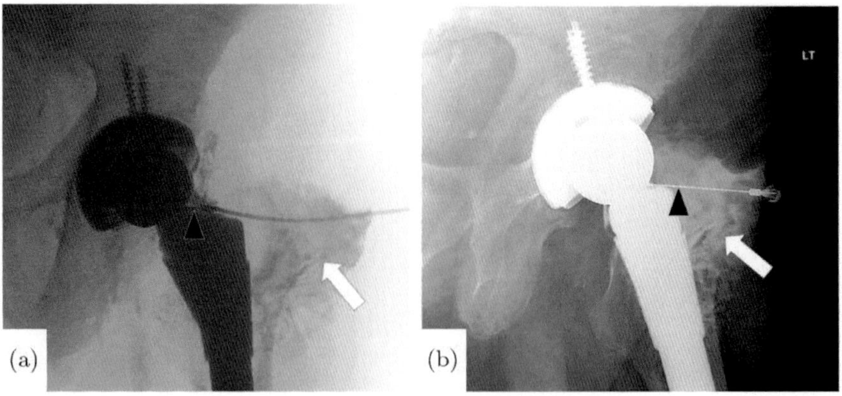

Fig. 10.3. Conventional arthrography demonstrates injection of contrast into joint space in a 60-year-old man status post-total hip arthroplasty (black arrowhead designates needle), with decompression of synovitis into the greater trochanteric bursa via a dehiscent capsule, where there is severe inflammatory synovitis as demonstrated by marked synovial irregularity and thickening; subsequent synovial fluid analysis demonstrated infection with Staph aureus.

outlines the synovial space, giving a rough demonstration of synovial processes such as thickening and proliferation (Fig. 10.3). Given the availability of much more sensitive modalities, however, conventional arthrography is typically performed only in the setting of imaging-guided interventional procedures, such as steroid injections.

10.3.1.3 *Computed tomography*

Computed tomography (CT) provides excellent cross-sectional depiction of osseous structures, and improved depiction of soft tissues relative to radiography, though direct evaluation of the synovium is limited. Given its superior depiction of fine osseous detail, CT is an optimal modality for assessing the extent and progression of osseous erosions, particularly in patients in whom MRI is contraindicated (Fig. 10.4). The downside of the use of CT is the relatively high dose of ionizing radiation relative to other modalities, though this is less of a consideration when imaging the extremities, as is often the case when evaluating patients with joint inflammation. Additionally, in patients with contraindications to MRI, CT arthrography may be utilized to obtain a gross overview of synovial inflammation and/or proliferation.[19,24]

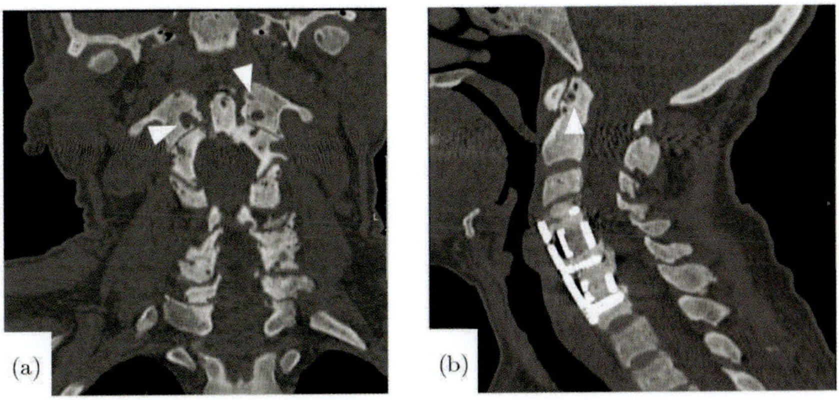

Fig. 10.4. Computed tomography in a 58-year-old woman with amyloid demonstrates numerous widespread well-defined osseous erosions (white arrowheads).

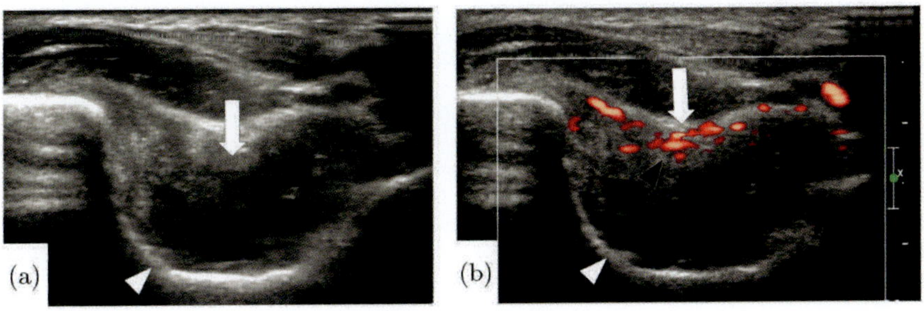

Fig. 10.5. Static sonographic images in a 22-year-old woman demonstrate severe inflammatory synovial thickening (white arrows) and synovial hyperemia (black arrowhead) on power Doppler images of the olecranon fossa (white arrowhead indicates the olecranon cortex) in a patient with known rheumatoid arthritis.

10.3.1.4 *Ultrasound*

Ultrasound (US) is an excellent modality for evaluation of patients with suspected joint inflammation, providing direct visualization of the synovium, as well as allowing for assessment of synovial hyperemia through utilization of Doppler scanning (Fig. 10.5).[19,24] Although evaluation of fine osseous detail and marrow edema is limited, erosions may also often be visualized, and the presence of synovitis on US has been shown to correlate with the presence of osteitis on MRI.[16] Shortcomings of this modality include relatively limited anatomic coverage, a greater degree of operator dependence

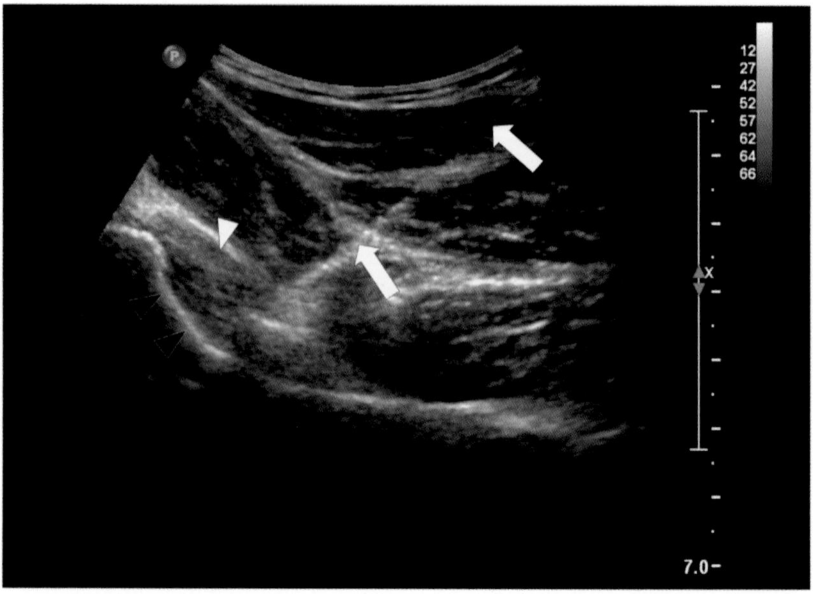

Fig. 10.6. Longitudinally oriented sonographic image of the hip obtained during therapeutic steroid injection in a 22-year-old woman with a history of rheumatoid arthritis demonstrates needle placement (white arrows) with tip along the femoral head-neck junction (black arrowheads) in the setting of inflammatory synovial expansion (white arrowhead).

relative to other modalities, and limited osseous evaluation. That being said, US is useful in the initial diagnosis and subsequent monitoring of inflammatory arthropathy, and has the added benefit of allowing concomitant imaging-guided therapeutic procedures such as steroid injection (Fig. 10.6). Both US and MRI have been shown to be superior to clinical examination in detection of joint inflammation, facilitating accurate disease monitoring.[18]

10.3.1.5 *Magnetic resonance imaging*

MRI offers superior evaluation of the synovium, as well as excellent detection of marrow edema and osseous erosions, making it an optimal modality for evaluation of patients with suspected joint inflammation.[34] At the author's institution, routine joint imaging incorporates three planes of high resolution proton density images plus an additional inversion recovery sequence in a single plane (example protocol in Table 10.1).

Table 10.1. MR imaging parameters for routine total hip arthroplasty at 1.5 T.

Parameter	Coronal MAVRIC IR	Axial FSE	Sagittal FSE	Coronal FSE	Axial FSE	Coronal MAVRIC
Imaged	*Whole pelvis*	*Whole pelvis*	*Affected hip*	*Affected hip*	*Affected hip*	*Whole pelvis*
TR (ms)	4000–5000	4500–5500	5500–6500	4500–5800	4500–5500	4000–5000
TE (ms)	40	21.4–32	23–30	24–30	24–30	40
T1 (ms)	150	na	na	na	na	na
BW (kHz)	±125	83–100	83–100	83–100	83–100	±125
NEX	0.5	4	4–5	4–5	4–5	0.5
FOV (cm)	40	32–36	17–18	18	17–19	40
Matrix	256 × 192	512 × 256	512 × 352	512 × 352	512 × 256–288	320–512 × 256–384
Slice/gap (mm)	5/0	5/0	2.5–3/0	4/0	4/0	3–4.5/0

IR = inversion recovery; FSE = fast spin echo; TR = repetition time; TE = echo time; TI = time to inversion; BW = receiver bandwidth; NEX = number of excitations; FOV = field of view.

Though contraindications may preclude some patients, such as those with pacemakers or claustrophobia, from obtaining MRI, the lack of radiation and sensitive evaluation of both osseous and soft tissues make MRI an excellent modality for diagnosis of early inflammatory disease. Additionally, an array of specialized pulse sequences exist, allowing the MR examination to be tailored to the specific clinical indication — for example, in a patient with suspected PVNS, the routine imaging protocol might be augmented by addition of a gradient echo sequence for detection of hemosiderin (Fig. 10.7), in order to differentiate this process from synovial chondromatosis, which may have a similar imaging appearance (Fig. 10.8). MRI readily demonstrates areas of osseous erosion and deposits

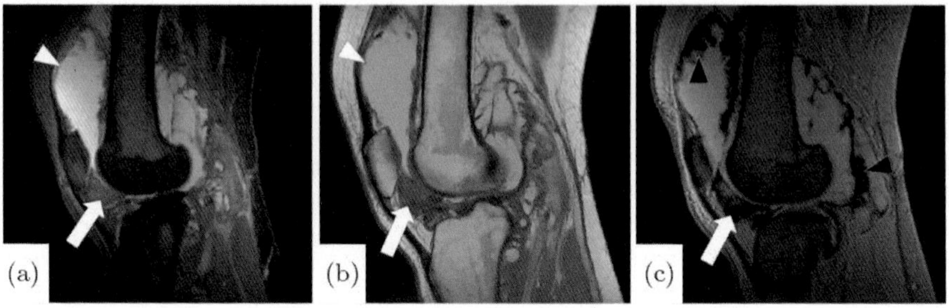

Fig. 10.7. Sagittal inversion recovery (a) and fast spin echo proton density (b) MR images in a 24-year-old woman with recurrent PVNS demonstrate marked synovial expansion (white arrowheads) and synovial proliferation (white arrows) with extensive blooming related to hemosiderin deposition (black arrowheads) on gradient echo (c) images.

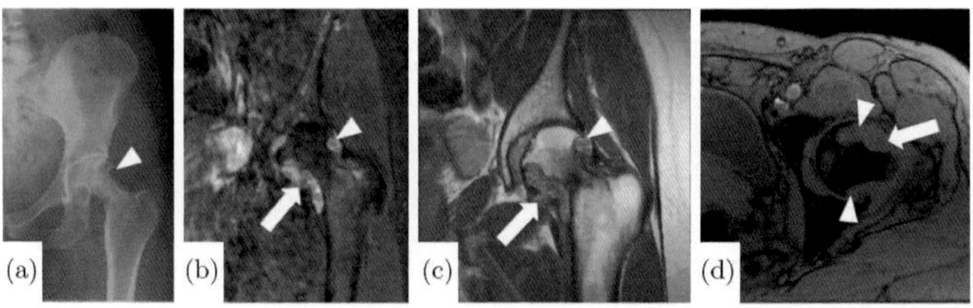

Fig. 10.8. Frontal radiograph of the left hip (a) in a 54-year-old woman with known synovial chondromatosis demonstrates extensive indolent osseous erosions (white arrowheads) related to chronic synovial expansion. Inversion recovery (b) and FSE PD (c) images demonstrate synovitis containing numerous uniformly sized intermediate signal intensity foci (white arrows), without evidence of blooming on gradient echo images (d) consistent with synovial chondromatosis.

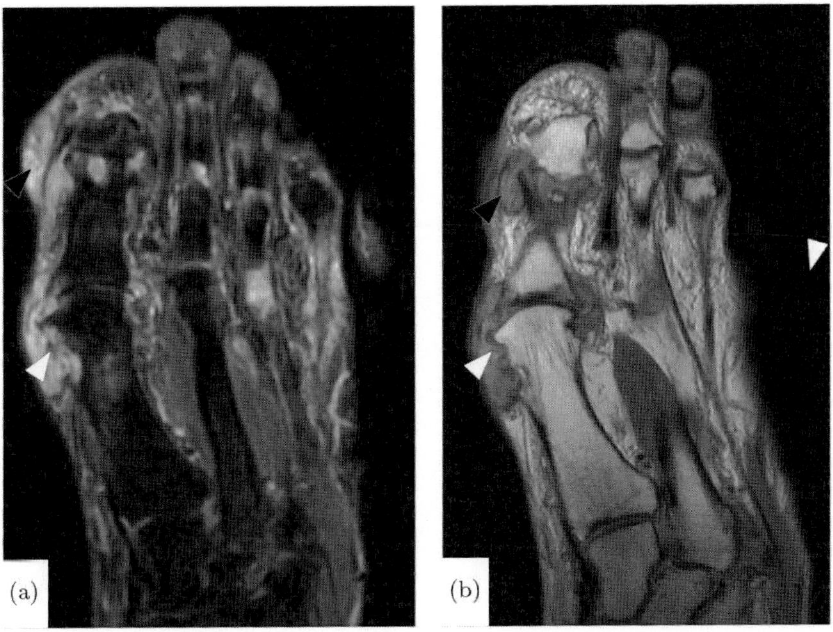

Fig. 10.9. MRI of the right foot in a 68-year-old man with gout demonstrates osseous erosions (white arrowheads) and soft tissue swelling (black arrowheads) related to tophaceous urate deposits.

in the setting of depositional diseases such as gout (Fig. 10.9) and amyloid (Fig. 10.10).[27] Additionally, MRI can provide excellent post-surgical evaluation with proper modification of pulse acquisition parameters, such as in these hip arthroplasty patients with adverse local tissue reaction to metal debris (Fig. 10.11) and periprosthetic infection (Fig. 10.12).

While synovitis is easily diagnosed on non-contrast MRI (Fig. 10.13), the administration of intravenous gadolinium-based contrast material may aid in increasing the conspicuity of inflamed synovium, and allows differentiation of joint fluid from hyperintense, thickened synovium. Additionally, the technique of dynamic contrast enhanced MRI allows a more quantitative assessment of synovitis, as discussed in the next section.

Rheumatoid arthritis magnetic resonance imaging score (RAMRIS) is a standardized assessment of soft tissue and bone involvement in patients with rheumatoid arthritis. The method involves scoring the severity of synovitis, edema, and erosions, typically at the wrist articulations and MP joints within the clinically dominant hand.[33] This technique provides

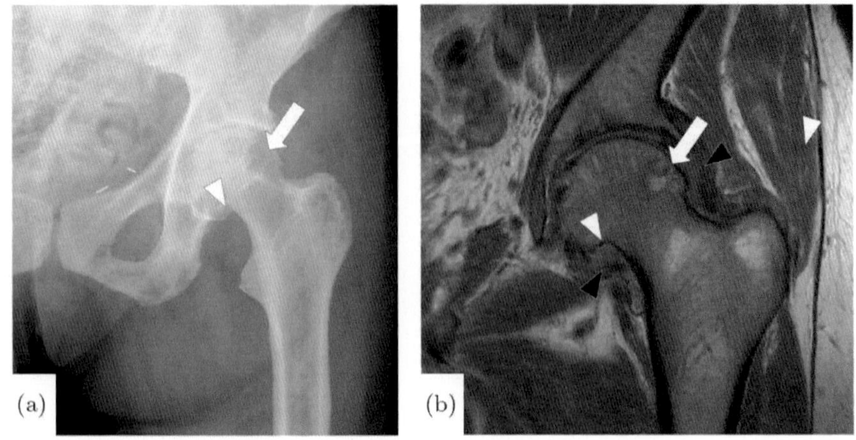

Fig. 10.10. Frontal radiograph (a) in a 58-year-old woman with amyloid demonstrates indolent osseous resorption (white arrowhead) and cystic change (white arrow), with corresponding findings on coronal FSE PD weighted MR image (b), as well as isointense synovial expansion (black arrowheads).

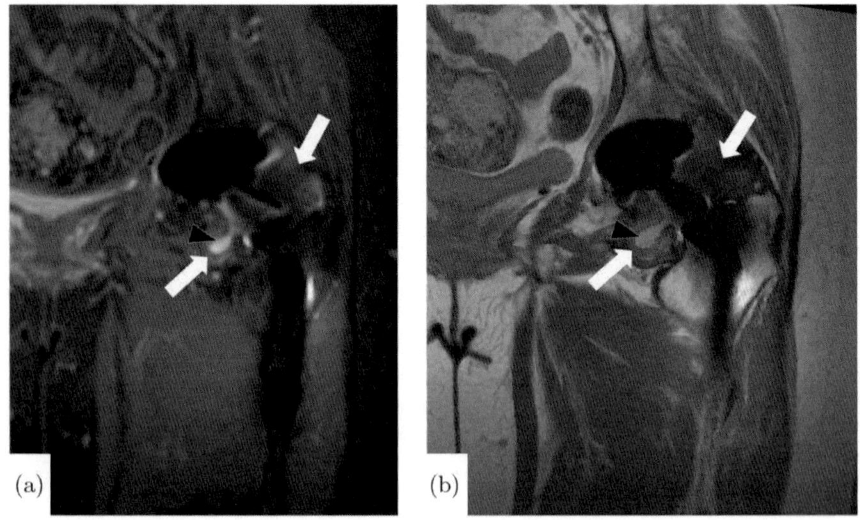

Fig. 10.11. Coronal MAVRIC inversion recovery (a) and FSE PD (b) images in a patient status post-total hip arthroplasty with dual taper modular stem demonstrate synovial expansion with both fluid (black arrowheads) and solid (white arrows) in a patient with adverse local tissue reaction to metal debris/corrosion products.

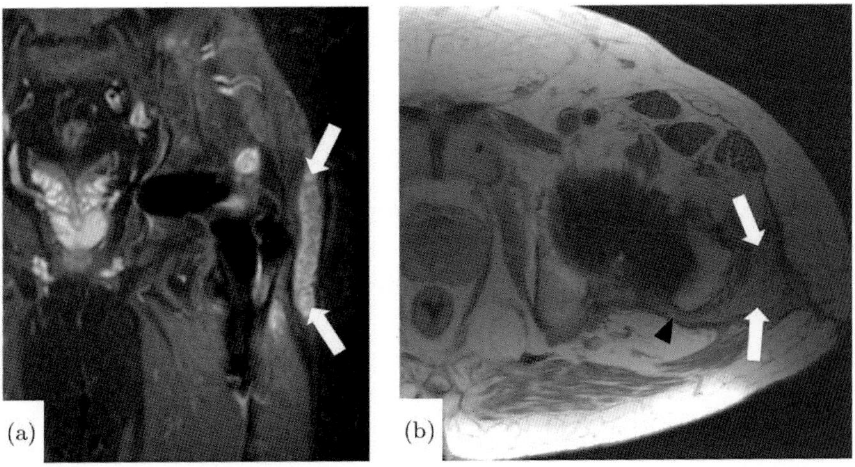

Fig. 10.12. Coronal inversion recovery (a) and FSE PD (b) images in a 60-year-old man with infected total hip arthroplasty demonstrate severe inflammatory synovitis decompressing into the greater trochanteric bursa (white arrows) via a lateral dehiscence in the posterior pseudocapsule (black arrowhead).

a standardized semi-quantitative method of scoring disease involvement, thereby facilitating assessment of disease progression and response to treatment.

10.3.2 *More advanced imaging techniques*

A variety of more advanced imaging techniques have been applied to the evaluation of joint inflammation and synovitis, though these are typically not currently in widespread clinical use.

10.3.2.1 *Whole body MRI*

Whole body MRI has been proposed as a method for overall assessment of disease activity throughout the body in patients with rheumatoid arthritis. Axelsen *et al.* utilized a protocol involving acquisition of STIR and pre- and post-contrast T1-weighted images of the whole body, with assessment of peripheral joints, entheses, and the spine.[1] The technique was found to provide higher sensitivity than clinical exam, with high inter-reader reliability and >70% readability for the majority of joints, though assessment of the most peripheral joints further from isocenter was limited.[1]

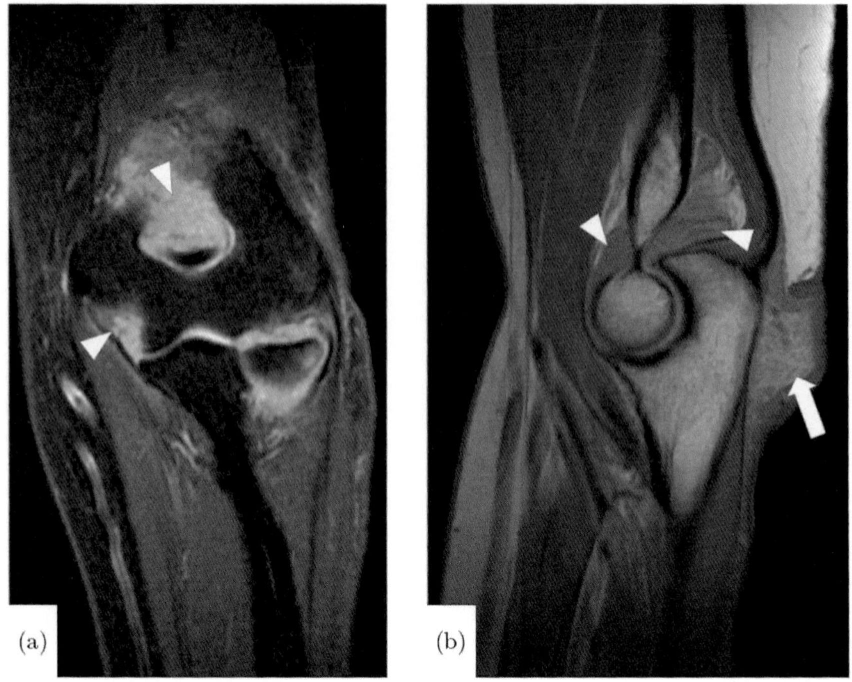

Fig. 10.13. Coronal inversion recovery (a) and FSE PD (b) images of the elbow in a 65-year-old woman with rheumatoid arthritis demonstrate marked inflammatory synovitis (white arrowheads) and severe olecranon bursitis (white arrow).

10.3.2.2 *Dynamic contrast-enhanced MRI, MRA*

Dynamic contrast-enhanced MRI, like MR angiography, involves the intravenous injection of gadolinium-based contrast, but provides an additional time-resolved element, allowing for assessment of time-dependent tissue contrast uptake, allowing for quantification of regional variability and changes in synovitis and marrow edema.[15,20,29] DCE MRI has been shown to provide sensitive detection of early manifestations of inflammation, such as synovitis and marrow edema, and to allow quantitative assessment of tissue enhancement associated with these phenomena. Additionally, DCE MRI findings have been demonstrated to correlate with the currently accepted method of quantifying synovitis on MRI, the rheumatoid arthritis MRI scoring system, RAMRIS.[29] Conventional MR angiography, while not quantitative, may also be useful in the evaluation of synovitis, for example, for assessment of hyperemia and associated vasculitides (Fig. 10.14), as well

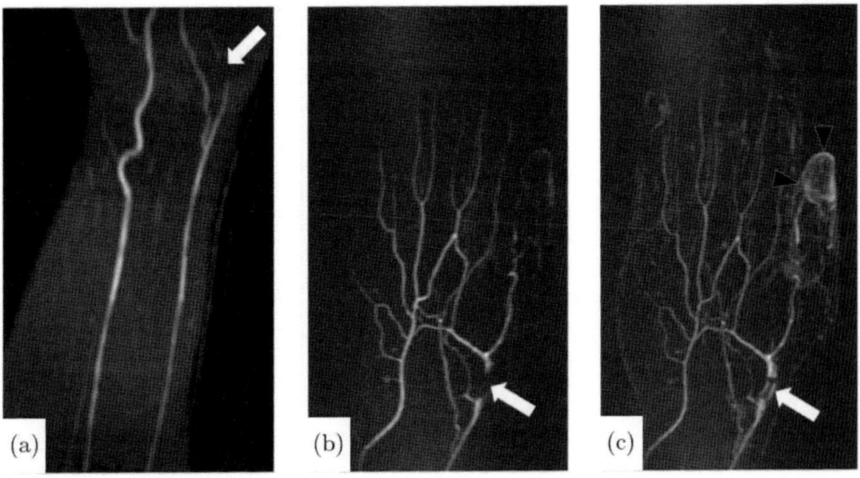

Fig. 10.14. Initial time of flight (a) MR angiographic images demonstrate probable filling defect (white arrow) within the radial artery. Subsequent early arterial time resolved imaging of contrast kinetics (TRICKS) MR angiographic image (b) demonstrates definite focal radial filling defect (white arrow); subsequent late arterial/early venous phase (c) image demonstrates focal thrombus in the area of previously identified filling defect (c), as well as focal vascular blush involving the distal thumb (black arrowheads) related to focal hyperemia.

as for evaluation of vascular injury in patients with recurrent hemarthrosis (Fig. 10.15).

10.3.2.3 *Contrast-enhanced ultrasound*

The use of contrast with ultrasound (CEUS) has been shown to improve the sensitivity of the modality for areas of subtle inflammation. Due to the sensitivity of this technique and the lack of ionizing radiation, CEUS is an excellent modality for both the diagnosis and post-treatment evaluation of patients with inflammatory arthrosis.[4]

10.3.2.4 *PET/PET CT*

Conventional positron emission tomography (PET) is based on the increased uptake of ^{18}F radiolabeled fluoro deoxyglucose (FDG) in areas of increased metabolic activity, such as about inflamed joints in patients with inflammatory arthropathy. While PET, as a whole body modality, may provide an overall assessment of disease activity and extent, ^{18}F FDG uptake is non-specific, and may be increased in a variety of conditions besides

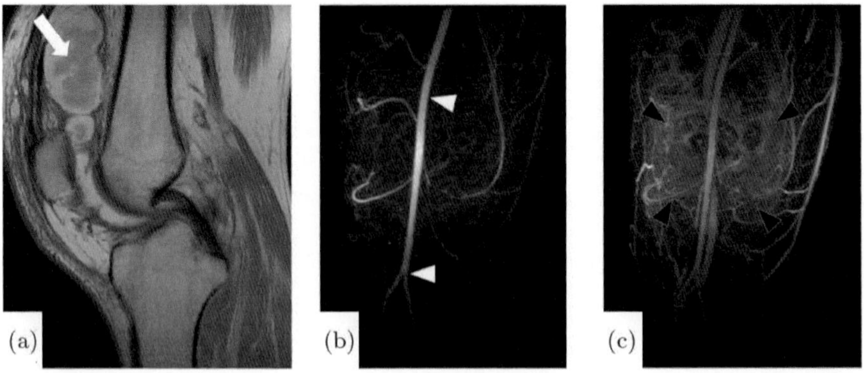

Fig. 10.15. Sagittal FSE PD image (a) in a patient with pain and swelling status post-arthroscopy demonstrates pronounced synovitis with mixed fluid signal and isointense foci, consistent with acute hemorrhage (white arrow). TRICKS angiographic MR image in the arterial phase (b) demonstrates normal flow-related enhancement of the popliteal artery and normal branching to anterior tibial artery and tibioperoneal trunk (white arrowheads). Delayed venous phase images (c) demonstrate pronounced synovial blush (black arrowheads) related to synovial inflammation in the setting of post-surgical hemarthrosis.

inflammatory arthrosis. ^{18}FDG PET is therefore not specific in terms of initially diagnosing inflammatory arthropathy; however, PET gives a good overall evaluation of distribution of inflammation, and may be useful in monitoring for changes in disease activity.[25]

10.3.3 *Experimental/preclinical imaging techniques*

10.3.3.1 *Near-infrared fluorescence optical imaging*

Fluorescence optical imaging is a technique that has been established as a marker of inflammation in animal models, which is emerging as a potential method of imaging patients with inflammatory arthritides in a clinical setting. This technique involves injection of a target fluorescence molecule (in this case, indocyanine green, which targets inflamed synovium), which is then excited by an external light source of appropriate wavelength.[31,37,38] The technique is limited due to limited tissue penetration; however, given that inflammatory arthroses commonly involve the distal extremities and digits, this is of less concern in these patients. Cross sectional scintigraphy may also be useful in evaluation of deeper joints and more precise localization of inflammation.[21] Werner *et al.* utilized indocyanine green Fluorescence optical imaging (FOI) in a cohort of 252 patients, correlating the findings with clinical examination, US, and MRI (RAMRIS score), finding statistically significant correlations with each.[38] Other molecular probes may be utilized for detection of inflammation, typically directed toward target proteins associated with cells such as macrophages. Labeled leukocytes have also been utilized with this technique.[22]

10.3.3.2 *Infrared thermography*

Because inflamed joints are typically warmer than normal joints, locally elevated skin surface temperature may be detected as an indicator of subjacent inflammation. This is the basis of infrared thermography, an optical imaging modality that detects regional variations in skin surface temperature. As with FOI, this technique is limited by the soft tissue envelope surrounding a given joint, and is therefore more useful in small joints. Benefits of this technique include relatively low cost, rapid acquisition, and lack of ionizing radiation.[22]

10.3.3.3 *Scintigraphy*

As previously mentioned, conventional ^{18}F FDG PET may be used to evaluate inflamed joints, but the ^{18}F FDG radiotracer is relatively non-specific. The utilization of other radiotracer probes specifically targeted to molecules associated with cellular processes involved in inflammation increases the specificity of PET for the detection of inflammation. These include tracers specific for angiogenesis, macrophage infiltration, B cell infiltration, extracellular matrix damage, and cell proliferation.[6,22,28] The performance of concurrent PETCT or PETMRI facilitates localization of areas of increased tracer uptake, as well as allowing correlation with any structural abnormalities visible on cross-sectional imaging.

10.4 Conclusion

Imaging features observed in patients with synovitis are related to underlying changes in the architecture and function of both synovial and non-synovial tissues within the joints. A wide variety of clinical entities may result in synovitis, and a wide variety of imaging modalities are available for evaluation of these conditions. Each of these modalities possesses various strengths and weaknesses, and in general, the modalities are largely complimentary to one another. While certain modalities, such as radiographs, ultrasound, and MRI, are currently in widespread clinical use for evaluation of patients with synovitis, a number of new and advanced techniques are currently being investigated with regard to their utility in evaluation of these conditions, many of which will likely become part of routine clinical imaging algorithms for patients with synovitis in the future.

References

1. Axelsen MB, Eshed I, Duer-Jensen A, Moller JM, Pedersen SJ, Ostergaard M (2014). Whole-body MRI assessment of disease activity and structural damage in rheumatoid arthritis: First step towards an MRI joint count. *Rheumatology*, 53(5), 845–853.
2. Becker M (2014). Clinical manifestations and diagnosis of gout. *Up To Date.* 08/20/2014.
3. Becker MA, Ryan LM, (2014). Clinical manifestations and diagnosis of calcium pyrophosphate crystal deposition (CPPD) disease. *Up To Date*, 08/20/2014.
4. Bonifati C, Elia F, Graceffa D, Ceralli F, Maiani E, De Mutiis C, *et al.* (2014). Clinical and contrast-enhanced ultrasound echography outcomes in psoriatic arthritis patients after one year of continuous therapy with anti-TNF drugs. *ISRN Dermatol*, 932721.
5. Dalbeth N, Haskard DO (2005). Mechanisms of inflammation in gout. *Rheumatology*, 44(9), 1090–1096.
6. Gent YY, Voskuyl AE, Kloet RW, van Schaardenburg D, Hoekstra OS, Dijkmans BA, *et al.* (2012). Macrophage positron emission tomography imaging as a biomarker for preclinical rheumatoid arthritis: Findings of a prospective pilot study. *Arthritis Rheum*, 64(1), 62–66.
7. Girish G, Glazebrook KN, Jacobson JA (2013). Advanced imaging in gout. *Am J Roentgenol*, 201(3), 515–525.
8. Gladman D, Ritchlin C (2014). Clinical Manifestations and Diagnosis of Psoriatic Arthritis. Available from: http://www.uptodate.com/contents/clinical-manifestations-and-diagnosis-of-psoriatic-arthritis.
9. Goldenberg DL, Sexton DJ (2014). Septic arthritis in adults. *Up To Date*, 08/20/214.
10. Hayter CL, Koff MF, Potter HG (2012). Magnetic resonance imaging of the postoperative hip. *J Magn Reson Imaging*, 35(5), 1013–1025.
11. Hayter CL, Koff MF, Shah P, Koch KM, Miller TT, Potter HG (2011). MRI after arthroplasty: Comparison of MAVRIC and conventional fast spin-echo techniques. *Am J Roentgenol*, 197(3), W405–W411.
12. Haywood L, Walsh DA (2001). Vasculature of the normal and arthritic synovial joint. *Histol Histopathol*, R16(1), 277–284.
13. Hoots WK, Shapiro AD (2014). Clinical manifestations and diagnosis of hemophilia. *Up To Date*, 08/20/14.
14. Huynh D, Kavanaugh A. Psoriatic arthritis: Current therapy and future approaches. *Rheumatology*, 54(1), 20–28.

15. Jans L, De Coninck T, Wittoek R, Lambrecht V, Huysse W, Verbruggen G, *et al.* (2013). 3 T DCE-MRI assessment of synovitis of the interphalangeal joints in patients with erosive osteoarthritis for treatment response monitoring. *Skeletal Radiol*, 42(2), 255–260.
16. Kawashiri SY, Suzuki T, Nakashima Y, Horai Y, Okada A, Nishino A, *et al.* (2014). Synovial inflammation assessed by ultrasonography correlates with MRI-proven osteitis in patients with rheumatoid arthritis. *Rheumatology*, 53(8), 1452–1456.
17. Khan MA, van der Linden SM (1990). A wider spectrum of spondyloarthropathies. *Seminars in arthritis and rheumatism*, 20(2), 107–113.
18. Mandl P, Kurucz R, Niedermayer D, Balint PV, Smolen JS (2014). Contributions of ultrasound beyond clinical data in assessing inflammatory disease activity in rheumatoid arthritis: Current insights and future prospects. *Rheumatology*. 53(12), 2136–2142.
19. McQueen FM (2013). Imaging in early rheumatoid arthritis: Best practice and research. *Clin Rheumatol*, 27(4), 499–522.
20. Meier R, Thuermel K, Noel PB, Moog P, Sievert M, Ahari C, *et al.* (2014). Synovitis in patients with early inflammatory arthritis monitored with quantitative analysis of dynamic contrast-enhanced optical imaging and MR imaging. *Radiology*, 270(1), 176–185.
21. Mohajerani P, Koch M, Thurmel K, Haller B, Rummeny EJ, Ntziachristos V, *et al.* (2014). Fluorescence-aided tomographic imaging of synovitis in the human finger. *Radiology*, 272(3), 865–874.
22. Mountz JM, Alavi A, Mountz JD (2012). Emerging optical and nuclear medicine imaging methods in rheumatoid arthritis. *Nat Rev Rheumatol*, 8(12), 719–728.
23. Nigrovic PA (2014). Hemathrosis. *Up To Date*, 08/20/2014.
24. Ohrndorf S, Werner SG, Finzel S, Backhaus M (2013). Musculoskeletal ultrasound and other imaging modalities in rheumatoid arthritis. *Curr Opin Rheumatol*, 25(3), 367–374.
25. Okabe T, Shibata H, Shizukuishi K, Yoneyama T, Inoue T, Tateishi U (2011). F-18 FDG uptake patterns and disease activity of collagen vascular diseases-associated arthritis. *Clin Nucl Med*, 36(5), 350–354.
26. Ottaviani S, Ayral X, Dougados M, Gossec L (2011). Pigmented villonodular synovitis: A retrospective single-center study of 122 cases and review of the literature. *Semin Arthritis Rheum*, 40(6), 539–546.
27. Popovich I, Dalbeth N, Doyle A, Reeves Q, McQueen FM (2014). Exploring cartilage damage in gout using 3-T MRI: Distribution and associations with joint inflammation and tophus deposition. *Skeletal Radiol*. 43(7), 917–924.
28. Pottier G, Bernards N, Dollé F, Boisgard R (2014). [(18)F]DPA-714 as a biomarker for positron emission tomography imaging of rheumatoid arthritis in an animal model. *Arthritis Res Ther*, 16(2), R69.
29. Rastogi A, Kubassova O, Krasnosselskaia LV, Lim AK, Satchithananda K, Boesen M, *et al.* (2013). Evaluating automated dynamic contrast enhanced wrist 3T MRI in healthy volunteers: One-year longitudinal observational study. *Eur J Radiol*, 82(8), 1286–1291.

30. Richette P, Bardin T, Doherty M (2009). An update on the epidemiology of calcium pyrophosphate dihydrate crystal deposition disease. *Rheumatology*, 48(7), 711–715.
31. Schafer VS, Hartung W, Hoffstetter P, Berger J, Stroszczynski C, Muller M, *et al.* (2013). Quantitative assessment of synovitis in patients with rheumatoid arthritis using fluorescence optical imaging. *Arthritis Res Ther*, 15(5), R124.
32. Schur PH. (2014) Arthritis associated with gastrointestinal disease. *Up To Date*, 08/20/14.
33. Sewerin P, Buchbender C, Vordenbaumen S, Scherer A, Miese F, Brinks R, *et al.* (2014). Advantages of a combined rheumatoid arthritis magnetic resonance imaging score (RAMRIS) for hand and feet: Does the RAMRIS of the hand alone underestimate disease activity and progression? *BMC Musculoskeletal Disorders*, 15, 104.
34. van Steenbergen HW, van Nies JA, Huizinga TW, Bloem JL, Reijnierse M, van der Helm-van Mil AH (2013). Characterising arthralgia in the preclinical phase of rheumatoid arthritis using MRI. *Ann Rheum Dis.*
35. Venebales P, Maini R (2014). Diagnosis and differential diagnosis of rheumatoid arthritis. Available from: http://www.uptodate.com/contents/topic.do?topicKey=RHEUM/7504.
36. Verspoor FG, Zee AA, Hannink G, van der Geest IC, Veth RP, Schreuder HW (2014). Long-term follow-up results of primary and recurrent pigmented villonodular synovitis. *Rheumatology*, 53(11), 2063–2070.
37. Werner SG, Langer HE, Ohrndorf S, Bahner M, Schott P, Schwenke C, *et al.* (2012). Inflammation assessment in patients with arthritis using a novel in vivo fluorescence optical imaging technology. *Ann Rheum Dis*, 71(4), 504–510.
38. Werner SG, Langer HE, Schott P, Bahner M, Schwenke C, Lind-Albrecht G, *et al.* (2013). Indocyanine green-enhanced fluorescence optical imaging in patients with early and very early arthritis: A comparative study with magnetic resonance imaging. *Arthritis Rheum*, 65(12), 3036–3044.
39. Yu D (2014). Reactive arthritis. Available from: http://www.uptodate.com/contents/reactive-arthritis? source= search_result&search= Reactive+Arthritis&selectedTitle= 1~105.

CHAPTER 11

CIRCULATORY PATHOLOGY IN OSTEOARTHRITIS

ROY K. AARON
Professor of Orthopaedic Surgery
The Warren Alpert Medical School of Brown University, Providence, RI

11.1 Introduction

Interest in the circulatory contributions to osteoarthritis (OA) has been stimulated by the demonstration that experimental venous occlusion of bone is accompanied by hallmarks of OA bone — intraosseous hypertension, focal avascular necrosis, trabecular remodeling, and thickening of the subchondral bone plate. Subsequent observations demonstrated that decreased perfusion, venous outflow obstruction, andvenous stasis, are associated with late-stage OA of the hip and that these circulatory changes can result in hypoxia in subchondral bone. Sophisticated imaging techniques including dynamic contrast-enhanced magnetic resonance imaging (DCE-MRI) and positron emission tomography (PET) with a variety of isotopes are demonstrating venous outflow obstruction resulting in intraosseous hypertension, reductions in perfusion, hypoxia, and remodeling of trabecular structure and architecture. In response to changes in pressure, perfusion, and oxygen content similar to that seen in OA, OA osteoblasts alter their expression of structural and signaling cytokines relevant to bone remodeling and cartilage breakdown. The changes in bone circulation may contribute to the initiation or progression of OA through associated changes in the physicochemical environment of osteocytes in subchondral bone.

11.2 Venous Stasis

11.2.1 *Experimental interruption of venous outflow*

The circulatory contributions to the pathology of OA have been emphasized by the venous ligation studies of Brookes.[9] After venous ligation, he observed decreased bone blood flow, pO_2, and pH. These changes were associated with trabecular remodeling and calcification of the deep cartilage zones. Other studies by this group demonstrated that venous obstruction is associated with increased intraosseous pressure and appeared causally related to the structural remodeling of bone. These studies were confirmed and extended some years later by Welch who showed in a caprine model that venous occlusion was associated with intraosseous hypertension and bone remodeling.[53] Metaphyseal bone formation was demonstrated with an increase of periosteal (+138%), endosteal (+286%), and trabecular (+889%) bone. Bone remodeling resulted in new bone volume of +376% with increases in the numbers of both osteoblasts and osteoclasts. Together, these and other studies of venous occlusion demonstrate an association of intraosseous hypertension with the histopathological features of OA bone — focal avascular necrosis, trabecular remodeling, thickening of the subchondral bone plate, endosteal and periosteal new bone formation, and sclerosis.

11.2.2 *Static imaging of human OA*

Studies of bone circulation of the human hip have been done by Arnoldi using static imaging with intraosseous venography.[3] The intraosseous injection of 5 ml of contrast filled the venous system of the proximal femur. In normal hips, blood exited within 3–6 minutes in a centrifugal pattern through retinacular veins at the femoral neck (Fig. 11.1).

OA hips were characterized by an absence of venous outflow through extraosseous retinacular veins and a centripetal pattern of venous drainage through diaphyseal intramedullary veins. Dilated intramedullary veins filled with contrast have been observed in OA.[6] Intramedullary venous stasis persisted in the OA hips for greater than 30 minutes after injection of contrast. This marked temporal and functional difference between normal and OA hips suggested the presence of venous stasis in OA (Fig. 11.2).

Venous stasis was suggested further by subtraction venography showing contrast accumulation around the trocar tip in OA hips that persisted

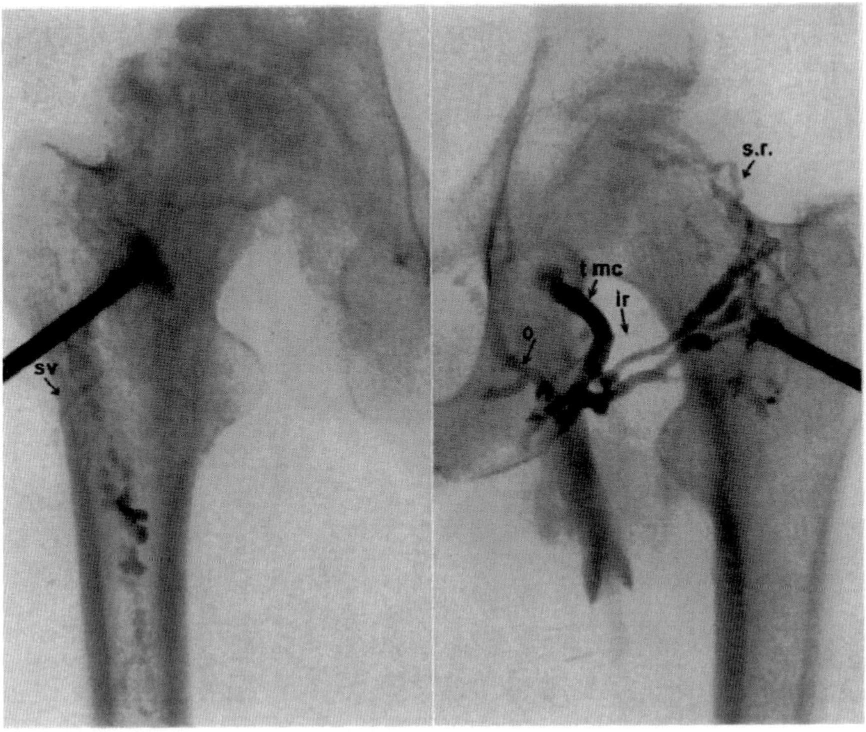

Fig. 11.1. Intraosseous venogram 30 seconds after contrast injection. Venous outflow of normal hips occurs through extraosseous retinacular veins at the femoral neck — s.r. = superior retinacular vein; i.r. = inferior retinacular vein. OA hips exhibit absence of retinacular venous flow and intramedullary venous drainage. (Reprinted from: Arnoldi CC, Linderholm H, Mussbichler H (1972). Venous engorgement and intraosseous hypertension in osteoarthritis of the hip. *J Bone Joint Surg Br*, 54(3), 409–421, with permission from The British Editorial Society of Bone & Joint Surgery.)

for 20 minutes, while in normal hips, clearance of contrast was prompt, occurring within minutes after injection of contrast (Fig. 11.3).

In summary, these studies demonstrate that venous drainage in the normal hip (femur) occurs in a *centrifugal* pattern through extraosseous veins with a short emptying time, under 10 minutes. Venous outflow in OA femora occurs in a *centripetal* pattern through diaphyseal intramedullary veins and is markedly delayed with a considerably longer emptying time, suggesting not only anatomic variance from normal but also outflow obstruction and venous stasis. Other studies have indicated the presence of intraosseous

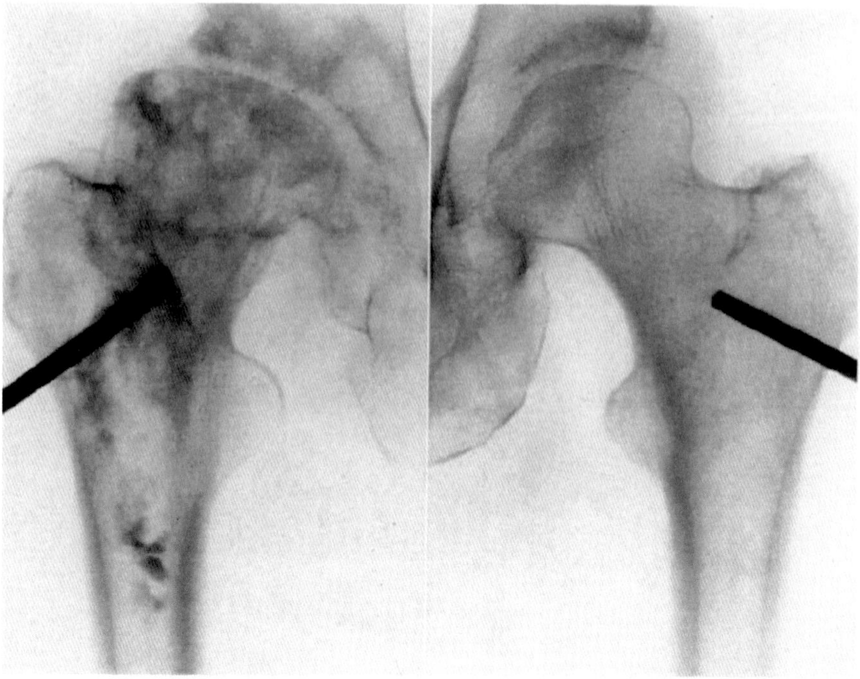

Fig. 11.2. Intraosseous venogram 30 minutes after contrast injection. All contrast has exited from the normal hip. Persistence of contrast in intramedullary veins is observed in the OA hips suggesting venous stasis. (Reprinted from: Arnoldi CC, Linderholm H, Mussbichler H (1972). Venous engorgement and intraosseous hypertension in osteoarthritis of the hip. *J Bone Joint Surg Br*, 54(3), 409–421, with permission from The British Editorial Society of Bone & Joint Surgery.)

hypertension in association with venous outflow obstruction, OA, and bone pain.[4,5,29]

11.2.3 *Dynamic imaging of OA*

While static imaging is useful for delineating anatomic patterns of blood flow, it cannot quantify perfusion characteristics. Dynamic imaging techniques with DCE-MRI and ^{18}F PET can be used to characterize changes in regional perfusion in subchondral bone and correlate that information with bone metabolism of interest to the pathophysiology of OA. Pharmacokinetic modeling techniques permit the characterization of perfusion kinetics and insight into physiology of blood flow in bone. DCE-MRI offers the opportunity to extract kinetic information on bone circulation including bone

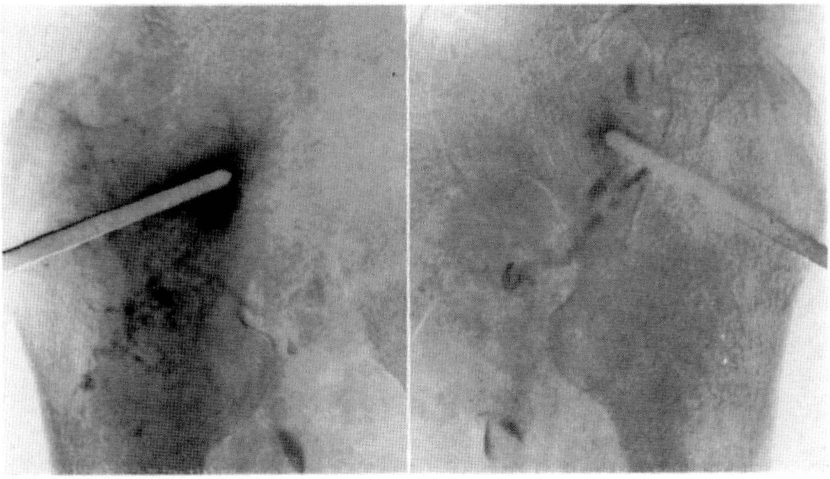

Fig. 11.3. Subtraction intraosseous venogram 1.5 minutes after injection of contrast. Accumulation of contrast is seen around the trochar tip in OA hips but not in normal hips reflecting venous stasis in OA. (Reprinted from: Arnoldi CC, Linderholm H, Mussbichler H (1972). Venous engorgement and intraosseous hypertension in osteoarthritis of the hip. *J Bone Joint Surg Br*, 54(3), 409–421, with permission from The British Editorial Society of Bone & Joint Surgery.)

blood flow, capillary permeability, and venous outflow.[13,31] PET using the bone-seeking isotope ^{18}F fluoride provides estimates of bone blood flow and bone formation.[35,40] These parameters have been compared to the severity of cartilage lesions and bone remodeling, and temporal and spatial relationships have been described. These functional imaging techniques provide insight into pathophysiologic mechanisms that are associated with bone remodeling and cartilage degeneration in OA, and put previous static vascular studies into functional pathophysiological contexts.

11.2.3.1 *DCE-MRI*

The techniques of DCE-MRI in subchondral bone include image acquisition, signal processing, and pharmacokinetic modeling, and have been described previously.[1,28] Briefly, signal enhancement in DCE-MRI is achieved with the use of a paramagnetic contrast medium, such as gadolinium, which causes local magnetic field fluctuations and signal enhancement in specific tissues. Signal enhancement and perfusion are proportional to the gadolinium concentration. Using pharmacokinetic models, the change in signal enhancement over time, described by signal intensity-time curves

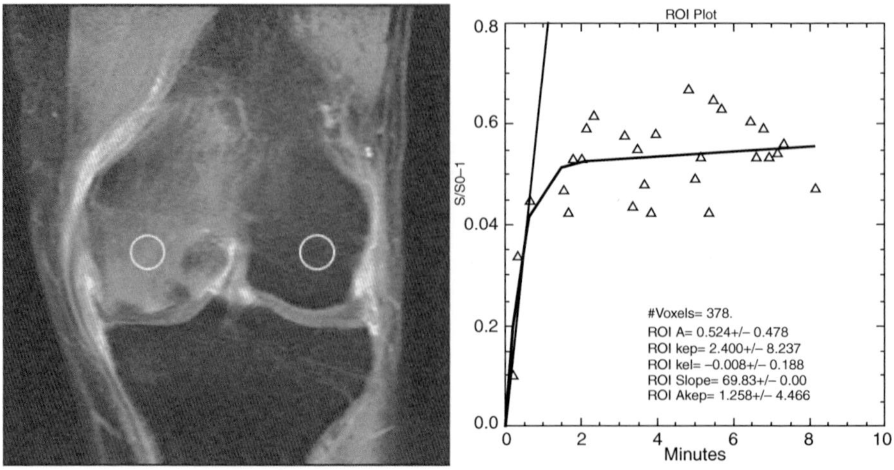

(a) (b)

Fig. 11.4. Signal enhancement of the human femoral condyle. (a) Regions of interest are identified for comparison. (b) Time-intensity curve of the MRI signal demonstrating inflow slope, amplitude, and clearance or washout phases of perfusion. (Reprinted from: Lee JH, Dyke JP, Ballon D, Ciombor DM, Tung G, Aaron RK. (1972). Assessment of bone perfusion with contrast-enhanced magnetic resonance imaging. *Orthop Clin North Am*, 40(2), 249–257, with permission from Elsevier.)

(Fig. 11.4), can be used to extract quantitative information concerning perfusion kinetics including the perfusion parameters, slope, amplitude (A), and elimination rate constant (kel).[8,48] These parameters reflect vascular inflow, extracellular contrast-agent retention, and vascular outflow in the perfused tissue. Regions of interest can be identified and kinetics measured for comparison.

We have used DCE-MRI with gadolinium to describe abnormalities in perfusion in subchondral bone in the Dunkin-Hartley guinea pig model of spontaneous OA. The hypothesis underlying these studies is that changes in circulatory dynamics in subchondral bone bear *functional* relationships to bone remodeling and cartilage degeneration.

One study explored relationships between perfusion in the subchondral bone and cartilage lesions of developing OA to characterize circulation kinetics and the time course of changes in perfusion in the developing arthritis.[28] Changes of OA in subchondral bone and cartilage begin at about 9 months of age and are well established by 12 months of age. This study

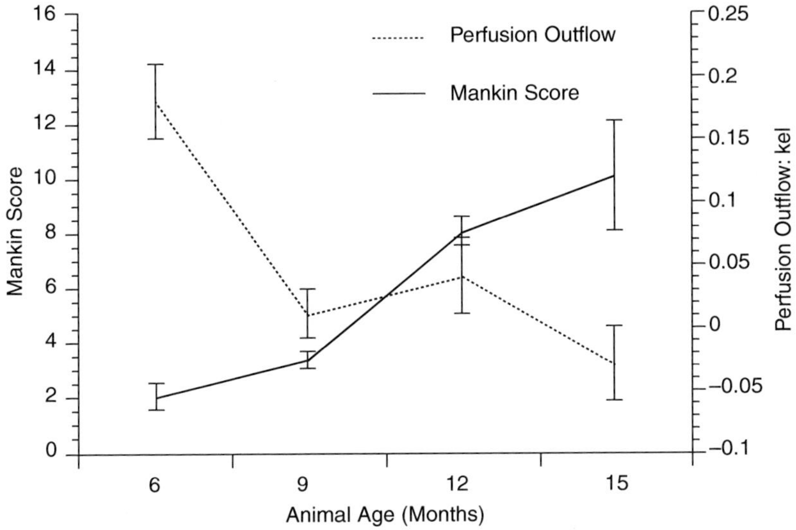

Fig. 11.5. Decreased venous outflow (kel) temporally preceding cartilage degeneration. Cartilage degeneration begins at about nine months of age (Mankin score). The kel is markedly reduced between six and nine months of age, reflecting venous outflow obstruction.

demonstrated a decrease in perfusion temporally preceding OA changes in cartilage (Fig. 11.5).

Decreased perfusion was only observed in the medial compartment at the site of eventual bone and cartilage lesions and, therefore, it was concluded that circulatory abnormalities spatially localized at the site of OA. Time intensity curves studies demonstrated that, at six months of age before the development of arthritis, bone circulation was normal with normal inflow, amplitude, and washout of contrast dye. By 12 months of age, lesions of OA in articular cartilage were visible. Time intensity curves demonstrated delayed venous outflow suggesting that the primary pathophysiological circulatory event was venous stasis (Fig. 11.6). These studies showed that decreased perfusion and venous stasis in developing guinea pig OA temporally preceded and spatially co-localized with the eventual morphological changes of bone and cartilage.

A second study, using DCE-MRI and ^{18}F PET, examined alterations in subchondral bone circulation and their relationships to bone structure and cartilage degeneration in the Dunkin-Hartley guinea pig with OA of varying severity.[14] DCE-MRI used small molecular contrast

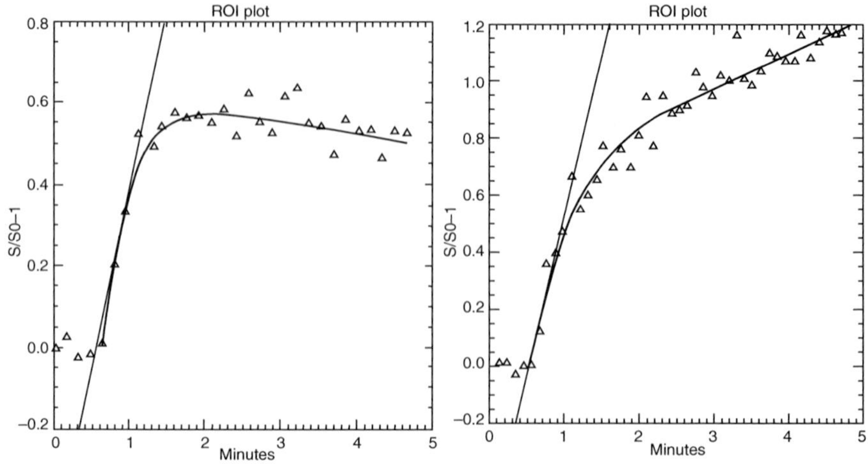

Fig. 11.6. Time-intensity curves in developing OA. At six months of age before OA, the kel = 0.06 indicating normal venous outflow. By 12 months of age, the kel = −0.11 reflecting venous outflow obstruction. (Reprinted from: Aaron RK, Dyke JP, Ciombor DM, Ballon D, Lee J, Jung E, Tung GA. (2007). Perfusion abnormalities in subchondral bone associated with marrow edema, osteoarthritis, and avascular necrosis. *Ann N Y Acad Sci*, 1117, 124–137, with permission from John Wiley and Sons.)

medium (gadolinium, 530 Da) to characterize perfusion. Prolongation of signal enhancement and delayed contrast clearance (kel) during the washout phase was correlated with the severity of OA ($p = 0.015$). Time intensity curves again suggested venous stasis in OA (Fig. 11.7).

To demonstrate that the changes in signal intensity were due to venous stasis, vascular permeability was measured with a macromolecular contrast medium (gadolinium-albumin, 92,000 Da). These studies showed no increase in vascular permeability with increasing severity of OA indicating that the increased signal intensity observed in OA is most likely not due to increased transvascular migration of gadolinium to the intraosseous extravascular space. These studies revealed a positive correlation of venous outflow obstruction with the severity of arthritis.

11.2.3.2 ^{18}F *PET*

^{18}F PET quantifies a perfusion phase within two minutes of radionuclide injection. The ^{18}F is then taken up into the hydroxyapatite crystal to provide a measure of mineralization and osteoblastic activity.

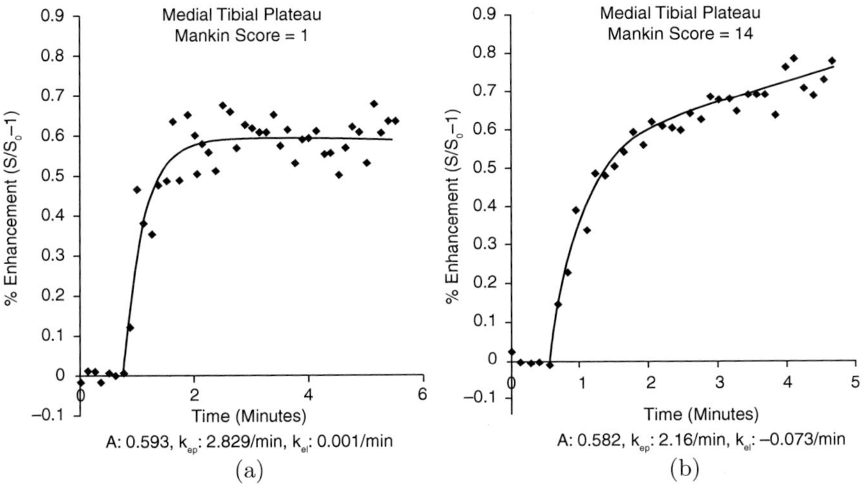

Fig. 11.7. Time-intensity curves in severe OA. Normal curve is seen with minimal OA (Mankin score of 1). Delayed contrast clearance is observed in severe OA (Mankin score of 14) reflecting venous stasis.

^{18}F PET scans have been used in the Dunkin-Hartley guinea pig model to demonstrate bone blood flow and bone formation at the site of OA morphological lesions.[14] The PET data have confirmed that decreased perfusion is related to the severity of OA and have extended that observation to show a relationship between changes in the circulatory environment in subchondral bone (decreased perfusion) and abnormal bone formation (decreased ^{18}F-fluoride influx) associated with the severity of cartilage degeneration (Mankin scores). Specifically, we observed in the medial tibial plateau: (1) a decrease in blood volume ($p = 0.005$) and blood flow ($p = 0.019$) with increasing cartilage degeneration; (2) a decrease in radionuclide incorporation into bone matrix reflecting decreased bone formation with increasing severity of cartilage lesions ($p = 0.05$); and (3) a correlation between blood flow and ^{18}F-fluoride in corporation into bone matrix ($p < 0.001$). These observations confirmed in functional terms associations among perfusion, bone remodeling, and cartilage lesions in OA.

DCE-MRI has the capability of extracting kinetic information on bone circulation including bone blood flow, capillary permeability, and venous outflow. ^{18}F PET, because it has both perfusion and osteogenic phases, can provide estimates of bone blood flow and correlate perfusion with bone

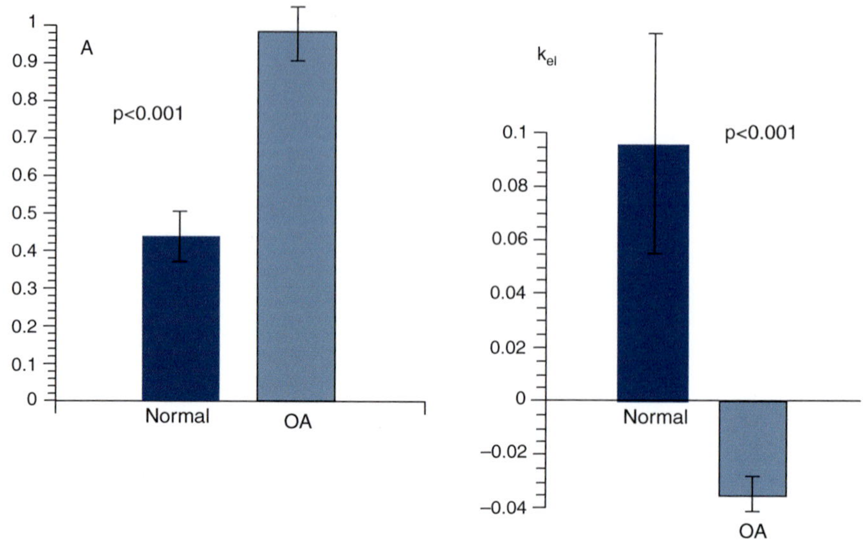

Fig. 11.8. Kinetic parameters of perfusion in normal OA knees. Data is derived from time-intensity curves. Signal amplitude (A) is greater in OA than in normal knees indicating accumulation of contrast media. The elimination constant (kel) is reduced in OA knees indicating venous outflow obstruction and stasis.

formation. To the extent that perfusion is related to OA, these functional imaging techniques provide insight into pathophysiologic mechanisms that are associated with, and may precede, structural changes of bone remodeling and cartilage degeneration in OA.

11.2.3.3 *DCE-MRI in human OA*

DCE-MRI has been used to characterize the circulation in human OA hips and knees, and similar delays in venous outflow have been observed as seen in the guinea pig OA model. Increased signal amplitude and decreased elimination constants have been observed in human OA knees (Fig. 11.8).

11.3 Venous Stasis and Hypoxia

The pathophysiological consequences of venous outflow obstruction may be related to its association with physiologically relevant reductions in perfusion and pO_2. Venous outflow obstruction reduces perfusion by a factor of 2, and also reduces pO_2 by 50%.[23] Associations have been

Table 11.1. Physiologic changes with venous occlusion (from Kaier).

Parameter	Pre	Post	Difference	p
pO_2 (mmHg)	45.6 ± 3.7	28.6 ± 4.4	17 (37%)	<0.002
pCO_2 (mmHg)	53.1 ± 2.9	64.8 ± 8.1	12 (18%)	0.23
Blood flow (ml/100g/min)	7.6 ± 1.2	4.3 ± 1.4	3.3 (43%)	<0.025

described between reduced perfusion and elevated intraosseous pressure resulting in hypoxia.[21,22] An elevation in intraosseous pressure from 26 to 45 mm Hg has been reported to result in a reduction of intraosseous perfusion of 60%.[22] Intraosseous hypertension with pressures of 43 ±3.7 mm Hg have been observed in late stage human OA hips compared to pressures of 26 ± 3.2 mmHg in normal hips ($p < 0.001$).[24,25] Several studies have demonstrated a two- to threefold increase in venous outflow obstruction and intraosseous pressure in late-stage OA of the hip.[3,6]

The physiologic consequences of venous stasis in bone have been studied by Kaier.[20,21] One study demonstrated the consequences of experimental venous occlusion. Reductions in pO_2 of 37% and in blood flow of 43% were observed (Table 11.1). A positive association between blood flow and pO_2 ($p < 0.006$) was also reported.

Other studies of the relationship of blood flow and pO_2 in the human OA bone revealed a pO_2 in normal bone of 63 ± 5.0 mm Hg compared to 43 ± 4.6 mm Hg in OA bone ($p < 0.05$).[24]

In summary, preclinical studies have demonstrated that venous outflow obstruction and decreased perfusion are associated with the severity of cartilage degeneration and bone remodeling. Clinical studies with static imaging have demonstrated an abnormal centripetal pattern through intramedullary veins, delayed venous drainage, and venous stasis with OA. Dynamic imaging has suggested that venous outflow obstruction appears to be a primary pathophysiologic event and supports a concept of vascular engorgement that has been termed a "venous outlet syndrome".[17,18,52] Venous stasis is associated with intraosseous hypertension, decreased blood flow, bone remodeling, and hypoxia. Therefore, static and dynamic imaging, together with physiologic and anatomic studies, strongly suggests venous stasis and a venous outlet syndrome with reduced perfusion and hypoxia as a pathophysiologic mechanism in OA.[3,14,24,25,38,52]

11.4 Potential Cellular Consequences of Hypoxia and Altered Blood Flow

Several observations of the responses of osteocytes suggest that alterations in the physicochemical environment of subchondral bone might be involved in the initiation or progression of OA. Osteocytes are responsive to changes in their physicochemical environment, especially to intraosseous pressure, fluid flow, and oxygen content.[12,16,45,51] Although the full mechanosensory mechanisms of bone are not yet fully understood, they probably involve, to a degree, fluid shear stress through osteocyte canaliculi.[11] Intraosseous pressure in OA subchondral bone is approximately 45 mmHg and oxygen content is 43 mmHg, within the range to which osteocytes are responsive.

Osteocytes can synthesize both signaling and structural cytokines of particular relevance to OA. A number of studies have described activation of cell signaling pathways in osteocytes in response to changes in perfusion and pressure including intracellular second messengers, transcription factors, enzymes, cfos, egr1, cox2, PGE2, and nitric oxide and MMP1, 3, and 13.[34,47,49] OA osteocytes express high levels of structural cytokines, alkaline phosphatase, osteocalcin, and IGF-1 that are related to bone production. OA osteocytes have been shown to accelerate remodeling of subchondral trabeculae and the subchondral plate, consistent with textural changes seen in OA.[10,26,27]

Osteocytes are particularly responsive to hypoxia. The cellular responses consist of alterations in the synthesis of cytokines and, in more severe environmental stress, of apoptosis and necrosis. Osteocytes can withstand only 2–4 hours of hypoxia before cell death occurs. Focal osteonecrosis is seen routinely in OA.[55] Using an avian ulna model of disuse osteopenia, one study found that 24 hours of unloading resulted in $8.4 \pm 1.8\%$ osteocyte hypoxia ($p = 0.03$ compared to control), approaching the 17% observed with venous occlusion.[12] In response to hypoxia, osteocytes upregulate the hypoxia-dependent transcription factor, HIF-1α. Osteocytes subjected to hypoxic conditions with pO_2 of 35–40 mmHg, markedly alter the expression profile of growth factors, including vascular endothelial growth factor (VEGF), IGF-II, TGFß-1 and its receptor, and type I collagen, that are associated with the pathologic findings of OA, increased bone remodeling, and cartilage degradation. Notably, the expression of tissue inhibitor of metalloproteinase (TIMP-1) was strikingly decreased in response to hypoxia.[51]

Osteocytes derived from OA bone express increased amounts and types of cytokines that could be related to cartilage breakdown. The hypothesis that abnormal OA osteocytes directly influence cartilage metabolism was initially based on *in vitro* studies showing that conditioned media from OA osteocytes enhanced glycosaminoglycan (GAG) release from normal cartilage.[54] Other studies have reported that OA osteocytes exhibit an altered cytokine expression profile, upregulating the fibrinolytic proteins, uPA and plasmin, as well as IGF-1.[15] Plasmin is a serine protease that activates cartilage matrix metalloproteases (MMPs) in OA including MMP-3, 9, 12, and 13. Elevated levels of plasmin have been found in OA cartilage and uPA and tPA have been found in both OA cartilage and subchondral bone, raising the possibility that activation of the fibrinolytic system occurs in OA subchondral bone and contributes to cartilage degradation.[15,33,39] OA osteocytes have also been shown to induce alterations in the pattern of gene expression in chondrocytes associated with the phenotypic shift toward hypertrophy and matrix mineralization associated with OA.[43] Co-cultures of OA osteocytes with chondrocytes induce a decrease in chondrocytic expression of COL 2, SOX 9, and PTHrP/PTH-R, and inhibit aggrecan synthesis but increase expression of osteoblast-stimulating factor (OSF-1) and the synthesis of MMP-3 and MMP-13.[42,43] Another study, also using co-cultures, confirmed that OA osteocytes induce a hypertrophic phenotype and matrix calcification by chondrocytes and demonstrated that this was due to suppression of p38 and ERK-1/2 phosphorylation in chondrocytes.[41]

11.5 Crossing the Tidemark: Is There a Communication between Bone and Cartilage in OA?

The subchondral plate and the calcified zone of cartilage have traditionally been thought of as impassable and blocking communication between bone and cartilage. A substantial body of data, however, is showing that several mechanisms of transport exist, providing opportunities for chemical communication by small proteins between bone and cartilage. Loss of osteochondral integrity, or osteochondral plasticity, reduces the barrier between articular cartilage and the subchondral bone and facilitates communication that may be a part of OA pathogenesis.[46]

Imhoff described the existence of a variety of vascular and non-vascular channels of communication from subchondral bone to cartilage.[17,18] They pointed out that intraosseous hypertension associated with venous outflow obstruction most likely facilitated the exchange of chemical mediators between cartilage and bone. Detailed 3D reconstructions of the chondro-osseous junction have demonstrated direct contact between cartilage and subchondral bone that could provide a pathway for diffusion and chemical communication.[30] These observations were interpreted as demonstrating "micro-anatomical pathways for molecular trafficking." The chondro-osseous junction has been shown to be permeable to saline under normal loading pressure providing a route for passage of "pathologic cytokines".[44] A detailed study using fluorescein and rhodamine tracers with fluorescence microscopy demonstrated an effective diffusivity of $9 \times 10^{-9}\,\mathrm{cm}^2\,\mathrm{s}^{-1}$.[2] This study showed that the tidemark and calcified cartilage are permeable to low molecular weight solutes, perhaps influenced by charge. Another study demonstrated the diffusivity of fluorescein (376 Da) from subchondral bone to cartilage.[37] Electron microscopic studies revealed that calcified cartilage contained unmineralized regions effectively creating pores that could serve as transport pathways. Calculations suggested that molecules similar in size to fluorescein such as prostaglandin E2, nitric oxide, or glucose, could readily perfuse through the chondro-osseous junction over a distance of $40\,\mu$m within 30 minutes. A review reported transit of TGF-β and IL-6 providing communication between subchondral bone and articular cartilage.[19]

Another mechanism of coupling of subchondral bone and cartilage, and providing opportunity for chemical signaling, is angiogenesis. Walsh has demonstrated blood vessels breaching the tidemark in normal and OA tibias.[50] These observations were confirmed by Mapp in both normal and OA human knees, and normal rat and guinea pig knees.[32] Osteochondral vascularity was greater in patients with OA and might be related to inflammation, hypoxia, or altered mechanics.[7] VEGF is a potent regulator of angiogenesis and itself is upregulated by hypoxia through activation of HIF-1α. Oxygen tension in articular cartilage is low, and studies referred to earlier in subchondral bone have shown hypoxia in human and preclinical models of OA. Hypoxia in OA is a prime stimulus for angiogenesis through HIF-1α and VEGF.[36,45] Therefore, a presumptive mechanism exists for subchondral hypoxia associated with reduced perfusion in OA to stimulate angiogenesis and contribute to breaching the subchondral plate and calcified cartilage and provide a pathway for destructive cytokines from subchondral bone to contribute to cartilage degeneration.

11.6 Conclusions

Anatomic, imaging, and physiologic studies have demonstrated in several models of OA, including humans, that venous outflow from bone is impeded, leading to a variety of pathologic conditions including intraosseous hypertension, reduced perfusion, and hypoxia. Intraosseous fluid flow may also be affected. Osteocytes in OA bone have been shown to express an altered pattern of cytokines, many of which contribute either to bone remodeling or cartilage degeneration and are of interest in the pathogenesis of OA. Because of the responsiveness of osteocytes to their physicochemical environment, it is reasonable to postulate that the changes observed in OA bone, especially hypoxia, can serve as stimuli to altered osteocyte synthesis of cytokines. Hypoxia can also serve to stimulate angiogenesis and may do so in the subchondral bone. Neovascularization, together with other channels through the subchondral plate and calcified cartilage, may permit transit of osteocyte-derived cytokines that can contribute to cartilage degeneration.

References

1. Aaron RK, Dyke JP, Ciombor DM, Ballon D, Lee J, Jung E, *et al.* (2007). Perfusion abnormalities in subchondral bone associated with marrow edema, osteoarthritis, and avascular necrosis. *Ann NY Acad Sci,* 1117, 124–137.
2. Arkill KP, Winlove CP (2008). Solute transport in the deep and calcified zones of articular cartilage. *Osteoarthritis Cartilage*, 16(6), 708–714.
3. Arnoldi CC (1994). Vascular aspects of degenerative joint disorders. A synthesis. *Acta Orthop Scand* Suppl, 261, 1–82.
4. Arnoldi CC, Djurhuus JC, Heerfordt J, Karle A (1980). Intraosseous phlebography, intraosseous pressure measurements and 99mTC-polyphosphate scintigraphy in patients with various painful conditions in the hip and knee. *Acta Orthop Scand*, 51(1), 19–28.
5. Arnoldi CC, Lemperg K, Linderholm H (1975). Intraosseous hypertension and pain in the knee. *J Bone Joint Surg Br*, 57(3), 360–363.
6. Arnoldi CC, Linderholm H, Mussbichler H (1972). Venous engorgement and intraosseous hypertension in osteoarthritis of the hip. *J Bone Joint Surg Br*, 54(3), 409–421.
7. Ashraf S, Walsh DA (2008). Angiogenesis in osteoarthritis. *Curr Opin Rheumatol*, 20(5), 573–580.
8. Brix G, Semmler W, Port R, Schad LR, Layer G, Lorenz WJ (1991). Pharmacokinetic parameters in CNS Gd-DTPA enhanced MR imaging. *J Comput Assist Tomogr*, 15(4), 621–628.
9. Brooks M, Revell, W (1998). *Blood Supply of Bone: Scientific Aspects.* London: Springer Verlag.

10. Burr DB (1998). The importance of subchondral bone in osteoarthrosis. *Curr Opin Rheumatol*, 10(3), 256–262.
11. Cowin SC (2002). Mechanosensation and fluid transport in living bone. *J Musculoskelet Neuronal Interact*, 2(3), 256–260.
12. Dodd JS, Raleigh JA, Gross TS (1999). Osteocyte hypoxia: Anovel mechanotransduction pathway. *Am J Physiol*, 277(3 Pt 1), C598–C602.
13. Dyke JP, Aaron RK (2010). Noninvasive methods of measuring bone blood perfusion. *Ann N Y Acad Sci*, 1192, 95–102.
14. Dyke JP, Synan M, Ezell P, Racine J, Aaron R. Characterization of bone perfusion by dynamic contrast-enhanced magnetic resonance imaging and positron emission tomography in the Dunkin-Hartley guinea pig model of advanced osteoarthritis. *J Orthop Res.* In press.
15. Hilal G, Martel-Pelletier J, Pelletier JP, Ranger P, Lajeunesse D (1998). Osteoblast-like cells from human subchondral osteoarthritic bone demonstrate an altered phenotype in vitro: Possible role in subchondral bone sclerosis. *Arthritis Rheum*, 41(5), 891–899.
16. Hillsley MV, Frangos JA (1994). Bone tissue engineering: The role of interstitial fluid flow. *Biotechnology and Bioengineering*, 43(7), 573–581.
17. Imhof H, Breitenseher M, Kainberger F, Trattnig S (1997). Degenerative joint disease: Cartilage or vascular disease? *Skeletal Radiol*, (7), 398–403.
18. Imhof H, Sulzbacher I, Grampp S, Czerny C, Youssefzadeh S, Kainberger F (2000). Subchondral bone and cartilage disease: Are discovered functional unit. *Invest Radiol*, (10), 581–588.
19. Karsdal MA, Leeming DJ, Dam EB, Henriksen K, Alexandersen P, Pastoureau P, *et al.* (2008). Should subchondral bone turnover be targeted when treating osteoarthritis? *Osteoarthritis Cartilage*, 16(6), 638–646.
20. Kiaer T (1994). Bone perfusion and oxygenation. Animal experiments and clinical observations. *Acta Orthop Scand* Suppl, 257, 1–41.
21. Kiaer T, Dahl B, Lausten G (1992). Partial pressures of oxygen and carbon dioxide in bone and their correlation with bone-blood flow: Effect of decreased arterial supply and venous congestion on intraosseous oxygen and carbon dioxide in an animal model. *J Orthop Res*, 10(6), 807–812.
22. Kiaer T, Dahl B, Lausten GS (1993). The relationship between inert gas wash-out and radioactive tracer microspheres in measurement of bone blood flow: Effect of decreased arterial supply and venous congestion on bone blood flow in an animal model. *J Orthop Res*, 11(1), 28–35.
23. Kiaer T, Gronlund J, Jensen B, Svalastoga E (1990). Effects of variation in systemic blood pressure on intraosseous pressure, PO2, and PCO2. *J Orthop Res*, 8(4), 618–622.
24. Kiaer T, Gronlund J, Sorensen KH (1988). Subchondral pO2, pCO2, pressure, pH, and lactate in human osteoarthritis of the hip. *Clin Orthop Relat Res*, 229, 149–155.
25. Kiaer T, Pedersen NW, Kristensen KD, Starklint H (1990). Intra-osseous pressure and oxygen tension in avascular necrosis and osteoarthritis of the hip. *J Bone Joint Surg*, 72B, 1023–1030.

26. Lahm A, Kreuz PC, Oberst M, Haberstroh J, Uhl M, Maier D (2006). Subchondral and trabecular bone remodeling in canine experimental osteoarthritis. *Arch Orthop Trauma Surg*, 126(9), 582–587.
27. Lavigne P, Benderdour M, Lajeunesse D, Reboul P, Shi Q, Pelletier JP, *et al.* (2005). Subchondral and trabecular bone metabolism regulation in canine experimental knee osteoarthritis. *Osteoarthritis Cartilage*, 13(4), 310–317.
28. Lee JH, Dyke JP, Ballon D, Ciombor DM, Rosenwasser MP, Aaron RK (2009). Subchondral fluid dynamics in a model of osteoarthritis: Use of dynamic contrast-enhanced magnetic resonance imaging. *Osteoarthritis Cartilage*, 17(10), 1350–1355.
29. Lemperg RK, Arnoldi CC (1978). The significance of intraosseous pressure in normal and diseased states with special reference to the intraosseous engorgement-pain syndrome. *Clin Orthop Relat Res*, 136, 143–156.
30. Lyons TJ, McClure SF, Stoddart RW, McClure J (2006). The normal human chondro-osseous junctional region: Evidence for contact of uncalcified cartilage with subchondral bone and marrow spaces. *BMC Musculoskelet Disord*, 7, 52.
31. Ma HT, Griffith JF, Yeung DK, Leung PC (2010). Modified brix model analysis of bone perfusion in subjects of varying bone mineral density. *J Magn Reson Imaging*, 31(5), 1169–1175.
32. Mapp PI, Avery PS, McWilliams DF, Bowyer J, Day C, Moores S, *et al.* (2008). Angiogenesis in two animal models of osteoarthritis. *Osteoarthritis Cartilage*, 16(1), 61–69.
33. Martel-Pelletier J, Faure MP, McCollum R, Mineau F, Cloutier JM, Pelletier JP (1991). Plasmin, plasminogen activators and inhibitor in human osteoarthritic cartilage. *J Rheumatol*, 18(12), 1863–1871.
34. McAllister TN, Frangos JA (1999). Steady and transient fluid shear stress stimulate NO release in osteoblasts through distinct biochemical pathways. *J Bone Miner Res*, 14(6), 930–936.
35. Messa C, Goodman WG, Hoh CK, Choi Y, Nissenson AR, Salusky IB, *et al.* (1993). Bone metabolic activity measured with positron emission tomography and [18F] fluoride ion in renal osteodystrophy: Correlation with bone histomorphometry. *J Clin Endocrinol Metab*, 77(4), 949–955.
36. Murata M, Yudoh K, Masuko K (2008). The potential role of vascular endothelial growth factor (VEGF) in cartilage: How the angiogenic factor could be involved in the pathogenesis of osteoarthritis. *Osteoarthritis Cartilage*, 16(3), 279–286.
37. Pan J, Wang B, Li W, Zhou X, Scherr T, Yang Y, *et al.* (2012). Elevated cross-talk between subchondral bone and cartilage in osteoarthritic joints. *Bone*, 51(2), 212–217.
38. Pedersen NW, Kiaer T, Kristensen KD, Starklint H (1989). Intraosseous pressure, oxygenation, and histology in arthrosis and osteonecrosis of the hip. *Acta Orthop Scand*, 60(4), 415–417.
39. Pelletier JP, Mineau F, Faure MP, Martel-Pelletier J (1990). Imbalance between the mechanisms of activation and inhibition of metalloproteases in the early lesions of experimental osteoarthritis. *Arthritis Rheum*, 33(10), 1466–1476.

40. Piert M, Zittel TT, Becker GA, Jahn M, Stahlschmidt A, Maier G, *et al.* (2001). Assessment of porcine bone metabolism by dynamic. *J Nucl Med*, 42(7), 1091–1100.
41. Prasadam I, van Gennip S, Friis T, Shi W, Crawford R, Xiao Y (2010). ERK-1/2 and p38 in the regulation of hypertrophic changes of normal articular cartilage chondrocytes induced by osteoarthritic subchondral osteoblasts. *Arthritis Rheum*, 62(5), 1349–1360.
42. Sanchez C, Deberg MA, Piccardi N, Msika P, Reginster JY, Henrotin YE (2005). Osteoblasts from the sclerotic subchondral bone downregulate aggrecan but upregulate metalloproteinases expression by chondrocytes. This effect is mimicked by interleukin-6, -1beta and oncostatin M pre-treated non-sclerotic osteoblasts. *Osteoarthritis Cartilage*, 13(11), 979–987.
43. Sanchez C, Deberg MA, Piccardi N, Msika P, Reginster JY, Henrotin YE (2005). Subchondral bone osteoblasts induce phenotypic changes in human osteoarthritic chondrocytes. *Osteoarthritis Cartilage*, 13(11), 988–997.
44. Simkin P, Peterson, J (2001). The cartilage/bone interface is permeable to saline under phsyiologic articular pressures. *Osteoarthritis Cartilage*, 9(Supp 2), S4.
45. Steinbrech DS, Mehrara BJ, Saadeh PB, Greenwald JA, Spector JA, Gittes GK, *et al.* (2000). Hypoxia increases insulinlike growth factor gene expression in rat osteoblasts. *Ann Plast Surg*, 44(5), 529–534.
46. Suri S, Walsh DA (2012). Osteochondral alterations in osteoarthritis. *Bone*, 51(2), 204–211.
47. Tanaka SM, Sun HB, Roeder RK, Burr DB, Turner CH, Yokota H (2005). Osteoblast responses one hour after load-induced fluid flow in a three-dimensional porous matrix. *Calcif Tissue Int*, 76(4), 261–271.
48. Tofts PS, Brix G, Buckley DL, Evelhoch JL, Henderson E, Knopp MV, *et al.* (1999). Estimating kinetic parameters from dynamic contrast-enhanced T(1)-weighted MRI of a diffusable tracer: Standardized quantities and symbols. *J Magn Reson Imaging*, 10(3), 223–232.
49. Wadhwa S, Choudhary S, Voznesensky M, Epstein M, Raisz L, Pilbeam C (2002). Fluid flow induces COX-2 expression in MC3T3-E1 osteoblasts via a PKA signaling pathway. *Biochem Biophys Res Commun*, 297(1), 46–51.
50. Walsh DA, Bonnet CS, Turner EL, Wilson D, Situ M, McWilliams DF (2007). Angiogenesis in the synovium and at the osteochondral junction in osteoarthritis. *Osteoarthritis Cartilage*, 15(7), 743–751.
51. Warren SM, Steinbrech DS, Mehrara BJ, Saadeh PB, Greenwald JA, Spector JA, *et al.* (2001). Hypoxia regulates osteoblast gene expression. *J Surg Res*, 99(1), 147–155.
52. Watt I (2009). Osteoarthritis revisited — again! *Skeletal Radiol*, 38(5), 419–423.
53. Welch RD, Johnston CE, 2nd, Waldron MJ, Poteet B (1993). Bone changes associated with intraosseous hypertension in the caprine tibia. *J Bone Joint Surg Am*, 75(1), 53–60.

54. Westacott CI, Webb GR, Warnock MG, Sims JV, Elson CJ (1997). Alteration of cartilage metabolism by cells from osteoarthritic bone. *Arthritis Rheum*, 40(7), 1282–1291.
55. Wong SY, Evans RA, Needs C, Dunstan CR, Hills E, Garvan J (1987). The pathogenesis of osteoarthritis of the hip: Evidence for primary osteocyte death. *Clin Orthop Relat Res*, 214, 305–312.

CHAPTER 12

OSTEOPOROSIS, CIRCULATION, AND FLUID DYNAMICS

BING ZHANG

Department of Orthopaedic Surgery,
University of California, San Diego, CA

JAIME MATEUS

Department of Aeronautics and Astronautics
Massachusetts Institute of Technology, Cambridge, MA

ALAN HARGENS

Department of Orthopaedic Surgery
University of California, San Diego, CA

12.1 Bone Development

The human skeleton, consisting of the craniofacial bones, the axial skeleton, and the appendicular skeleton, arises from cells of three distinct embryonic lineages. Only the development of the axial and appendicular skeleton will be discussed here.

Development of the axial skeleton can be divided into three stages that begin at week 4 after gestation.[173] During the "pre-cartilaginous stage" (weeks 4–6), cells from the paraxial mesoderm condense to first form somites, or bilateral progenitor bodies, and then sclerotomes which surround the notochord and become precursors for the vertebral bodies and most of the skull. Sclerotomes also differentiate into chondrocytes, which migrate around the notochord to form the neural arches, ribs, and transverse processes. During the "cartilaginous stage" (week 7), the embryonic structures, or *anlagen*, are replaced by cartilage produced by the chondrocytes. In the final "bony stage" (week 7 to year 25), three primary ossification centers from each cartilaginous vertebra play different roles in forming the bony spine. One ventral ossification center becomes the vertebral body, while two dorsal ones fuse together to form the two vertebral arches by the third to fifth year of life. Secondary ossification centers ensure that vertebral development continues well into puberty.

The appendicular skeleton is formed by cells that originate from the lateral plate mesoderm.[129] The shaping of limbs during development depends on growth factors from specialized cells in the environment. Fibroblast growth factor (FGF) directs specialized epithelial cells in the apical ectodermal ridge[58] at the tips of limb buds to undergo proximodistal outgrowth, while anteroposterior growth is directed by the sonic hedgehog (SHH) chemokine. The limb bones are formed in an orderly fashion with the humerus/femur first taking shape. Phalangeal *anlagen* are formed last, and segmentation and formation of joints are produced by apoptotic cell death. During limb development, cells from the somite migrate to the embryonic appendages and develop into nerves, blood vessels, and muscles.

12.2 Osteoporosis

12.2.1 *Background and definitions*

The terms "osteoporosis" and "osteopenia" refer to the loss of bone mass and strength, resulting in an increased risk of fractures. The World Health Organization (WHO) defines the two terms using a T-score, which describes the bone mass of an individual relative to a comparative population of age 20.[170] A T-score<-1.0 means having a bone mass less than 1.0 standard deviations[44] below the mean for young healthy adults of the same gender, defined by the NHANES reference database on Caucasians 20–29 years old.[102] A T-score<-2.5 represents having a bone mass of 2.5 standard deviations below the benchmark population. The reference site of bone mass density (BMD) measured by dual-energy x-ray absorptiometry (DEXA) scan is the femoral neck, but other central sites (lumbar spine, total hip) may be used for clinical diagnosis.

Osteoporosis is separated into two broad categories. Primary or idiopathic osteoporosis typically refers to age-related changes in bone remodeling that are exaggerated and pathologic.[63] Two types of primary osteoporosis are post-menopausal osteoporosis and senile osteoporosis. Post-menopausal osteoporosis occurs in women between 51 and 75 years old, and is linked to estrogen deficiency accompanying menopause. Senile osteoporosis usually occurs in those older than 60 years old, affects both men and women, and has a different pathophysiology of reduced bone turnover due to reduction in the number of osteoblasts. Secondary osteoporosis describes bony degenerative changes not directly related to age. Some common causes include medications such as diuretics, endocrine disorders, and congenital abnormalities.[77] Up to one-third of those with idiopathic osteoporosis also have a co-existing condition contributing to bone loss, which exacerbates the expected decrease in BMD that accompanies age.

12.2.2 *Epidemiology*

The worldwide prevalence of osteoporosis is estimated to be over 200 million.[34] In the United States alone, at least 8 million women and 2 million men have osteoporosis. An additional 18 million people have osteopenia, which put them at increased risk of continuing to lose BMD.[101] The US Preventive Services Task Force (USPSTF) estimates that half of all post-menopausal women are expected to have at least one osteoporosis-related fracture in their lifetime, of which 25% will suffer from a vertebral deformity and 15% will experience a hip fracture.[101] This tremendous prevalence contributes to at least 1.5 million fractures each year, with an estimated annual cost of $17 billion.[47] As the population continues to age, the rate and burden of osteoporosis and osteopenia will continue to increase.

12.2.3 *Pathophysiology*

Osteoporosis is essentially a consequence of imbalance between bone resorption and formation during bone remodeling.[63, 138] Osteoclasts, which are macrophage-like cells found in the lacunae, initiate the resorption process by initially acidifying the extracellular compartment causing demineralization. The process continues with degradation of the organic matrix by cysteine proteases. After fulfilling their function, osteoclasts undergo apoptosis and are subsequently replaced by osteoblasts, fibroblast-like cells that replete the resorbed bone by first depositing osteoid (unmineralized bone matrix), which then undergo mineralization to maintain bone density and strength.

Bone density is well maintained during young adulthood, when bone resorption is slightly less than bone growth. However, after the ages of 30–45, resorption exceeds formation and ultimately leads to osteopenia/osteoporosis and increased fracture risk. The degree of bone loss depends on multiple factors including age, gender, medical history, lifestyle, and body sites, all of which determine signaling regulators controlling this dynamic process.[101, 111] In recent years, genome-wide association studies have identified specific loci and genes associated with BMD, which has historically been observed to be highly heritable.[12, 44, 145]

Non-Modifiable	Potentially Modifiable
History of fracture as adult	Current cigarette smoking
History of fracture in first-degree relative	Alcoholism
Female gender	Impaired eyesight despite adequate correction
Advanced age	Recurrent falls
White ethnicity	Inadequate physical activity
Dementia	Poor health/frailty
	Low body weight (<58 kg, or <127 lbs)
	Estrogen deficiency
	Early menopause (<45 years) or bilateral ovariectomy
	Low calcium intake

12.2.4 *Clinical consequences*

The most common fractures sites from osteoporosis are the vertebrae, the hips, and the wrist, with incidences of 700,000, 300,000, and 250,000 cases per year, respectively.[101] Vertebral compression fractures can cause kyphosis, height loss, and other changes in body habitus that may result in decreased ambulatory abilities and further trigger pulmonary and gastrointestinal dysfunctions.[63] Hip fractures lead to permanently diminished mobility in 50% of all patients, dramatically increase the incidence of deep vein thrombosis and pulmonary embolism, and are associated with a mortality rate of 5–20% in the post-surgical year. Pain, the most common symptom of osteoporosis-related fractures, reduces ability to work, limits social activities, and reduces the general quality of life.[33] Elderly patients' abilities to carry out activities of daily living are greatly diminished even after recovery from fractures, while their mortality risk is increased by 5–10 years with each low-impact fracture.[20]

12.2.5 *Contributing and preventative factors*

Preservation of BMD is crucial in the prevention of pathological fractures. In a study of post-menopausal women older than 50 years, fractures were associated with approximately 4- and 1.8-fold increase with osteoporosis and osteopenia, respectively.[170] More importantly, almost half of the population had undetected low BMD. The USPSTF recommends that all women over 65 be routinely screened.[47]

Osteoporosis is the endresult of an interplay between non-modifiable (i.e. age, gender, ethnicity, genetics) and modifiable factors. Current recommendations are to consume 1,000 mg of calcium and 600 units of vitamin D daily in men older than 50, 1,200 mg of calcium and 600 units of vitamin D daily in women older than 50, and 1,200 mg of calcium and 800 units of vitamin D daily in those older than 70.[2] Additionally, increase in protein intake and decreases in alcohol and caffeine intake are associated with decreasing fracture risks.[62, 85, 119] Mediations such as steroids, heparin, certain anti-epileptics and many others may exacerbate bone loss, so preventive measures are especially important for these patients.[117] Regular high-impact exercise and smoking cessation have been correlated with higher BMD.[35, 68]

12.3 Bone Fluid Flow and Cellular Physiology

Regulation of bone density and strength was first postulated in 1892 by Julius Wolff, whose "law" attributed bone growth to proportional mechanical loading.[196] *In vitro* and *in vivo* studies of bone remodeling, partly encouraged by the need to elucidate measures to prevent severe osteoporosis in astronauts from prolonged space travel,[1] led to the recognition of fluid flow as another important regulator of the dynamic process.[70, 142] Rather than two distinct forces, mechanical stress exerts its effect through altering fluid flow to regulate remodeling and growth.[130]

12.3.1 *Bone remodeling*

Bone remodeling is a five-step process based on the intricate dynamics of three cell types.[138] The *activation phase* begins with the detection of remodeling signals by osteocytes, which compose more than 95% of all skeletal bone cells and have long dendrites that extend to bone marrow and surface.[23] Signals take on many forms, from mechanical stress causing structural damage to hormones (e.g., PTH or estrogen) induced by homeostatic changes. In the *resorption phase*, osteocytes and their precursor osteoblasts respond to molecular signals (e.g., parathyroid hormone) by producing cytokines, notably monocyte chemoattractant protein-1 (MCP-1, chemoattractant for osteoclast precursors), colony stimulating factor 1

(CSF-1) and receptor activator of nuclear factor κB ligand (RANKL, which works to promote survival, proliferation, and differentiation of osteoclast precursors into osteoclasts), and reducing the production of OPG (which inhibits osteoclast proliferation).[75,99,107] These molecular changes increase the presence of both precursor and mature osteoclasts, which then attach to the leading front of a basic multicellular unit (BMU), a temporary structure created from the aforementioned cell types during bone remodeling. The *reversal phase* thenensues with the digestion of demineralized collagen matrix by "reversal cells," likely of osteoblastic lineage. Transition from bone resorption to formation within the BMU is orchestrated by coupling signals. The *formation phase* is defined by the production mainly of collagen type I, the main organic bone component, and non-collagenous proteins such as proteoglycans, by activated osteoblasts.[114,124] These molecules conjugate together to form osteoid, which is the foundation for subsequent hydroxylapatite deposition of an unknown mechanistic nature. In the final step, the *termination/quiescence phase*, mature osteoblasts cease activity, undergo apoptosis, or differentiate into osteocytes after being surrounded in mineralized bone matrix.[138]

12.3.2 *Mechanical loading and fluid flow*

Alteration of intramedullary fluid flow by mechanical loading to assist diffusion in delivering nutrients to bone cells was first proposed by Piekarski& Munro in 1977, from the observations that diffusion was a slow process and bones undergoing cyclic loading grew thicker and healthier while immobilization resulted in atrophy.[81,134] Subsequent studies attempted to decipher the mechanism of nutrient delivery in relation to fluid flow, focusing on aspects of bone porosity, protein penetration, and response to fluid shear stress.[44,156,157] *In vitro* experiments demonstrated the ability of bone cells to detect flow stimulation and respond by moderating gene expression, similar to endothelial cells.[91,140–142] Flow-induced mechanotransduction depends both on the cell type (i.e., osteocytes, osteoblasts, osteoclasts) and the type of flow dynamics (i.e., steady, oscillating, or pulsing).[78]

The characteristics of strain experienced by bones depend on the nature of physical activity. On minor exertion such as standing, bones experience continuous extremely low-magnitude, high-frequency stress as a product of constant muscle contractions to maintain posture and encourage blood and lymphatic flow.[74] Under heavy stress, bones can withstand approximately 0.7% deformation before irreversible damage. During these times, they will experience peak loading with low frequencies.[4,48] The importance of mechanical loading in retaining skeletal integrity is demonstrated by rapid bone loss experienced even from the lack of static or holding posture, such as chronic bed rest or cast immobilization.[86,96] Bone loss is proportional to muscle atrophy, which is why strength training is encouraged as a means of preventing osteoporosis.[74]

Load stresses experienced by bone cells are amplified by the extensive network of canaliculi and interstitial fluid surrounding them. Movement of intraosseous fluid from positional changes and muscular contractions generates dynamic fluid movement to induce shear stress. Oscillating fluid flow appears to generate more biochemical responsiveness in bone cells compared to constant flow, suggesting that dynamic mechanical signals are required for bone remodeling and adaptation.[30,36,189,201] Interestingly, chronic unloading can reduce the ability of blood vessels to increase blood flow by inducing increased vascular resistance.[175] This leads to reduced nutrient delivery, possibly by limiting canalicular flow velocity, the existence of which has been shown to enhance the transport of sodium compared to diffusion alone.[137]

12.4 Bone-Blood Circulation

Bones are made up of two different layers, an outer layer made of compact bone (the cortex) and an inner spongy bone layer that encloses a network of trabeculae in a honeycomb-like structure. Long bones all have a similar structure: a long shaft or diaphysis, and round ends which typically have larger diameters than the shaft and are called epiphyses. Compact bone makes up the thick outer layer of the diaphysis, and at the center is the medullary cavity, which contains either yellow (fatty) or red (hemopoietic) bone marrow. The interiors of the epiphyses and the ends of the diaphysesare composed of trabecular bone. The outer layer of the epiphyses is made up of a layer of compact bone that is much thinner than the layer found around the diaphysis. The region in between the diaphysis (shaft) and epiphyses (ends) of the bone is the metaphysis and is separated from the epiphysis by the physisin growing bone, which gradually disappears as the bone matures. The outer surface of the bone is lined with a thin membrane called the periosteum.[28,112]

12.4.1 *Vascular anatomy of the long bone*

The vascular anatomy of a typical long bone can be divided into three separate systems: afferent vessels, the microvascular network, and efferent vessels. Blood supply to the bone comes from the afferent vessels, which include the nutrient artery, epiphyseal arteries, metaphyseal arteries, and periosteal arteries.[28,118] Ion exchange between the blood and bone marrow occurs only in the microvascular network, which is composed of capillaries and sinusoids. The venous system includes the large central sinuses, as well as the epiphyseal, metaphyseal, periosteal, and nutrient veins.[27,93]

The nutrient artery is one of the main blood supplies to long bone; it typically enters the bone halfway along the diaphysis at a shallow angle.[37,118] Once it reaches the medullary cavity, it splits into central ascending and descending longitudinal arteries that run parallel to the shaft, along the central longitudinal axis of the marrow, and alongside the central venous sinus. Small branches come off the longitudinal artery and run radially outward into both the marrow and into the encasing compact bone where they eventually branch off into small vessels that supply blood to the Haversian canals.[103,190] Nutrient veins accompany the nutrient artery through the central sinus and into the smaller radial branches into the cortex.[127]

Compact bone is made up of many osteons, which are long cylindrical units that run parallel to the bone shaft. At the center of the osteon is the Haversian canal, which contains both arterial and venous blood vessels as well as nerve fibers. Capillaries have also been observed inside the Haversian canals, representing the exchange vessels within the cortical bone. Oriented roughly perpendicular to the Haversian canals are Volkmann's canals which connect the Haversian canals and the medullary cavity to the nerves and blood vessels outside of the bone.[112] Arterial flow through healthy bone is centrifugal, coming from the nutrient arteries in the medullary cavity and going outward through the cortex.[27,118]

In addition to the main nutrient artery, there are numerous smaller epiphyseal and metaphyseal arteries supplying blood to the ends of the bone.[28,37,93] On the periosteum, a network of small periosteal vessels surrounds the bone. The extent to which the periosteal vessels supply blood to the bone is not clear; some have argued a "dual supply" theory where periosteal flow complements the centrifugal blood flow from the medullary cavity, while others have argued against this. While the full extent of the function of the periosteal vessels is not fully understood, they appear to supply blood at least to the outer surface of the bone.[127,187] Some evidence suggests that in certain conditions such as peripheral artery disease, where arterial supply to the medulla may be impaired, the periosteal arterial supply may be enhanced. The increased periosteal blood supply acts as a compensatory mechanism and may effectively reverse the typical centrifugal blood flow direction.[27]

The venous or vascular sinuses are thin vessels that connect to the central venous sinus, which runs parallel to the longitudinal artery in the marrow. The central venous sinus collects the venous flow from the many smaller veins in the diaphyseal marrow.[93] It connects directly with the nutrient vein as well as numerous metaphyseal and epiphyseal veins, and it appears to also be connected to the periosteal veins.[13] It is thought that the cortical capillaries, on the other hand, connect with the periosteal capillaries, which drain to intramuscular veins.[28]

While this classification of the vascular system in bone is helpful in understanding the overlying structure, it is important to realize that in reality the vascular network has numerous anastomoses that create interconnections between various branches of the vascular tree.[28,93] Additionally, there is still some debate as to the relative importance of the different vascular branches as well as to their functional anatomy.[118]

12.4.2 *Mechanisms regulating bone circulation*

Bone blood circulation is under the control of several different mechanisms including neural, humoral, and metabolic processes.[167,168] Bone is highly innervated with sympathetic fibers, and while nerve fibers are found throughout, they are denser in the periosteum, metaphyses, and epiphyses than in cortical bone.[67,118,162] Electrical stimulation of bone nerve fibers has been shown to result in vasoconstriction and reduced blood flow in different mammals such as cats, dogs,[21,22,41,42] and rabbits[167] as measured by decreased outflow from the bone or a decrease in intramedullary pressure. A drop in the intramedullary pressure is known to correlate with a decrease in blood flow through the bone, as the pressure difference that drives the centrifugal flow is decreased.[166] Additionally, increased bone flow has been observed after complete sciatic nerve section in rabbits.[167]

Bone blood vessels have been shown to respond to a number of vasoactive substances. Early studies have shown a fall in blood flow and intramedullary pressure in response to injection of adrenaline.[13,161,166] More recent studies have demonstrated vasodilation in response to nitroglycerin and nitric oxide release, and vasoconstriction in response to endothelin.[26,115] Overall, it appears that bone is more sensitive to vasoconstrictors than to vasodilators.[26,46,118] There are several metabolic factors such as blood pH, oxygen concentration, carbon dioxide concentration, and acid metabolites that have been shown to affect bone blood flow. In general, decreasing the oxygen concentration or increasing the carbon dioxide content results in increased arterial flow. Reactive hyperemic responses have also been observed in bone, and these remained even after cutting the nerves, suggesting a strong metabolic control mechanism that does not depend on neural innervation.[28,166]

The myogenic effect, first reported by Bayliss in 1902, describes the natural tendency of blood vessels to vasodilate in response to a decrease in transmural pressure and to vasoconstrict in response to an increase in transmural pressure.[16] Although the exact mechanism is not yet fully understood,[38,69,159] it has been shown to be an important mechanism regulating blood flow in skin, muscle, and many other organs.[24,25,79] While the myogenic effect may be enhanced during sympathetic stimulation, it is a separate mechanism that can be seen even when all innervation has been cut.[22,41,42,166] Since the blood vessels inside the bone are encased in the stiff bone structure, it is unclear exactly how a transmural pressure difference that activates the myogenic effect might be transmitted to these vessels. Yet some recent data indicate that the myogenic effect may indeed also occur in bone blood vessels, though the mechanism by which it is activated has only been hypothesized.[116]

12.5 Animal Studies of Bone Loss

12.5.1 *Ground-based experiments*

Prolonged weightlessness experienced by astronauts during space missions leads to rapid and severe osteoporosis of normally weight-bearing bones, of which many are not completely reversible.[71,72] To develop countermeasures, both ground-based and space-flight animal models have been utilized to better understand bone adaptation. These *in vivo* studies elucidated the effect of perfusion and interstitial fluid flow on bone remodeling.

One of the most widely used rodent models to simulate microgravity is hindlimb unloading.[120,121] Developed in the mid-1970s by the National Aeronautics and Space Agency (NASA) Ames Research Center, the model has been widely accepted as a valid simulation of microgravity. Rodents are suspended by attaching their tails to a pulley, allowing them mobility, grooming, and feeding using their forelimbs. This model offers a variety of advantages. First, a head-down position generates cephalic fluid shift, which occurs in absence of gravity.[122] Second, forearms bear normal load and provide internal control.[64] Third, hindlimb suspension enables further manipulation.[120] Fourth, the model does not induce extra stress on the animals, as determined by corticosteroid levels and weight gain.[60, 199]

Unloading of the hindlimb leads to diminishing skeletal mass and bone mineral content as expected.[56, 61, 185] Particularly, bone radius is diminished in both the metaphysis and the diaphysis; cortical and cancellous bones are similarly affected.[56] Bone length remains unaffected, suggesting that factors other than load determine longitudinal growth.[110, 174, 181, 182] The observed changes in bone structure may be mediated by decreases in osteoblast proliferation, maturation, and activity.[19, 109, 206] Influences on osteoclast number and bone resorption are not consistent, and increases may reflect the amount of stress felt by the animals rather than the lack of load stimulus.[61, 108, 110, 184, 186, 199] Decrements in bone mass increase the risk of fracture or bending, even at lower loads and in as little as two weeks.[3, 113, 165, 182] Finally, unloading for 14 days followed by equal or longer duration of reloading may not adequately reverse the remodeling, despite rapid activating of bone formation rate at the initiation of reloading.[163, 185]

Studies assessing the significance of fluid dynamics on bone remodeling independent of weight bearing have demonstrated the ability to alter bone remodeling through perfusion alone. In early experiments, it was discovered that fractures healed at an accelerated rate distal to a venous tourniquet, presumably due to increased interstitial fluid flow.[70, 92] Unloading of the hindlimbs immediately decreased mean arterial flow, which continued to diminish until a steady state of ~60% control value was reached in five days. When unloading was stopped, blood flow returned to pre-suspension levels, suggesting a possible role of blood flow in the etiology of both muscle atrophy and bone loss.[148] Ligation of one femoral vein in hindlimb unloaded animals, while using the other femur as control, resulted in increased bone mineral content, length, and distal femur width. Vein ligation significantly elevated interstitial fluid flow (IFF) in the affected limb compared to the control.[18] The difference in bone structure was attributed to (IFF), which is the movement of intramedullary fluid surrounding osteocytes, osteoclasts, and osteoblasts.

Further evidence demonstrating the effect of perfusion and IFF on bone remodeling comes from following changes in structure and composition in bones that are normally partial or non-weight-bearing. Tailsuspension induces bodily fluid redistribution, resulting in cephalad fluid shift from the lower extremities to the head and upper body.[64,160,193,194] The mass of lower extremities substantially diminished as expected. Correspondingly, increases in the mass of bones in the upper bodies were observed. Hindlimb unloading alters only fluid flow without the addition of external pressure.[31,147] Since cranial bones are normally non-loaded while the humerus are partial-loaded compared to bones of the lower body, the observed increasesare solely attributable to the head-ward fluid shift and increased perfusion.

12.6 Clinical and Regenerative Medicine

12.6.1 *Bed-rest studies*

Bed-rest studies in humans are designed to simulate physiological changes that accompany prolonged stay in microgravity.[133] Many studies tilt the head of the bed downward by 3–6° to better simulate space travel. Maintaining a supine position for an extended time period induces similar physiological effects as seen in astronauts returning from missions. Specific to the effects on bone demineralization, extended immobilization and decreased lower-body fluid pressure induced muscle atrophy especially in the lower extremities, increased fatigability, increased calcium excretion, and mineral loss of the weight-bearing bones.[88,136,146,171] Comparison of the results from previous bed-rest studies and actual spaceflight demonstrates that the simulated microgravity model actually underestimates the magnitude of bone loss from spaceflight.[14,96,97,172]

Gravity exerts a tremendous influence on the body's fluid dynamics. Fluid and blood shift from the lowers legs was observed immediately in transition from upright to supine position with significant decreases in thigh and calf cross-sectional area after only 120 minutes.[17] After only eight hours of 5° of head-down tilt, cephalic fluid movement induced facial edema and nasal congestion. Interstitial fluid pressure of the lower-extremity muscle and subcutaneous tissue fell significantly, as did calf girth and lower leg volume.[65] Further duration of head-down bed rest could increase leg venous distension by up to 50%, increase emptying-time, and decrease arterial flow by up to 50%. Elevated fluid stasis reflects diminished flow rate of the lower extremities that correlated with muscle atrophy.[104–106]

Normal muscular tone is crucial for the prevention of osteopenia, as both weight-bearing and fluid flow rely on muscular activity to exert effect on bone cells. The largest forces experienced by the bones are not from gravity, but are from muscle action that works against gravity.[132] Prolonged disuse from bedrest induces muscle atrophy, especially of the anti-gravity muscles in the lower limbs, while back muscles are affected to a lesser degree. The effects of muscle disuse are rapid and profound — a 3% reduction in the cross-sectional area of thigh muscles was observed in only seven days of bed rest, and significant decreases in the maximal torque generated by ankle and knee flexors and extensors in the magnitude of 8–16% occurred after 20 days.[5–7] Force and velocity of the upper extremities were not affected by bedrest, which is similar to studies on the effect of actual and simulated microgravity on bone remodeling of the upper limbs.[51]

As expected, longer periods of bed rest produce more dramatic effects of lower-limb muscular atrophy and function, although the decrements do not continue at a linear rate. After 90 days, knee extensor and plantar flexor muscle mass decreased by 18% and 29%, respectively.[8,9] Power of the lower-extremity muscle groups can decrease from 30% to 55%.[146] Calf muscle atrophy increased to 25%, while forearm cross-sectional area still remained unchanged. Muscle biopsies show the muscles with the most composition of slow-twitch fibers undergo the most atrophy, while the composition of fast-twitch fibers in these muscles increase, leading to higher contraction velocity.[45,179,191,192]

Bone remodeling and metabolism complemented muscle changes from inactivity. In 17-week bed-rest studies of healthy volunteers, the largest decrements in bone mineral density were observed at the lumbar spine, femoral neck, trochanter, tibia, and calcaneus.[97,164] These bones usually bear the most amount of weight under normal gravity, and serve as attachments for slow-twitch fibers that serve to maintain posture against gravity. The sites most affected were the femoral neck (3.9%), a common site for pathological fractures in osteoporosis, and the tibia (4.6%). Surprisingly, DEXA analysis did not reveal changes for shorter durations of bedrest, suggesting that bone remodeling is less reactive compared to skeletal muscle atrophy, both in the duration until change occurs and the total magnitude of change.[95,177,180]

12.6.2 *Bone fracture recovery studies*

Fluid dynamics also play a crucial role in clinical recovery from injury, since increases in vascular flow and tissue perfusion accompanying post-fracture recovery are crucial to bone healing. Several experiments from the 1960s in which fractures were experimentally produced in animals initiated higher blood flow toward both the fractured bone and the surrounding muscles and skin.[139,143,144,166,197,198] This change was induced by vasodilation of the associated blood vessels, also responsible for the associated edema of the fracture site.[197,198] Subsequent clinical studies following the recovery of patients suffering from fractures confirmed higher perfusion of the injured sites.[139] This reactive hyperemia can be seen as early as five minutes of the trauma,[197] and regresses to normal after the fracture has healed.[89]

Experiments and clinical outcomes have proven that inadequate re-establishment of bone blood supply will result in necrosis.[80,166] However, in cases where only some arteries are damaged, compensatory hyper-vascularization of adjacent functional vasculature occurs.[94,143,144] Angiogenesis also occurs in the post-fracture state as a physiological response,[54,84,90,176] which contributes to the site-specific hyperemia together with increased perfusion by the existing vasculature. The establishment of these new vessels is important to bone healing, as animal models have demonstrated that inhibiting angiogenesis can lead to "atrophic non-union," or failed fracture healing.[29,66]

Clinically, early physical activity has been encouraged after reduction and fixation of bone fractures. Ambulation after hip fracture has led to a lower risk of developing post-surgical pneumonia and other complications, shortening the length of hospital stay.[83] Ambulation within 48-hours after hip fracture surgery has also resulted in more discharges directly to home and fewer to skilled nursing or rehabilitation facilities.[128] Early post-operative exercise programs are well tolerated, lead to significant improvements in hip range of motion and stiffness,and are associated with earlier functional recovery.[55] Tailored exercise without overexertion of the healing bone likely induces higher blood flow to the anatomical location, and muscle contraction encourages the shift of fluid into the intramedullary space, aiding in nutrient delivery and bone recovery.

12.7 Diagnosis and Treatment of Osteoporosis

12.7.1 *Non-invasive measurement of bone perfusion*

Adequate perfusion of osseous tissue is required to maintain a healthy skeleton, yet there are still some significant challenges in directly measuring or assessing the state of circulation in the skeletal system. Many of the available tools require invasive approaches, the use of destructive methods or radioactive isotopes that are usually not suitable for *in vivo* measurement in humans. Development of non-invasive techniques for assessing the vascular health of bones is an active area of research that may lead to innovative and clinically valuable diagnostic tools.

Most of the non-invasive methods that have been explored include the use of light in the near-infrared (IR) spectrum, taking advantage of the fact that light in the "biological window" wavelength of around 800–1,100 nm can penetrate through both bone and skin with little attenuation, yet is highly absorbed by blood.[11, 15, 100, 125, 135] A greater amount of light will be absorbed if there is more blood, and vice-versa.[10, 82] These approaches focus on illuminating tissue with a light source (e.g., a laser or light-emitting diodes) and measuring the reflected or backscattered light signal with a photodetector. This is a fundamental concept behind one of the most commonly used medical devices, the pulse oximeter, where signal processing of the reflected light spectrum is used to obtain tissue O_2 saturation data. The core technology behind this and other similar devices is often referred to as photoplethysmography (PPG), or in some cases near-infrared spectroscopy (NIRS). These devices often share very similar underlying hardware, though they can differ substantially in their signal processing depending on the desired end-use and the parameter they are designed to measure. Besides pulse oximetry, PPG has also been used in various research studies to assess microvascular skin and muscle hemodynamics.[40, 49, 50, 52, 158, 202–205] Yet only recently has PPG been used to measure perfusion in skeletal tissue with some preliminary validation provided by a study with measurements on the human patella.[126] Experiments measuring the skin and tibial bone tissue perfusion responses of humans to various stimuli have provided further validation of PPG as a non-invasive technique for assessing bone hemodynamics.[115]

However, not all bone tissues are suitable for PPG measurements of bone perfusion. The penetration depth of the IR light is limited and may not be able to reach very deep tissues. Certain bones such as the tibia, patella, or calcaneus are close to the surface and have little or no muscle tissue in between the skin and the surface of the bone, making them ideal sites for measurement. Deeper bone tissues may not be practical sites for PPG-based bone perfusion measurements. Even in the regions with only a thin layer of skin between the bone and the measurement probe, care must be taken to ensure that the deep-tissue signals are not being significantly affected by changes in the hemodynamics of the thin skin layer. In many cases, this can be adequately addressed by the design parameters of the device probe, signal processing, and experimental validation of the apparatus.

The biggest limitation of PPG is that the data it produces are only reliably expressed in relative units, such as a change from a baseline measurement. This makes long-term monitoring or comparison of intra-patient measurements difficult or impossible. Converting the PPG data into an absolute scale of measurement with a tangible physiological interpretation would be of enormous value, and is perhaps the greatest challenge in this line of research. Reaching this goal would allow for the direct comparison of signals from different subjects, enabling the systematic exploration of differences in bone perfusion across patient populations.

12.7.2 *Physical management of osteoporosis*

Current prevention and treatment of osteoporosis are widely categorized into non-pharmacologic modalities or pharmacotherapy. Of the different strategies available, exercise is the most accessible and highly recommended for several different reasons. Unloading leads to loss of bone mass, while stress from exercise can increase bone mineral density, improve quality of life, decrease pain, and improve physical function in post-menopausal women.[43, 98] Improved muscle strength, balance, coordination, and reaction time may also reduce falls and fractures.[87] Particularly, muscle-bearing exercises can increase BMD at weight-bearing sites that are prone to osteopenic fractures such as the lumbar spine and femoral neck.[32] However, not all studies have demonstrated a positive relationship between exercise and prevention of osteoporosis.[123, 169, 195] And even if activity leads to increased bone mineral density, its protective effect on fractures is not absolute.[57]

The effect of fluid flow in regulating bone mineral density independent of boneloading has generated interest in the development of novel non-pharmacologic therapies for managing osteoporosis.[188] The role of bone fluid flow as an intermediary in translation of mechanical load into intramedullary signals that stimulate bone cells demonstrates possible non-invasive intervention to counter osteopenia and osteoporosis.[73] One area of research is the utilization of mechanical vibration to prevent or reverse osteoporosis. Low-intensity and high-frequency vibration can prevent bone loss in rats treated with glucocorticoids.[39] Other animal studies have confirmed the response of bone cells to low-magnitude, high-frequency stimuli.[53, 131, 150–154, 200] However, in older adults and postmenopausal women, the utility of whole-body vibration to maintain BMD or reverse its loss has proven inconclusive. Three studies showed no positive changes after six or 12 months of treatment, while other studies suggest it may be an effective non-pharmacological intervention in maintaining bone density.[59,76,149,155,183] Inconsistencies in study design, characteristics of vibration, duration and length of treatment, and participant characteristics and results have prevented the widespread adoption of this technique.[178]

12.8 Conclusion

Bone is composed of an outer layer made of compact bone (cortex), and an inner spongy bone layer that encloses a network of trabeculae. The cortex is made up of many osteons, long cylindrical units that run parallel to the bone shaft. At the center of the osteon is the Haversian canal, which contains both arterial and venous blood vessels as well as nerve fibers. Arterial flow through healthy bone is centrifugal, coming from the nutrient arteries in the medullary cavity and going outward through the cortex. Depending on bone microvascular flow, interstitial fluid stimulates osteoblasts and importantly affects bone growth independent of weight-bearing. For example, fractures heal at an accelerated rate distal to a venous tourniquet, presumably due to increased interstitial fluid flow. On the other hand, unloading of the rodent hindlimbs decreases arterial flow, reducing bone quantity and strength.

References

1. (2001) In: Ball JR, Evans CH, eds., *Safe Passage: Astronaut Care for Exploration Missions.* Washington, DC: National Academies Press.
2. (2011) In: Ross AC, Taylor CL, Yaktine AL, Del Valle HB, eds., *Dietary Reference Intakes for Calcium and Vitamin D.* Washington, DC: National Academies Press.
3. Abram AC, Keller TS, Spengler DM (1988). The effects of simulated weightlessness on bone biomechanical and biochemical properties in the maturing rat. *J Biomech*, 21, 755–767.
4. Adams DJ, Spirt AA, Brown TD, Fritton SP, Rubin CT, *et al.* (1997). Testing the daily stress stimulus theory of bone adaptation with natural and experimentally controlled strain histories. *J Biomech*, 30, 671–678.
5. Akima H, Kubo K, Kanehisa H, Suzuki Y, Gunji A, *et al.* (2000). Leg-press resistance training during 20 days of 6 degrees head-down-tilt bed rest prevents muscle deconditioning. *Eur J Appl Physiol*, 82, 30–38.
6. Akima H, Kuno S, Suzuki Y, Gunji A, Fukunaga T (1997). Effects of 20 days of bed rest on physiological cross-sectional area of human thigh and leg muscles evaluated by magnetic resonance imaging. *J Gravit Physiol*, 4, S15–S21.

7. Akima H, Ushiyama J, Kubo J, Tonosaki S, Itoh M, *et al.* (2003). Resistance training during unweighting maintains muscle size and function in human calf. *Med Sci Sports Exerc*, 35, 655–662.
8. Alkner BA, Tesch PA (2004). Efficacy of a gravity-independent resistance exercise device as a countermeasure to muscle atrophy during 29-day bed rest. *Acta Physiol Scand*, 181, 345–357.
9. Alkner BA, Tesch PA (2004). Knee extensor and plantar flexor muscle size and function following 90 days of bed rest with or without resistance exercise. *Eur J Appl Physiol*, 93, 294–305.
10. Allen J (2007). Photoplethysmography and its application in clinical physiological measurement. *Physiol Meas*, 28, R1–R39.
11. Anderson RR, Parrish JA (1981). The optics of human skin. *J Invest Dermatol*, 77, 13–19.
12. Arden NK, Baker J, Hogg C, Baan K, Spector TD (1996). The heritability of bone mineral density, ultrasound of the calcaneus and hip axis length: Astudy of postmenopausal twins. *J Bone Miner Res*, 11, 530–534.
13. Arlet J, Mazieres B (1987). Bone circulation and bone necrosis. Proceedings of the IVth International Symposium on Bone Circulation, Toulouse (France), 17th–19th September 1987. Toulouse, France: Springer Verlag.
14. Baecker N, Tomic A, Mika C, Gotzmann A, Platen P, *et al.* (2003). Bone resorption is induced on the second day of bed rest: Results of a controlled crossover trial. *J Appl Physiol* (1985), 95, 977–982.
15. Bashkatov AN, Genina EA, Kochubey VI, Tuchin VV (2006). Optical properties of human cranial bone in the spectral range from 800 to 2000 nm. Saratov Fall Meeting 2005: Optical Technologies in Biophysics and Medicine VII.
16. Bayliss WM (1902). On the local reactions of the arterial wall to changes of internal pressure. *J Physiol*, 28, 220–231.
17. Berg HE, Tedner B, Tesch PA (1993). Changes in lower limb muscle cross-sectional area and tissue fluid volume after transition from standing to supine. *Acta Physiol Scand*, 148, 379–385.
18. Bergula AP, Huang W, Frangos JA (1999). Femoral vein ligation increases bone mass in the hindlimb suspended rat. *Bone*, 24, 171–177.
19. Bikle DD, Harris J, Halloran BP, Morey-Holton E (1994). Altered skeletal pattern of gene expression in response to spaceflight and hindlimb elevation. *Am J Physiol*, 267, E822–E827.
20. Bliuc D, Nguyen ND, Milch VE, Nguyen TV, Eisman JA, *et al.* (2009). Mortality risk associated with low-trauma osteoporotic fracture and subsequent fracture in men and women. *JAMA*, 301, 513–521.
21. Boegehold MA, Johnson PC (1988). Periarteriolar and tissue PO2 during sympathetic escape in skeletal muscle. *Am J Physiol*, 254, H929–H936.
22. Boegehold MA, Johnson PC (1988). Response of arteriolar network of skeletal muscle to sympathetic nerve stimulation. *Am J Physiol*, 254, H919–H928.
23. Bonewald LF (2007). Osteocytes as dynamic multifunctional cells. *Ann NY Acad Sci*, 1116, 281–290.

24. Bouskela E, Wiederhielm CA (1979). Microvascular myogenic reaction in the wing of the intact unanesthetized bat. *Am J Physiol*, 237, H59–H65.
25. Breit GA, Watenpaugh DE, Ballard RE, Murthy G, Hargens AR (1993). Regional cutaneous microvascular flow responses during gravitational and LBNP stresses. *Physiologist*, 36, S110–S111.
26. Brinker MR, Lippton HL, Cook SD, Hyman AL (1990). Pharmacological regulation of the circulation of bone. *J Bone Joint Surg Am*, 72, 964–975.
27. Brookes M, Elkin A, Harrison R, Heald C (1961). A new concept of capillary circulation in bone cortex. *Lancet*, 277, 1078–1081.
28. Brookes M, Revell WJ (1998). *Blood Supply of Bone: Scientific Aspects.* London: Springer Verlag.
29. Carano RA, Filvaroff EH (2003). Angiogenesis and bone repair. *Drug Discov Today*, 8, 980–989.
30. Case N, Sen B, Thomas JA, Styner M, Xie Z, *et al.* (2011). Steady and oscillatory fluid flows produce a similar osteogenic phenotype. *Calcif Tissue Int*, 88, 189–197.
31. Colleran PN, Wilkerson MK, Bloomfield SA, Suva LJ, Turner RT, *et al.* (2000). Alterations in skeletal perfusion with simulated microgravity: Apossible mechanism for bone remodeling. *J Appl Physiol* (1985), 89, 1046–1054.
32. Colletti LA, Edwards J, Gordon L, Shary J, Bell NH (1989). The effects of muscle-building exercise on bone mineral density of the radius, spine, and hip in young men. *Calcif Tissue Int*, 45, 12–14.
33. Cook DJ, Guyatt GH, Adachi JD, Epstein RS, Juniper EF, *et al.* (1999). Development and validation of the mini-osteoporosis quality of life questionnaire (OQLQ) in osteoporotic women with back pain due to vertebral fractures. Osteoporosis Quality of Life Study Group. *Osteoporos Int*, 10, 207–213.
34. Cooper C, Campion G, Melton LJ, 3rd (1992). Hip fractures in the elderly: Aworld-wide projection. *Osteoporos Int*, 2, 285–289.
35. Cornuz J, Feskanich D, Willett WC, Colditz GA (1999). Smoking, smoking cessation, and risk of hip fracture in women. *Am J Med*, 106, 311–314.
36. Cowin SC, Weinbaum S, Zeng Y (1995). A case for bone canaliculi as the anatomical site of strain generated potentials. *J Biomech*, 28, 1281–1297.
37. Crock HV (1996). *An Atlas of Vascular Anatomy of the Skeleton and Spinal Cord.* London: Martin Dunitz.
38. Davis MJ (1988). Control of bat wing capillary pressure and blood flow during reduced perfusion pressure. *Am J Physiol*, 255, H1114–H1129.
39. de Oliveira ML, Bergamaschi CT, Silva OL, Nonaka KO, Wang CC, *et al.* (2010). Mechanical vibration preserves bone structure in rats treated with glucocorticoids. *Bone*, 46, 1516–1521.
40. Dorlas JC, Nijboer JA (1985). Photo-electric plethysmography as a monitoring device in anaesthesia: Application and interpretation. *Br J Anaesth*, 57, 524–530.
41. Driessens M, Vanhoutte PM (1979). Vascular reactivity of the isolated tibia of the dog. *Am J Physiol*, 236, H904–H908.

42. Drinker CK, Drinker KR (1916). A method for maintaining an artificial circulation through the tibia of the dog, with a demonstration of the vasomotor control of the marrow vessels. *Am J Physiol*, 40, 514–521.
43. Ernst E (1998). Exercise for female osteoporosis: A systematic review of randomised clinical trials. *Sports Med*, 25, 359–368.
44. Estrada K, Styrkarsdottir U, Evangelou E, Hsu YH, Duncan EL, *et al.* (2012). Genome-wide meta-analysis identifies 56 bone mineral density loci and reveals 14 loci associated with risk of fracture. *Nat Genet*, 44, 491–501.
45. Fitts RH, Riley DR, Widrick JJ (2001). Functional and structural adaptations of skeletal muscle to microgravity. *J Exp Biol*, 204, 3201–3208.
46. Fleming JT, Barati MT, Beck DJ, Dodds JC, Malkani AL, *et al.* (2001). Bone blood flow and vascular reactivity. *Cells Tissues Organs* 169, 279–284.
47. Force USPST (2011). Screening for osteoporosis: Recommendation statement. *Am Fam Physician*, 83, 1197–1200.
48. Fritton SP, McLeod KJ, Rubin CT (2000). Quantifying the strain history of bone: Spatial uniformity and self-similarity of low-magnitude strains. *J Biomech*, 33, 317–325.
49. Fronek A (1995). Photoplethysmography in the diagnosis of venous disease. *Dermatol Surg*, 21, 64–66.
50. Fronek A, DiTomasso DG, Allison M (2007). Noninvasive assessment of endothelial activity in patients with peripheral arterial disease and cardiovascular risk factors. *Endothelium*, 14, 199–205.
51. Funato K, Matsuo A, Yata H, Akima H, Suzuki Y, *et al.* (1997). Changes in force-velocity and power output of upper and lower extremity musculature in young subjects following 20 days bed rest. *J Gravit Physiol*, 4, S22–S30.
52. Gailite L, Spigulis J, Lihachev A (2008). Multilaser photoplethysmography technique. *Lasers MedSci*, 23, 189–193.
53. Garman R, Gaudette G, Donahue LR, Rubin C, Judex S (2007). Low-level accelerations applied in the absence of weight bearing can enhance trabecular bone formation. *J Orthop Res*, 25, 732–740.
54. Geris L, Gerisch A, Sloten JV, Weiner R, Oosterwyck HV (2008). Angiogenesis in bone fracture healing: Abioregulatory model. *J Theor Biol*, 251, 137–158.
55. Gilbey HJ, Ackland TR, Wang AW, Morton AR, Trouchet T, *et al.* (2003). Exercise improves early functional recovery after total hip arthroplasty. *Clin Orthop Relat Res*, 408, 193–200.
56. Globus RK, Bikle DD, Morey-Holton E (1986). The temporal response of bone to unloading. *Endocrinology*, 118, 733–742.
57. Greendale GA, Barrett-Connor E, Edelstein S, Ingles S, Haile R (1995). Lifetime leisure exercise and osteoporosis. The Rancho Bernardo study. *Am J Epidemiol*, 141, 951–959.
58. Griffin TA, Nandi D, Cruz M, Fehling HJ, Kaer LV, *et al.* (1998). Immunoproteasome assembly: cooperative incorporation of interferon gamma (IFN-gamma)-inducible subunits. *J Exp Med*, 187, 97–104.

59. Gusi N, Raimundo A, Leal A (2006). Low-frequency vibratory exercise reduces the risk of bone fracture more than walking: a randomized controlled trial. *BMC Musculoskelet Disord*, 7, 92.
60. Halloran BP, Bikle DD, Cone CM, Morey-Holton E (1988). Glucocorticoids and inhibition of bone formation induced by skeletal unloading. *Am J Physiol*, 255, E875–E879.
61. Halloran BP, Bikle DD, Wronski TJ, Globus RK, Levens MJ, *et al.* (1986). The role of 1,25-dihydroxyvitamin D in the inhibition of bone formation induced by skeletal unloading. *Endocrinology*, 118, 948–954.
62. Hallstrom H, Wolk A, Glynn A, Michaelsson K (2006). Coffee, tea and caffeine consumption in relation to osteoporotic fracture risk in a cohort of Swedish women. *Osteoporos Int*, 17, 1055–1064.
63. Duque G, Troen BR (2009). Chapter 117. Osteoporosis. In Halter JB, Ouslander JG, Tinetti ME, Studenski S, High KP, Asthana S (Eds), *Hazzard's Geriatric Medicine and Gerontology*, sixth ed. US: The McGraw-Hill Companies, Inc.
64. Hargens AR, Steskal J, Johansson C, Tipton CM (1984). Tissue fluid shift, forelimb loading, and tail tension in tail suspended rats. *Physiologist*, 27, S37–38.
65. Hargens AR, Tipton CM, Gollnick PD, Mubarak SJ, Tucker BJ, *et al.* (1983). Fluid shifts and muscle function in humans during acute simulated weightlessness. *J Appl Physiol Respir Environ Exerc Physiol*, 54, 1003–1009.
66. Hausman MR, Schaffler MB, Majeska RJ (2001). Prevention of fracture healing in rats by an inhibitor of angiogenesis. *Bone*, 29, 560–564.
67. He JY, Jiang LS, Dai LY (2011). The roles of the sympathetic nervous system in osteoporotic diseases: A review of experimental and clinical studies. *Ageing Res Rev*, 10, 253–263.
68. Heinonen A, Kannus P, Sievanen H, Oja P, Pasanen M, *et al.* (1996). Randomised controlled trial of effect of high-impact exercise on selected risk factors for osteoporotic fractures. *Lancet*, 348, 1343–1347.
69. Hill MA, Sun Z, Martinez-Lemus L, Meininger GA (2007). New technologies for dissecting the arteriolar myogenic response. *Trends Pharmacol Sci*, 28, 308–315.
70. Hillsley MV, Frangos JA (1994). Bone tissue engineering: The role of interstitial fluid flow. *Biotechnol Bioeng*, 43, 573–581.
71. Holick MF (1998). Perspective on the impact of weightlessness on calcium and bone metabolism. *Bone*, 22, 105S–111S.
72. Holick MF (2000). Microgravity-induced bone loss: Will it limit human space exploration? *Lancet*, 355, 1569–1570.
73. Hu M, Serra-Hsu F, Bethel N, Lin L, Ferreri S, *et al.* (2013). Dynamic hydraulic fluid stimulation regulated intramedullary pressure. *Bone*, 57, 137–141.
74. Huang RP, Rubin CT, McLeod KJ (1999). Changes in postural muscle dynamics as a function of age. *J Gerontol A Biol Sci Med Sci*, 54, B352–B357.

75. Insogna KL, Sahni M, Grey AB, Tanaka S, Horne WC, *et al.* (1997). Colony-stimulating factor-1 induces cytoskeletal reorganization and c-src-dependent tyrosine phosphorylation of selected cellular proteins in rodent osteoclasts. *J Clin Invest*, 100, 2476–2485.
76. Iwamoto J, Takeda T, Sato Y, Uzawa M (2005). Effect of whole-body vibration exercise on lumbar bone mineral density, bone turnover, and chronic back pain in post-menopausal osteoporotic women treated with alendronate. *Aging Clin Exp Res*, 17, 157–163.
77. Bethel M, Lohr KM, Carbone, LD, Machua W. (2015, February 26). Osteoporosis. Retrieved June 19, 2015, from http://emedicine.medscape.com/article/330598-overview.
78. Jacobs CR, Yellowley CE, Davis BR, Zhou Z, Cimbala JM, *et al.* (1998). Differential effect of steady versus oscillating flow on bone cells. *J Biomech*, 31, 969–976.
79. Johnson PC (1989). The myogenic response in the microcirculation and its interaction with other control systems. *J Hypertens*, Suppl 7, S33–S39, discussion S40.
80. Johnson RW Jr (1968). A physiological study of the blood supply of the diaphysis. *Clin Orthop Relat Res*, 56, 5–11.
81. Jones HH, Priest JD, Hayes WC, Tichenor CC, Nagel DA (1977). Humeral hypertrophy in response to exercise. *J Bone Joint Surg Am*, 59, 204–208.
82. Kamal AA, Harness JB, Irving G, Mearns AJ (1989). Skin photoplethysmography: A review. *Comput Methods Programs Biomed*, 28, 257–269.
83. Kamel HK, Iqbal MA, Mogallapu R, Maas D, Hoffmann RG (2003). Time to ambulation after hip fracture surgery: Relation to hospitalization outcomes. *J Gerontol A Biol Sci Med Sci*, 58, 1042–1045.
84. Kanczler JM, Oreffo RO (2008). Osteogenesis and angiogenesis: The potential for engineering bone. *Eur Cell Mater*, 15, 100–114.
85. Kanis JA, Johansson H, Johnell O, Oden A, De Laet C, *et al.* (2005). Alcohol intake as a risk factor for fracture. *Osteoporos Int*, 16, 737–742.
86. Kannus P, Jarvinen M, Sievanen H, Oja P, Vuori I (1994). Osteoporosis in men with a history of tibial fracture. *J Bone Miner Res*, 9, 423–429.
87. Karlsson MK, Nordqvist A, Karlsson C (2008). Physical activity, muscle function, falls and fractures. *Food Nutr Res*, 52.
88. Kawashima S, Akima H, Kuno SY, Gunji A, Fukunaga T (2004). Human adductor muscles atrophy after short duration of unweighting. *Eur J Appl Physiol*, 92, 602–605.
89. Kellerova E, Delius W, Olerud S, Strom G (1970). Changes in the muscle and skin blood flow following lower leg fracture in man. *Acta Orthop Scand*, 41, 249–260.
90. Keramaris NC, Calori GM, Nikolaou VS, Schemitsch EH, Giannoudis PV (2008). Fracture vascularity and bone healing: Asystematic review of the role of VEGF. *Injury*, 39(Suppl 2), S45–S57.
91. Klein-Nulend J, van der Plas A, Semeins CM, Ajubi NE, Frangos JA, *et al.* (1995). Sensitivity of osteocytes to biomechanical stress in vitro. *FASEB J*, 9, 441–445.

92. Kruse RL, Kelly PJ (1974). Acceleration of fracture healing distal to a venous tourniquet. *J Bone Joint Surg Am*, 56, 730–739.
93. Laroche M (2002). Intraosseous circulation from physiology to disease. *Joint Bone Spine*, 69, 262–269.
94. Larson RL, Kelly PJ, Janes JM, Peterson LF (1961). Suppression of the perosteal and nutrient blood supply of the femora of dogs: A histologic, microangiographic and roentgenologic study. *Clin Orthop*, 21, 217–225.
95. LeBlanc A, Schneider V, Krebs J, Evans H, Jhingran S, *et al.* (1987). Spinal bone mineral after 5 weeks of bed rest. *Calcif Tissue Int*, 41, 259–261.
96. LeBlanc A, Schneider V, Shackelford L, West S, Oganov V, *et al.* (2000). Bone mineral and lean tissue loss after long duration space flight. *J Musculoskelet Neuronal Interact*, 1, 157–160.
97. Leblanc AD, Schneider VS, Evans HJ, Engelbretson DA, Krebs JM (1990). Bone mineral loss and recovery after 17 weeks of bed rest. *J Bone Miner Res*, 5, 843–850.
98. Li WC, Chen YC, Yang RS, Tsauo JY (2009). Effects of exercise programmes on quality of life in osteoporotic and osteopenic postmenopausal women: Asystematic review and meta-analysis. *Clin Rehabil*, 23, 888–896.
99. Li X, Qin L, Bergenstock M, Bevelock LM, Novack DV, *et al.* (2007). Parathyroid hormone stimulates osteoblastic expression of MCP-1 to recruit and increase the fusion of pre/osteoclasts. *J Biol Chem*, 282, 33098–33106.
100. Lindberg LG, Oberg PA (1991). Photoplethysmography: Part 2. Influence of light source wavelength. *Med Biol Eng Comput*, 29, 48–54.
101. Lindsay R, Cosman F (2012). Chapter 354. Osteoporosis. In Longo DL, Fauci AS, Kasper DL, Hauser SL, Jameson J, Loscalzo J (Eds), *Harrison's Principles of Internal Medicine*, 18th ed. The McGraw-Hill Companies. Retrieved September 28, 2014 from http://accessmedicine.mhmedical.com/content.aspx?bookid=331&Sectionid=40727160.
102. Looker AC, Wahner HW, Dunn WL, Calvo MS, Harris TB, *et al.* (1998). Updated data on proximal femur bone mineral levels of US adults. *Osteoporos Int*, 8, 468–489.
103. Lopez-Curto JA, Bassingthwaighte JB, Kelly PJ (1980). Anatomy of the microvasculature of the tibial diaphysis of the adult dog. *J Bone Joint Surg Am*, 62, 1362–1369.
104. Louisy F, Berry P, Marini JF, Guell A, Guezennec CY (1995). Characteristics of the venous hemodynamics of the leg under simulated weightlessness: Effects of physical exercise as countermeasure. *Aviat Space Environ Med*, 66, 542–549.
105. Louisy F, Gaudin C, Oppert JM, Guell A, Guezennec CY (1990). Haemodynamics of leg veins during a 30-days-6 degrees head-down bedrest with and without lower body negative pressure. *Eur J Appl Physiol Occup Physiol*, 61, 349–355.
106. Louisy F, Schroiff P, Guell A (1997). Changes in leg vein filling and emptying characteristics and leg volumes during long-term head-down bed rest. *J Appl Physiol* (1985), 82, 1726–1733.

107. Ma YL, Cain RL, Halladay DL, Yang X, Zeng Q, *et al.* (2001). Catabolic effects of continuous human PTH (1-38) in vivo is associated with sustained stimulation of RANKL and inhibition of osteoprotegerin and gene-associated bone formation. *Endocrinology*, 142, 4047–4054.
108. Machwate M, Zerath E, Holy X, Hott M, Godet D, *et al.* (1995). Systemic administration of transforming growth factor-beta 2 prevents the impaired bone formation and osteopenia induced by unloading in rats. *J Clin Invest*, 96, 1245–1253.
109. Machwate M, Zerath E, Holy X, Hott M, Modrowski D, *et al.* (1993). Skeletal unloading in rat decreases proliferation of rat bone and marrow-derived osteoblastic cells. *Am J Physiol*, 264, E790–E799.
110. Machwate M, Zerath E, Holy X, Pastoureau P, Marie PJ (1994). Insulin-like growth factor-I increases trabecular bone formation and osteoblastic cell proliferation in unloaded rats. *Endocrinology*, 134, 1031–1038.
111. Manolagas SC, Jilka RL (1995). Bone marrow, cytokines, and bone remodeling. Emerging insights into the pathophysiology of osteoporosis. *N Engl J Med*, 332, 305–311.
112. Marieb EN, Hoehn K (2012). *Human Anatomy and Physiology*. US: Pearson.
113. Martin RB (1990). Effects of simulated weightlessness on bone properties in rats. *J Biomech*, 23, 1021–1029.
114. Martin TJ, Sims NA (2005). Osteoclast-derived activity in the coupling of bone formation to resorption. *Trends Mol Med*, 11: 76–81.
115. Mateus J, Hargens AR (2012). Photoplethysmography for non-invasive in vivo measurement of bone hemodynamics. *Physiol Meas*, 33, 1027–1042.
116. Mateus J, Hargens AR (2013). Bone hemodynamic responses to changes in external pressure. *Bone*, 52, 604–610.
117. Mazziotti G, Canalis E, Giustina A (2010). Drug-induced osteoporosis: Mechanisms and clinical implications. *Am J Med*, 123, 877–884.
118. McCarthy I (2006). The physiology of bone blood flow: A review. *J Bone Joint Surg Am*, 88(Suppl 3), 4–9.
119. Misra D, Berry SD, Broe KE, McLean RR, Cupples LA, *et al.* (2011). Does dietary protein reduce hip fracture risk in elders? The Framingham Osteoporosis Study. *Osteoporos Int*, 22, 345–349.
120. Morey-Holton ER, Globus RK (1998) Hindlimb unloading of growing rats: a model for predicting skeletal changes during space flight. Bone 22: 83S-88S.
121. Morey-Holton ER, Globus RK (2002). Hindlimb unloading rodent model: technical aspects. *J Appl Physiol* (1985), 92, 1367–1377.
122. Morey ER (1979). Spaceflight and bone turnover: Correlation with a new rat model of weightlessness. *Bioscience*, 29, 168–172.
123. Mundy GR (2001). Osteoporosis: Pathophysiology and non-pharmacological management. *Best Pract Res Clin Rheumatol*, 15, 727–745.
124. Murshed M, Harmey D, Millan JL, McKee MD, Karsenty G (2005). Unique coexpression in osteoblasts of broadly expressed genes accounts for the spatial restriction of ECM mineralization to bone. *Genes Dev*, 19, 1093–1104.

125. Nadya Ugryumova, Matcher SJ, Attenburrow DP (2004). Measurement of bone mineral density via light scattering. *Phys Med Biol*, 49, 469–483.
126. Naslund J, Pettersson J, Lundeberg T, Linnarsson D, Lindberg LG (2006). Non-invasive continuous estimation of blood flow changes in human patellar bone. *Med Biol Eng Comput*, 44, 501–509.
127. Nelson GE Jr, Kelly PJ, Peterson LF, Janes JM (1960). Blood supply of the human tibia. *J Bone Joint Surg Am*, 42-A, 625–636.
128. Oldmeadow LB, Edwards ER, Kimmel LA, Kipen E, Robertson VJ, *et al.* (2006). No rest for the wounded: Early ambulation after hip surgery accelerates recovery. *ANZ J Surg*, 76, 607–611.
129. Olsen BR, Reginato AM, Wang W (2000). Bone development. *Annu Rev Cell Dev Biol*, 16, 191–220.
130. Owan I, Burr DB, Turner CH, Qiu J, Tu Y, *et al.* (1997). Mechanotransduction in bone: Osteoblasts are more responsive to fluid forces than mechanical strain. *Am J Physiol*, 273, C810–C815.
131. Ozcivici E, Garman R, Judex S (2007). High-frequency oscillatory motions enhance the simulated mechanical properties of non-weight bearing trabecular bone. *J Biomech*, 40, 3404–3411.
132. Özkaya N, Özkaya N (2012). *Fundamentals of Biomechanics: Equilibrium, Motion, and Deformation.* New York: Springer Verlag, xvii, 275.
133. Pavy-Le Traon A, Heer M, Narici MV, Rittweger J, Vernikos J (2007). From space to Earth: Advances in human physiology from 20 years of bed rest studies (1986–2006). *Eur J Appl Physiol*, 101, 143–194.
134. Piekarski K, Munro M (1977). Transport mechanism operating between blood supply and osteocytes in long bones. *Nature*, 269, 80–82.
135. Pifferi A, Torricelli A, Taroni P, Bassi A, Chikoidze E, *et al.* (2004). Optical biopsy of bone tissue: Astep toward the diagnosis of bone pathologies. *J Biomed Optics*, 9, 474–480.
136. Portero P, Vanhoutte C, Goubel F (1996). Surface electromyogram power spectrum changes in human leg muscles following fourweeks of simulated microgravity. *Eur J Appl Physiol Occup Physiol*, 73, 340–345.
137. Price C, Zhou X, Li W, Wang L (2011). Real-time measurement of solute transport within the lacunar-canalicular system of mechanically loaded bone: Direct evidence for load-induced fluid flow. *J Bone Miner Res*, 26, 277–285.
138. Raggatt LJ, Partridge NC (2010). Cellular and molecular mechanisms of bone remodeling. *J Biol Chem*, 285, 25103–25108.
139. Ray RD, Kawabata M, Galante J (1967). Experimental study of peripheral circulation and bone growth: An experimental method for the quantitative determination of bone blood flow. *Clin Orthop Relat Res*, 54, 175–185.
140. Reich KM, Frangos JA (1991). Effect of flow on prostaglandin E2 and inositol trisphosphate levels in osteoblasts. *Am J Physiol*, 261, C428–C432.
141. Reich KM, Frangos JA (1993). Protein kinase C mediates flow-induced prostaglandin E2 production in osteoblasts. *Calcif Tissue Int*, 52, 62–66.

142. Reich KM, Gay CV, Frangos JA (1990). Fluid shear stress as a mediator of osteoblast cyclic adenosine monophosphate production. *J Cell Physiol*, 143, 100–104.
143. Rhinelander FW, Baragry R (1962). Microangiography in bone healing: I. Undisplaced closed fractures. *J Bone Joint Surg Am*, 44-A, 1273–1298.
144. Rhinelander FW, Phillips RS, Steel WM, Beer JC (1968). Microangiography in bone healing: II. Displaced closed fractures. *J Bone Joint Surg Am*, 50, 643–662 passim.
145. Richards JB, Zheng HF, Spector TD (2012). Genetics of osteoporosis from genome-wide association studies: Advances and challenges. *Nat Rev Genet*, 13, 576–588.
146. Rittweger J, Frost HM, Schiessl H, Ohshima H, Alkner B, *et al.* (2005). Muscle atrophy and bone loss after 90 days'bed rest and the effects of flywheel resistive exercise and pamidronate: Results from the LTBR study. *Bone*, 36, 1019–1029.
147. Roer RD, Dillaman RM (1990). Bone growth and calcium balance during simulated weightlessness in the rat. *J Appl Physiol*, (1985) 68, 13–20.
148. Roer RD, Dillaman RM (1994). Decreased femoral arterial flow during simulated microgravity in the rat. *J Appl Physiol*(1985), 76, 2125–2129.
149. Rubin C, Recker R, Cullen D, Ryaby J, McCabe J, *et al.* (2004). Prevention of postmenopausal bone loss by a low-magnitude, high-frequency mechanical stimuli: Aclinical trial assessing compliance, efficacy, and safety. *J Bone Miner Res*, 19, 343–351.
150. Rubin C, Turner AS, Bain S, Mallinckrodt C, McLeod K (2001). Anabolism: Low mechanical signals strengthen long bones. *Nature*, 412, 603–604.
151. Rubin C, Turner AS, Mallinckrodt C, Jerome C, McLeod K, *et al.* (2002). Mechanical strain, induced noninvasively in the high-frequency domain, is anabolic to cancellous bone, but not cortical bone. *Bone*, 30, 445–452.
152. Rubin C, Turner AS, Muller R, Mittra E, McLeod K, *et al.* (2002). Quantity and quality of trabecular bone in the femur are enhanced by a strongly anabolic, noninvasive mechanical intervention. *J Bone Miner Res*, 17, 349–357.
153. Rubin C, Xu G, Judex S (2001). The anabolic activity of bone tissue, suppressed by disuse, is normalized by brief exposure to extremely low-magnitude mechanical stimuli. *FASEB J*, 15, 2225–2229.
154. Rubin CT, Sommerfeldt DW, Judex S, Qin Y (2001). Inhibition of osteopenia by low magnitude, high-frequency mechanical stimuli. *Drug Discov Today*, 6, 848–858.
155. Russo CR, Lauretani F, Bandinelli S, Bartali B, Cavazzini C, *et al.* (2003). High-frequency vibration training increases muscle power in postmenopausal women. *Arch Phys Med Rehabil*, 84, 1854–1857.
156. Salzstein RA, Pollack SR (1987). Electromechanical potentials in cortical bone: II. Experimental analysis. *J Biomech*, 20, 271–280.
157. Salzstein RA, Pollack SR, Mak AF, Petrov N (1987). Electromechanical potentials in cortical bone: I. A continuum approach. *J Biomech*, 20, 261–270.

158. Sandberg M, Lindberg LG, Gerdle B (2004). Peripheral effects of needle stimulation (acupuncture) on skin and muscle blood flow in fibromyalgia. *Eur J Pain*, 8, 163–171.
159. Schubert R, Mulvany MJ (1999). The myogenic response: established facts and attractive hypotheses. *Clin Sci (Lond)*, 96, 313–326.
160. Seliger WG (1970). Tissue fluid movement in compact bone. *Anat Rec*, 166, 247–255.
161. Semb H (1971). Effect of vasoactive drugs on the bone marrow blood flow. *Acta Orthop Scand*, 42, 10–17.
162. Serre CM, Farlay D, Delmas PD, Chenu C (1999). Evidence for a dense and intimate innervation of the bone tissue, including glutamate-containing fibers. *Bone*, 25, 623–629.
163. Sessions ND, Halloran BP, Bikle DD, Wronski TJ, Cone CM, *et al.* (1989). Bone response to normal weight bearing after a period of skeletal unloading. *Am J Physiol*, 257, E606–E610.
164. Shackelford LC, LeBlanc AD, Driscoll TB, Evans HJ, Rianon NJ, *et al.* (2004). Resistance exercise as a countermeasure to disuse-induced bone loss. *J Appl Physiol* (1985), 97, 119–129.
165. Shaw SR, Zernicke RF, Vailas AC, DeLuna D, Thomason DB, *et al.* (1987). Mechanical, morphological and biochemical adaptations of bone and muscle to hindlimb suspension and exercise. *J Biomech*, 20, 225–234.
166. Shim SS (1968). Physiology of blood circulation of bone. *J Bone Joint Surg Am*, 50, 812–824.
167. Shim SS, Copp DH, Patterson FP (1966). Bone blood flow in the limb following complete sciatic nerve section. *Surg Gynecol Obstet*, 123, 333–335.
168. Sim FH, Kelly PJ (1970). Relationship of bone remodeling, oxygen consumption, and blood flow in bone. *J Bone Joint Surg Am*, 52, 1377–1389.
169. Singh JA, Schmitz KH, Petit MA (2009). Effect of resistance exercise on bone mineral density in premenopausal women. *Joint Bone Spine*, 76, 273–280.
170. Siris ES, Miller PD, Barrett-Connor E, Faulkner KG, Wehren LE, *et al.* (2001). Identification and fracture outcomes of undiagnosed low bone mineral density in postmenopausal women: Results from the National Osteoporosis Risk Assessment. *JAMA*, 286, 2815–2822.
171. Smith SM, Davis-Street JE, Rice BL, Nillen JL, Gillman PL, *et al.* (2001). Nutritional status assessment in semiclosed environments: Ground-based and space flight studies in humans. *J Nutr*, 131, 2053–2061.
172. Smith SM, Nillen JL, Leblanc A, Lipton A, Demers LM, *et al.* (1998). Collagen cross-link excretion during space flight and bed rest. *J Clin Endocrinol Metab*, 83, 3584–3591.
173. Sommerfeldt DW, Rubin CT (2001). Biology of bone and how it orchestrates the form and function of the skeleton. *Eur Spine J*, 10(Suppl 2), S86–S95.
174. Spengler DM, Morey ER, Carter DR, Turner RT, Baylink DJ (1983). Effects of spaceflight on structural and material strength of growing bone. *Proc Soc Exp Biol Med*, 174, 224–228.

175. Stabley JN, Prisby RD, Behnke BJ, Delp MD (2013). Chronic skeletal unloading of the rat femur: Mechanisms and functional consequences of vascular remodeling. *Bone*, 57, 355–360.
176. Street J, Bao M, deGuzman L, Bunting S, Peale FV, Jr., *et al.* (2002). Vascular endothelial growth factor stimulates bone repair by promoting angiogenesis and bone turnover. *Proc Natl Acad Sci USA*, 99, 9656–9661.
177. Suzuki Y, Akima H, Igawa S, Fukunaga T, Kawakub K, *et al.* (1996). Decrease of bone mineral density and muscle and/or strength in the leg during 20 days horizontal bed rest. *J Gravit Physiol*, 3, 42–43.
178. Totosy de Zepetnek JO, Giangregorio LM, Craven BC (2009). Whole-body vibration as potential intervention for people with low bone mineral density and osteoporosis: Areview. *J Rehabil Res Dev*, 46, 529–542.
179. Trappe SW, Trappe TA, Lee GA, Widrick JJ, Costill DL, *et al.* (2001). Comparison of a space shuttle flight (STS-78) and bed rest on human muscle function. *J Appl Physiol* (1985), 91, 57–64.
180. Uebelhart D, Bernard J, Hartmann DJ, Moro L, Roth M, *et al.* (2000). Modifications of bone and connective tissue after orthostatic bedrest. *Osteoporos Int*, 11, 59–67.
181. Vailas AC, Deluna DM, Lewis LL, Curwin SL, Roy RR, *et al.* (1988). Adaptation of bone and tendon to prolonged hindlimb suspension in rats. *J Appl Physiol* (1985), 65, 373–376.
182. van der Meulen MC, Morey-Holton ER, Carter DR (1995). Hindlimb suspension diminishes femoral cross-sectional growth in the rat. *J Orthop Res*, 13, 700–707.
183. Verschueren SM, Roelants M, Delecluse C, Swinnen S, Vanderschueren D, *et al.* (2004). Effect of six-month whole body vibration training on hip density, muscle strength, and postural control in postmenopausal women: Arandomized controlled pilot study. *J Bone Miner Res*, 19, 352–359.
184. Vico L, Bourrin S, Novikov V, Very JM, Chappard D, *et al.* (1991). Adaptation of bone cellular activities to tail suspension in rats. *Cells and Materials*, 143–150.
185. Vico L, Bourrin S, Very JM, Radziszowska M, Collet P, *et al.* (1995). Bone changes in six-month-old rats after head-down suspension and a reambulation period. *J Appl Physiol* (1985), 79, 1426–1433.
186. Vico L, Novikov VE, Very JM, Alexandre C (1991). Bone histomorphometric comparison of rat tibial metaphysis after 7-day tail suspension vs 7-day spaceflight. *Aviat Space Environ Med,* 62, 26–31.
187. Wallace AL, Draper ER, Strachan RK, McCarthy ID, Hughes SP (1991). The effect of devascularisation upon early bone healing in dynamic external fixation. *J Bone Joint Surg Br*, 73, 819–825.
188. Warriner AH, Saag KG (2013). Osteoporosis diagnosis and medical treatment. *Orthop Clin North Am*, 44, 125–135.

189. Weinbaum S, Cowin SC, Zeng Y (1994). A model for the excitation of osteocytes by mechanical loading-induced bone fluid shear stresses. *J Biomech*, 27, 339–360.
190. Weiss L (1984). *The Blood Cells and Hematopoietic Tissues.* New York: Elsevier.
191. Widrick JJ, Knuth ST, Norenberg KM, Romatowski JG, Bain JL, *et al.* (1999). Effect of a 17-day spaceflight on contractile properties of human soleus muscle fibres. *J Physiol*, 516(Pt 3), 915–930.
192. Widrick JJ, Romatowski JG, Norenberg KM, Knuth ST, Bain JL, *et al.* (2001). Functional properties of slow and fast gastrocnemius muscle fibers after a 17-day spaceflight. *J Appl Physiol* (1985), 90, 2203–2211.
193. Wilkerson MK, Lesniewski LA, Golding EM, Bryan RM, Jr., Amin A, *et al.* (2005). Simulated microgravity enhances cerebral artery vasoconstriction and vascular resistance through endothelial nitric oxide mechanism. *Am J Physiol Heart Circ Physiol*, 288, H1652–H1661.
194. Wilkerson MK, Muller-Delp J, Colleran PN, Delp MD (1999). Effects of hindlimb unloading on rat cerebral, splenic, and mesenteric resistance artery morphology. *J Appl Physiol* (1985), 87, 2115–2121.
195. Wolff I, van Croonenborg JJ, Kemper HC, Kostense PJ, Twisk JW (1999). The effect of exercise training programs on bone mass: A meta-analysis of published controlled trials in pre- and postmenopausal women. *Osteoporos Int*, 9, 1–12.
196. Wolff J (1892). *Das Gesetz der Transformation der Knochen.* Berlin: A Hirshwald.
197. Wray JB (1964). Acute changes in femoral arterial blood flow after closed tibial fracture in dogs. *J Bone Joint Surg Am*, 46, 1262–1268.
198. Wray JB, Lynch CJ (1959). The vascular response to fracture of the tibia in the rat. *J Bone Joint Surg Am*, 41-A, 1143–1148.
199. Wronski TJ, Morey-Holton ER (1987). Skeletal response to simulated weightlessness: Acomparison of suspension techniques. *Aviat Space Environ Med*, 58, 63–68.
200. Xie L, Jacobson JM, Choi ES, Busa B, Donahue LR, *et al.* (2006). Low-level mechanical vibrations can influence bone resorption and bone formation in the growing skeleton. *Bone*, 39, 1059–1066.
201. You L, Cowin SC, Schaffler MB, Weinbaum S (2001). A model for strain amplification in the actin cytoskeleton of osteocytes due to fluid drag on pericellular matrix. *J Biomech*, 34, 1375–1386.
202. Zhang Q, Andersson G, Lindberg LG, Styf J (2004). Muscle blood flow in response to concentric muscular activity vs passive venous compression. *Acta Physiol Scand*, 180, 57–62.
203. Zhang Q, Ericson K, Styf J (2003). Blood flow in the tibialis anterior muscle by photoplethysmography during foot-transmitted vibration. *Eur J Appl Physiol*, 90, 464–469.

204. Zhang Q, Lindberg LG, Kadefors R, Styf J (2001). A non-invasive measure of changes in blood flow in the human anterior tibial muscle. *Eur J Appl Physiol*, 84, 448–452.
205. Zhang Q, Styf J (2004). Abnormally elevated intramuscular pressure impairs muscle blood flow at rest after exercise. *Scand J Med Sci Sports*, 14, 215–220.
206. Zhang R, Supowit SC, Klein GL, Lu Z, Christensen MD, *et al.* (1995). Rat tail suspension reduces messenger RNA level for growth factors and osteopontin and decreases the osteoblastic differentiation of bone marrow stromal cells. *J Bone Miner Res*,10, 415–423.

CHAPTER 13

CIRCULATION OF THE PEDIATRIC AND ADOLESCENT HIP

JEREMY DOAK

Associate Professor of Clinical Orthopaedics
School of Medicine Biomedical Sciences
State University of New York, Buffalo, NY

JONATHAN SCHILLER

Assistant Professor of Orthopaedic Surgery
The Warren Alpert Medical School of Brown University, Providence, RI

CRAIG EBERSON

Associate Professor of Orthopaedic Surgery
The Warren Alpert Medical School of Brown University, Providence, RI

13.1 Development of the Vascularity of the Hip

Managing disorders affecting the vascularity of the hip remains a challenging dilemma for orthopaedic surgeons. From pediatric patients afflicted with Legg-Calve-Perthes disease or slipped capital femoral epiphysis to adults with post-traumatic avascular necrosis (AVN) of the femoral head, conditions injuring the blood supply to the femoral head continue to result in long-term poor clinical outcomes.

In order to better understand this pathology, we must first understand the natural anatomy of the hip, and in particular, its vascular supply.

13.1.1 *Embryology of the hip*

The embryonic stage of human development encompasses approximately the initial eight weeks of development following fertilization of the oocyte. During the latter half of the embryonic stage, a majority of joint differentiation is completed. The remaining period of gestations is termed the fetal stage. It is during this time that the limbs and joints undergo continuing growth, maturation, and differentiation in preestablished spatial orientations.[82]

Limb formation begins at four weeks of intrauterine life with protrusions of the ventro-lateral wall of the embryo, or terminal buds.The limb buds consist of an outer ectoderm shell and an inner cellular mass of mesoderm. Bone, cartilage, muscle, tendon, and the joints arise from the mesoderm layer.[59] The ectoderm gives rise to the skin, nails, and hair of the developing limb. At about six weeks following fertilization, the lower limb buds have continued to elongate and form terminal footplates. From these structures, cellular multiplication and differentiation continue to form a club-shaped cartilage model of the future femur. Chondroblasts condense at the proximal, central, and distal ends of the femoral template. Continued chondrification of precursor cells and fusion of the primitive chondrification centers leads to formation of the complete cartilaginous model of the femur by about seven weeks of gestation.

Similarly, the acetabulum develops concurrently with the fusion of the primitive ilium, pubis, and ischium. The ilium and ischium are first to fuse, followed by the ilium and pubis. This occurs in rapid progression until finally the pubis and ischium coalesce during the seventh week of embryonic development. These two ossification centers leave a small opening laterally that results in formation of the acetabular fossa.[84] At this stage in the late embryonic period, both the femoral and acetabular cartilaginous models have been fully formed. The mass of cells between these models now undergoes apoptosis to yield the beginning of the future synovial hip joint.[84]

During the eighth week of development, the primary ossification center of the femur appears in its shaft. Ossification proceeds both distally and proximally from this center. Concurrently, the arterial supply to the proximal femur begins its development with the appearance of the primary ossification center.[82]

13.1.2 *Fetal development of the arterial supply to the hip*

At about the time of the transition from the embryonic to fetal stages of development, the primary ossification center of the femoral shaft has fully developed. Concurrently, capillaries deliver fibroblastic and hematopoietic cells into the marrow by breaking through the periosteum at the middle third of the femoral shaft cartilaginous *anlage*. This corresponds to the level of the adult nutrient artery. For the next four to six weeks, this remains the only feeding vasculature for the entire femur.[82] At about 12 to 14 weeks, a vasculature ring forms around the neck of the femur, giving rise to the future medial and lateral circumflex vessels. The obturator and superior and inferior gluteal vessels also arise from this early vascular ring.[59] Blood vessels connected to this ring invade the head and neck of the femur to give rise to the future retinacular vessels vital to the perfusion of the fully developed proximal femur.

The formation of the blood supply to the acetabulum, similar to the development of the cartilaginous model, proceeds just after initiation of the arterial supply to the proximal femur. This occurs at 12–14 weeks of development. There is evidence of capillary invasion into the pulvinar and ligamentum teres at around eight weeks. However, the significance of this blood flow to the future development of the hip is controversial. The contribution of the ligamentum teres and pulvinar to the blood flow to the hip remains a disputed topic throughout the development and the life of the hip joint. No anastomosis with the arterial terminals in the femoral head was observed by Strayer until around age 15.[82] At this stage, ossification of the femoral head is generally nearly complete, if not fully complete. Only one out of seven fetuses that he examined demonstrated vessels entering the femoral head from the ligamentum teres.These findings suggest that the artery of the ligamentum teres does not seem to contribute significantly to the development of the femoral head. Clinically, this holds true in the treatment of the dysplastic hip undergoing osteotomy and open reduction of the hip joint itself. During the procedure, the ligamentum teres is routinely sectioned as it has become elongated and redundant due to lateral subluxation of the femoral head from the acetabulum. This increased size and length make it a block to concentric reduction of the femoral head into the acetabulum. Routinely, the ligamentum teres is completely excised. Clinically, this has not been reported to cause adverse consequences to the further development of the femoral head.

13.1.3 *Childhood arterial supply to the hip*

The arterial supply to the proximal femur and acetabulum established during fetal life largely endures throughout remaining childhood. Chung demonstrated this in a perfusion study of fetuses and children aged 26 weeks to 14 years.[18]

An extracapsular arterial ring formed by the conjoining of branches from the medial and lateral circumflex arteries gives rise to ascending retinacular or cervical vessels that enter the proximal aspect of the hip joint capsule. These retinacular vessels ascend the femoral neck intra-articularly toward the femoral head. They are divided into four groups based upon their location on the femoral neck: lateral, posterior, medial, and anterior. Branches of the retinacular arteries enter the femoral neck to supply the greater trochanter laterally and the femoral neck medially, or anastomose with the ascending nutrient vessels from the femoral shaft.[59] As the cervical vessels continue to track proximally, they form another anastomosis at the junction of the femoral neck and the articular cartilage of the femoral head.[59] This gives rise to an intra-articular subsynovial ring. This ring in turn gives rise to epiphyseal and metaphyseal branches which provide arterial nourishment to the most proximal portion of the femur. The metaphyseal branches invade the femoral neck and proceed distally. The epiphyseal branches gain access to the epiphysis by crossing the perichondrial ring superficially and then entering the cartilaginous femoral head. None of these vessels directly transverse the physeal plate.

The subsynovial ring can sometimes be incomplete. This is more common in males and may have implications in the predilection of Legg-Calve-Perthes disease in the male gender. The ring is also typically more robust on the medial and lateral aspects of the femoral neck as compared to the anterior and posterior surfaces.[18]

The overall redundancy of the blood supply of the acetabulum makes pathologic conditions resulting from interruption of blood flow to this area far less of a clinical concern. The adult blood supply of the acetabulum is established early in development and has no significant alterations from childhood anatomy. Branches of the superior gluteal artery supply the acetabular dome with blood flow, whereas the inferior gluteal artery provides nutrient vessels to the medial acetabulum. Finally, a posterior branch of the obturator artery provides nourishment to the inferior acetabular bone (Fig. 13.1).[72] An extensive network of intra- and extraosseous anastomoses between these vessels makes AVN of the acetabulum extremely rare.[59] This is true even in the setting of various methods of pelvic osteotomy done for the treatment of any number of hip disorders in the young child.

The physeal plate provides the main anatomic variation in the proximal femur of children as compared to mature adults. This cartilaginous growth plate serves as a barrier to vessels, which do not cross it. As discussed above, the ephiphyseal branches of the subsynovial ring formed from the anastomosis of the ascending cervical arteries, reach the femoral head by

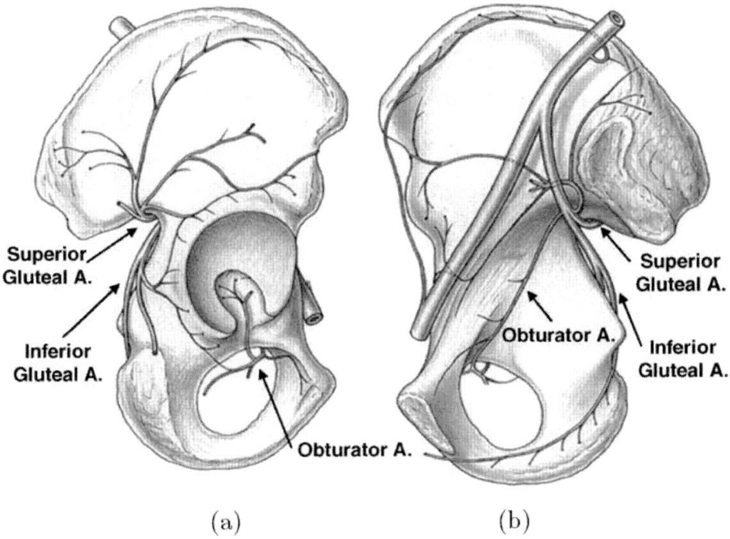

Fig. 13.1. Lateral (a) and medial (b) views of the right acetabulum with its associated vascular supply. Note the clockwise arrangement of the superior gluteal artery, obturator artery, and inferior gluteal artery contributions to the acetabulum. *Source*: Beck M, Leunig M, Ellis T, Sledge B, Ganz R (2003). The acetabular blood supply: Implications for periacetabular osteotomies. *Surg Radiol Anat*, 361–367. Reproduced with permission.

tracking along the periphery of the physis at the perichondrial ring. There is, however, an extraosseous anastomosis of the intraosseous circulation of the neck and head of the femur at the subsynovial ring. When the physis closes at maturity, vessels can then course through the femoral neck to the femoral head and form an intraosseous connection.[20]

It is widely recognized that in the mature adult, the medial circumflex artery and its terminal branch, the lateral portion of the extracapsular arterial ring, provide the majority of the blood supply to the femoral head, neck, and great trochanter.[18] Gautier *et al.* described the anatomy of the medial circumflex artery in great detail by examining 24 cadaveric hips.[31] They described five consistent branches: deep, descending, acetabular, ascending, and superficial. The deep branch was found to enter the hip capsule and divide into terminal branches termed the lateral epiphyseal arteries. These arteries would in turn course beneath the synovial sheath of the reflected capsule posterosuperiorly to insert into the neck of the femur.[31,79] A maturation process occurs in the circulation of the proximal femur throughout childhood to result in this supply. Whereas the number of lateral and posterior ascending cervical arteries remains constant through maturation, the number of vessels along the anterior and medial femoral neck decreases by about 50%.[18] This was confirmed in a separate study by Lauritzen that demonstrated that the lateral retinacular arteries supply the majority of blood supply to the femoral head by the age of ten.[58] Also during the course of development, independent vascular territories in the femoral head defined by the epiphyseal branches supplying their blood flow coalesce into a larger network via anastomoses between the vascular zones. This network may not be complete, and therefore occlusion of specific ascending retinacular arteries may cause necrosis of specific defined anatomic zones.[59]

With a clearer understanding of the normal vascular supply to the hip, we can understand more fully the clinical conditions that cause injury to this system of vasculature and the resulting pathology.

13.2 Traumatic Clinical Conditions Related to Pathologic Vascularity

13.2.1 *Femoral neck fractures*

AVN following femoral neck fractures in children is a known and feared phenomenon.There is no general consensus on the exact causative factor in the development of interrupted blood flow following trauma to the femoral neck. More likely, a combination of factors plays a role in the development of AVN. Moon and Mehlman performed a systematic review of 360 cases of femoral neck fracture in children aged 1 to 16 years old and found that fracture type, displacement, age of the patient, and treatment type were all independent predictors of AVN.[66] However, after performing logistic regression analysis, fracture type and age were the only two statistically significant variables with regard to the development of AVN. Transphyseal and transcervical fractures were associated with the highest rates of AVN. Intracapsular fractures were demonstrated to have a 14-fold increase in the frequency of AVN as compared to extracapsular fractures (Table 13.1). Extracapsular fractures likely cause less direct injury to the subsynovial ring, which provides blood flow to the proximal femoral epiphysis.

In addition, with each advancing year of age, the older child was 1.14 times more likely to develop AVN.[66] A number of studies have supported higher rates of AVN in older children as compared to their younger counterparts.[50, 66, 73] With the changing vascularity of the proximal femur discussed

Table 13.1. AVN risk as related to location of femoral neck fracture.

Fracture Location	% Cases	AVN %
Transepiphyseal	8.1	38
Transcervical	40.3	28
Cervicotrochanteric	33.3	18
Intertrochanteric	18.3	5

Adapted from Moon ES, Mehlman CT. (2006). Risk factors for avascular necrosis after femoral neck fractures in children: 25 Cincinnati cases and meta-analysis of 360 cases. *J Orthop Trauma*, 323–329. Reprinted with permission.

above, this may be a predictable consequence. The physis remains open, thus inhibiting intraosseous blood supply to the femoral head. Also, the number of retinacular vessels decreases, particularly those along the anterior and medial femoral neck. The younger child seems to have an increased ability to revascularize and remodel the femoral head, possibly due to the more abundant collateral blood flow to the femoral head during earlier ages in childhood prior to the loss of those ascending cervical vessels originating from the lateral circumflex artery.

There is a general consensus that displacement of a femoral neck fracture is an important predictor in the development of AVN.[66] This would seem to be consistent with the hypothesis that AVN results from direct trauma to the retinacular vessels supplying the proximal femur. However, this does not offer an explanation as to the development of AVN following non-displaced femoral neck fractures. It has been hypothesized that increased intracapsular pressure following an acute hemarthrosis from an intracapsular fracture, can cause a tamponade effect and compromise blood flow to the femoral epiphysis. It has been suggested by some authors that treatment of acute femoral neck fractures should include a decompression of the hip joint capsule. However, the protective nature of this procedure has not been convincingly demonstrated in the literature to date. By the above rationale, a displaced fracture could be somewhat protective by causing a rupture of the hip joint capsule and thus preventing this tamponade effect.

There is conflict in the existing literature relating to the role of surgical intervention in the development of AVN. This is clearly very difficult to assess due to the constantly evolving surgical techniques, implantable devices available for fixation, and treatment protocols utilized to treat the acute femoral neck fracture. Currently, it is generally felt that obtaining an anatomic reduction and providing stable fixation is the standard of care in treating these fractures. This provides the appropriate anatomic scaffolding that the vascularity of the hip depends upon. Displaced fractures may cause spasm or occlusion of retinacular vessels and thereby diminish blood flow to the femoral head. By restoring proper anatomy, the spasm or occlusion of injured, but not ruptured; vessels may resolve and re-establish blood flow to the femoral head. Conversely, there is literature demonstrating that repeated reduction attempts or the use of internal fixation can cause further damage to the blood supply to the femoral head and increase the risk of AVN.[25,73] However, there is significant selection bias in many of the studies demonstrating poor outcomes in operatively treated patients. The operatively treated patients tended to have more displaced fractures that could certainly have had more damage to the retinacular vessels even prior to surgical intervention. More recent studies have shown better outcomes with early reduction and fixation of displaced femoral neck fractures, sometimes with arthrotomy of the hip capsule as well.[17,26,81] Dendane *et al.* demonstrated that a delay in reduction greater than 48 hours was an independent risk factor for the development of AVN as well.[22]

The data outlined above, as well as the vast amounts of data existing in the orthopedic literature, do not associate the development of AVN following a femoral neck fracture with one specific risk factor. Rather, progression to AVN likely develops due to the interrelationship of a number of factors including the location of the fracture, the age of the patient, and non-iatrogenic and iatrogenic trauma to the retinacular vessels supplying the femoral head. Our understanding of the anatomy of the blood supply to the proximal femur can help the physician counsel patients about the risks of developing AVN after a femoral neck fracture. Unfortunately, the currently available knowledge base does not offer a reliable method of preventing AVN or successfully treating AVN after it develops.

13.2.2 *Slipped capital femoral epiphysis*

Although not technically the same as a transphyseal fracture of the femoral neck, a slipped capital femoral epiphysis (SCFE) has similarities to an acute femoral neck fracture, particularly as it pertains to the development of AVN. Unlike a femoral neck fracture, which results from acute high-energy trauma, a SCFE is thought to occur through a diseased and weakened physis with minimal to no trauma. The femoral head remains in the acetabulum, retroverted from the femoral neck and shaft, which have displaced anteriorly. Much research has been directed to the study of AVN resulting from SCFE due to reports that the treatment of SCFE resulted in iatrogenic disruption of the blood flow to the proximal femur during manipulation of displaced SCFEs.[14,16] This has numerous medical legal implications to the practicing orthopaedic surgeon.

A differentiation must be made between an unstable and stable slipped capital femoral epiphysis. This classification first described by Loder has important treatment and prognostic implications. A stable SCFE is defined by Loder as an SCFE upon which the child can bear weight, with or without the use of assistive devices. The patient with an unstable slip cannot bear weight at all on the injured extremity. The practical implications of this classification system are that the stable SCFE tends to be the result of a slowly progressive and chronic developing deformity. In contrast, the unstable SCFE is more of an acute event involving significant deformity, which develops nearly instantaneously. The ramifications for the development of AVN cannot be overstated. Whereas the stable SCFE has a very low rate of AVN approaching zero,[16,38,69] the unstable SCFE has rates of AVN reported as high as 50%.

The pathoanatomy of an unstable SCFE is likely quite similar to that of an acute femoral neck fracture, particularly as it pertains to the development of AVN. An angiographic study performed by Maeda *et al.* elegantly described the vascular anatomy of the retinacular vasculature as it relates to SCFE.[63] They demonstrated via selective angiography of the medial circumflex artery that the posterior ascending cervical branch was filled in all stable SCFE hips. The superior retinacular artery branching off the posterior ascending cervical artery formed an acute angle with that feeding vessel as it coursed posteromedially to the retroverted femoral head. However, all five stable SCFEs studied had intact perfusion of both of these vessels. This was found independent to the degree of slip, or amount of deformity that occurred as a result of the SCFE. Of the five unstable SCFE hips examined, the posterior ascending cervical artery was filled in two out of the five hips. Of the three hips that did not show filling of the posterior ascending cervical artery, one went on to develop AVN. Interestingly, an angiographic exam was conducted on one unstable slip before and after a gentle manipulation to correct the alignment of the proximal femur. In that particular hip, there was no flow in the posterior ascending cervical artery prior to manipulation. However, there was reconstitution of flow following gentle manipulation into correct anatomy. These findings seem to suggest that the vascular insult occurs at the time of an acute unstable slip due to interruption of blood flow through the ascending cervical arteries. This is similar to the likely pathoanatomy in the acute fracture of the femoral neck. This interruption, at least in some patients, can be due to a kinking of the vessels, which can be relieved by manipulation back into correct anatomy. It is important to note, however, that this does not take into account possible surgical damage to the vasculature caused by an open approach to the hip.

Many studies have demonstrated much lower rates of femoral head AVN in stable as opposed to unstable SCFEs.[16, 38, 69] This is in concordance with the findings of Maeda *et al.* that demonstrated intact superior retinacular vessel flow in all stable slips.[63] This was independent of the degree of deformity noted and thought to be related to the slow development of femoral head retroversion in stable SCFEs. This theoretically gives the retinaculum and the retinacular vessels time to slowly stretch and accommodate the deformity. The angle between the posterior ascending cervical branch and the superior retinacular artery was found to be much more acute in stable SCFEs when compared to normal hips.[63]

13.2.3 *Fractures of the greater trochanter*

A rare complication of a rare injury provides more insight into the tenuous vascular supply to the proximal femur. As discussed previously, injury to the posterolateral branches of the medial circumflex artery has been associated with the development of AVN of the femoral head. There have been a few case reports in the literature describing AVN of the femoral head following greater trochanteric fracture of the proximal femur.[49, 62, 70]

In the developing child, the femoral capital epiphysis and greater trochanteric apophysis share a common physeal plate. The differential growth rates between the medial and lateral aspects of this physis during development leads to the final formation of the adult proximal femur. To review, Chung demonstrated that the greatest arterial supply to the femoral head originated from a branch of the medial circumflex femoral artery at the posterosuperior aspect of the hip capsule at the junction of the greater trochanter and the base of the femoral neck.[18] He termed this artery the lateral ascending cervical artery. This artery was often found to be a single artery crossing the base of the capsule prior to branching into multiple posterosuperior epiphyseal vessels and supplying the majority of blood to the growing femoral epiphysis.[18, 70] As the contribution from medial epiphyseal vessels decreases in the growing child, the lateral ascending cervical artery takes on much more importance. This is particularly true since Chung found only two of the 26 specimens that he examined had an anastomosis between the medial and lateral circumflex vessels.[18] Therefore, injury to the isolated lateral ascending cervical artery prior to closing of the proximal femoral physis causes an interruption to the majority of femoral head blood supply as there is no intraosseous route for blood flow into the proximal femoral epiphysis.

When the greater trochanter is fractured, particularly with anterior avulsion by the hip abductors, the medial circumflex artery can be disrupted.[70] At this terminal location, it is tethered by the lateral ascending cervical artery and the descending metaphyseal arteries piercing the femoral neck proximal to the physis, making it susceptible to injury.

13.2.4 *Hip dislocation*

The mechanism by which dislocation of the femoroacetabular joint results in AVN of the femoral head is thought to be similar to those discussed in relation to femoral neck fracture, SCFE, and greater trochanteric fracture. A direct traumatic injury, by longitudinal stretch and resulting vessel spasm or avulsion, limits blood flow to the susceptible femoral head circulation resulting in AVN.

13.3 Histology of Avascular Necrosis

The earliest histologic change noted in AVN is diffuse cell death in the marrow space, disorganization of the marrow stroma, and loss of osteoblasts lining the trabeculae.[55] Empty lacunae appear in the necrotic bone within a few weeks. Chondronecrosis of the deep layer of articular cartilage surrounding the secondary ossification center occurs shortly after the onset of necrosis.[53] The physis, however, shows limited cell death; what cell death does occur, happens on the epiphyseal side of the physis.[52] The vascularity of the metaphysis and femoral neck is well maintained by the anastomoses with the femoral shaft circulation. Revascularization of the femoral head occurs via fibrovascular tissue invasion of the necrotic marrow and bone.[54] Osteoclast activity is then observed to return in this area; however, osteoblastic bone formation does not seem to immediately return. The mechanical failure allowing collapse of the femoral head may likely involve the loss of normal bone metabolism as evidenced by the loss of normal balanced osteoblastic and osteoclastic activity.

The clear understanding of the vasculature of the proximal femur in the normal hip as well as the anatomy of the vasculature in the traumatized hip can aid in the medical decision-making process for patients suffering from these injuries. This can help aid in treatment as well as in patient education about treatment options and prognosis following these conditions.

13.4 Non-Traumatic Clinical Conditions Related to Pathologic Vascularity

13.4.1 *Legg-Calve-Perthes disease*

Legg-Calve-Perthes (Perthes) disease is a self-limiting idiopathic condition of the hip in young children leading to osteonecrosis of the femoral head, which progresses through four distinct radiographic stages. During the first, or initial, stage the femoral head ossific nucleus appears more radiodense and smaller than the unaffected side. The medial joint space also appears wider, likely due to hypertrophy of the epiphyseal cartilage. During the second, or fragmentation, stage, the ossific nucleus has areas of increased radiodensity and radiolucency giving the appearance of a "fragmenting" femoral head. The third, or reparative, stage is characterized by re-ossification of the ossific nucleus of the femoral head with return of more normal radiographic appearance of the bone density. In the final, or healed, stage, the process is completed and the proximal femur is left with any residual deformity. The spherecity of the femoral head and the congruency of the hip joint, at this stage ultimately determine the long-term prognosis as it relates to function of the hip, pain, and development of future osteoarthritis. Perthes disease cannot be compared with AVN following femoral neck fracture or slipped capital femoral epiphysis. Healing from these processes occurs rapidly without progressing through the prolonged stages of fragmentation and repair seen in Perthes disease.[76]

The presumed etiology of Perthes disease has gone through many iterations throughout the years of advancing medical knowledge. Most early theories centered on an inflammatory or infectious etiology.[74,75] Congenital and traumatic etiologies have also been proposed. However, most recent theories suggest some form of vascular embarrassment to the proximal femur. Hemodynamic alterations, endothelial injury, and hypercoagulability or hypofibrinolysis have all been proposed as possible pathogenic factors.[4]

Perthes disease is most common between the ages of four and eight, and also more common in the male gender by a 4:1 ratio when compared to females. These tendencies correlate well with Chung's findings of an incomplete subsynovial articular ring more commonly found in boys.[18] Also, as the child continues to mature, fewer vessels are present along the anterior and medial neck of the proximal femur to provide collateral flow to the femoral head, which could explain why Perthes is rarely seen prior to age four. The epiphyseal and metaphyseal branches of the lateral ascending cervical artery, which contribute the majority of the blood supply to the proximal femoral epiphysis, originate from a single vessel that crosses the trochanteric notch to pierce the hip capsule.[82] The space between the femoral neck and the trochanter is extremely narrow in children under the age of eight,[82] which results in this single artery being vulnerable to occlusion at this point as it crosses into the hip joint. Whatever blood supply to the femoral head arises from the ligamentum teres likely does not affect Perthes disease, as it has not been shown to vary by age or sex.[82]

Shore *et al.* examined 22 hips in 19 children with healed Perthes disease with high-resolution contrast-enhanced magnetic resonance imaging (MRI) to visualize the path of the medial circumflex artery and the lateral epiphyseal arterial branches supplying the femoral head.[79] That study demonstrated a significant decrease in lateral epiphyseal arteries inserting into the femoral head (2.63 on average) when compared to controls with developmental dysplasia of the hip (5.2 on average). In Chung's work, he identified an average of 4.1 lateral vessels in 150 pediatric specimens.[18] Shore also found that despite the fewer number of lateral epiphyseal vessels, their caliber also was diminished when compared to controls. These results were consistent with previous angiographic work done by Atsumi *et al.*, which demonstrated 68% of patients with Perthes disease had disruption of the true lateral epiphyseal artery at its origin at the joint capsule.[6] Their work also found that in the healing phase, the lateral epiphyseal arteries were small in caliber and in an irregular pattern.

A scintographic classification system based upon reperfusion of the lateral epiphyseal arteries has been proposed by Conway.[19] He and others hypothesize that the prognosis for children with Perthes disease is related to the reperfusion of the lateral epiphyseal arteries. In his classification system, he describes that revascularization can occur via two methods: either recanalization of the existing vessels which is a quick process, or by slower neovascularization through the development of new vessels. "Lateral column" visualization on bone scintography carries a good prognosis. However, neovascularization is demonstrated by a "mushroom filling" appearance and is associated with a poorer prognosis.[79] This system has clear parallels with the lateral pillar classification proposed by Herring that has widespread acceptance as an important prognostic indicator in Perthes disease. The Herring classification is based upon the radiographic maintenance of the height of the lateral pillar (lateral third) of the femoral head throughout the stages of Perthes disease.

Diffusion MRI has also been utilized to evaluate the changes in vascularity in the pathologic femoral neck of Perthes disease. It has been demonstrated that there is an early and significant increase in the apparent diffusion coefficient (ADC) in the femoral neck of a Perthes hip, when compared to normal controls.[13,43,60,65] This relates to an increase in neovascularization and revascularization occurring through the osseous femoral neck as opposed to through the lateral epiphyseal arteries (Fig. 13.2).

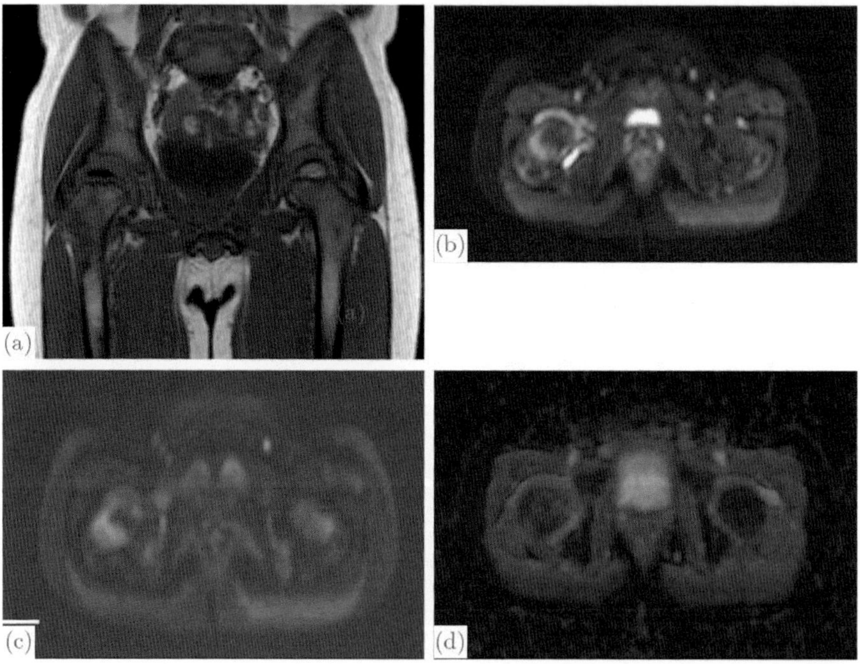

Fig. 13.2. Seven-year-old child, four months after the onset of symptoms: (a) T1 sequence LCPD on the right side in the fragmentation stage; (b) DWI: b0 cut passing through the necks of the femurs; (c) DWI: b1000 cut for the same area; (d) corresponding ADC cartography showing a hypersignal of the pathological side compared to the left side (ADC increase by 95%). *Source*: Boutault JR, Baunin C, Berard E, Vial J, Labarre D, Domenech C, Sales de Gauzy J, Sans N(2012). Diffusion MRI of the neck of the femur in Legg-Calve-Perthes disease: A preliminary study. *Diagn Interv Imaging*, 78–83. Reproduced with permission.

Much like Conway's scintographic data, higher ADCs are associated with more neovascularization of the femoral neck. This in turn correlates with decreased recanalization of the lateral epiphyseal arteries and a worse prognosis. Boutault *et al.* demonstrated a correlation between increase in ADC and the Catterall classification.[13] This classification system is based upon the radiographic appearance of femoral head involvement with hips having more complete epiphyseal involvement having higher scores and, therefore, worse prognoses.

An ultrasound study, demonstrated vascularity present in the pathologic epiphyseal cartilage of Perthes disease. When compared to asymptomatic hips with no evidence of Perthes disease, there was vascularity in the physeal cartilage but none in the normal epiphyseal cartilage. This seems to support the hypothesis that vascular channels permeate from the metaphysis, across the physeal cartilage, and into the epiphysis in symptomatic Perthes disease.[23] This would seemingly occur in an apparent attempt to supply nourishment to the epiphyseal cartilage that is normally supplied by the lateral epiphyseal arteries in the non-Perthes hip.

Alpaslan *et al.* were able to recreate the histology noted in Perthes disease by embolization causing one single infarct in the femoral arteries of dogs.[4] Dogs are a useful model for Perthes disease because of similarities in the vascularity of their proximal femurs to that of humans as well as the natural occurrence of Perthes disease in dogs.[11,41] Importantly in this work, revascularization was verified by angiography prior to obtaining histologic specimens at as early as one week post-embolization. The study demonstrated necrosis in bone trabeculae obtained from the subchondral area as well as pyknosis of cartilage cells adjacent to the subchondral bone with empty lacunae. Enchondral ossification is known to destroy the cartilage found closer to the joint surface that is responsible for secretion of the interstitial substance. The interruption of enchondral ossification allowed for the proliferation of this cartilage, which obtains its nutrition through the synovium and not the lateral epiphyseal arteries. The apparent radiographic widening of the joint space was in fact determined to be hypertrophy of this cartilage layer supplied nutrients by the synovium, and not due to hyperemia of the ligamentum which had previously been hypothesized.[4] This would seem to explain the coxa magna that is generally a late finding in the healed Perthes hip. Concurrently, the physis, and in particular the hypertrophic area, were markedly thinned, whereas the resting cartilage zone was thickened. The study demonstrated that a non-recurrent artificial embolism caused changes in the femoral head similar to changes observed during the course of Perthes disease. This suggests that the chronic changes characteristic of Perthes disease can result after one vascular insult, and chronic interruption of the blood supply may not be necessary.[4]

The same study group had previously demonstrated increased levels of fibrinolytic capacity, thrombomodulin, and tissue factor pathway inhibitor suggesting that alteration of the normal clotting cascade may play an important role in the development of Perthes disease. Immunological and inflammatory processes, along with malfunction of damaged endothelium, may play a role in the microvascular compromise associated with Perthes disease as well.[87] At some point in the disease process, all Perthes hips will develop synovitis to some degree. Transient synovitis has been implicated in the future development of Perthes disease by some authors,[48,68] although this belief is not commonly subscribed to. Histopathological and electron microscopy has demonstrated perivascular collections of plasma cells and lymphocytes in the synovial tissue of the Perthes hip.[46,56] Inflammation is known to have prothrombotic effects, upregulating procoagulant factors and downregulating anti-coagulants, as well as inhibiting fibrinolytic activity.[4] There is, however, no clear understanding as to whether the synovitis and inflammatory response is a cause, or an effect, of the loss of blood supply to the femoral epiphysis with resulting necrosis. In fact, both mechanisms may occur as the development of Perthes disease is very likely multifactorial.

13.4.1.1 *Coagulopathies in relation to Perthes disease*

There is general consensus in the current literature that Legg-Calve-Perthes is a disorder that in some way involves decreased perfusion of the femoral epiphysis through the lateral epiphyseal vessels. However, there is no significant agreement on the exact cause of this vascular insult. The role of thrombophilia in the development of Perthes disease may not be limited to arterial blockage of the lateral epiphyseal arteries. The formation of venous thrombi can block the outflow from the femoral head resulting in increased intraosseous pressure and subsequent osteonecrosis as well.[9] There has been considerable attention given to the possibility that hypercoagulable and thrombophilic states could play a role in the Perthes disease process. This is likely due to the fact that Perthes disease is generally not related to any specific traumatic event that would otherwise cause such a vascular disruption. Occlusion of the epiphyseal arteries could be precipitated by any number of factors including passive cigarette smoke,[21,30] inherited thrombophilia, or fibrinolytic coagulopathy.[33,36] Much of the early work on the affiliation of thrombophilia with Perthes disease was done by Glueck *et al.*,[33,36] who implicated protein C and S deficiencies in the pathogenesis of Perthes disease. In 2001, Eldridge *et al.* found a statistically significant increased risk of Perthes disease with decreasing levels of protein C and a nearly significant increased risk with decreasing levels of protein S.[24] They concluded that "abnormalities of the coagulation system leading to thrombophilic state play a role in Legg-Perthes disease." Antiphospholipid antibodies, anticardiolipin, factor V Leiden, prothrombin II and methylenetetrahydrofolate reductase (MTHFR) have also all been implicated as hypercoagulable states that could play a role in the development of Perthes disease.[87] Glueck *et al.*[32–36] demonstrated an association between the G1691A Leiden mutation of the factor-V gene and Perthes disease. This mutation resists activated protein C degradation which removes one of the regulators of the coagulation cascade.[57] They went so far to say that screening for thrombotic disorders was indicated for patients with Perthes disease and their families. Their results were duplicated by many other investigators.[5,39,83]

However, the results linking factor-V Leiden mutation with Perthes disease reported by the above authors were refuted by others (Fig. 13.3). Hresko *et al.*[40] found that the proportion of children with the factor-V Leiden mutation and Perthes did not differ significantly from the expected population frequency of 5%.[9] Many investigations favored that there was no correlation between the factor-V Leiden mutation and Perthes disease.[27,40,47,80]

Balasa *et al.* performed a study involving a non-selected and consecutive series of 72 patients with Perthes disease and compared them with 197 controls.[9] Their results demonstrated a positive correlation between thrombophilic states and Perthes disease. Specifically, they performed assays for factor-V Leiden, prothrombin G20210A, MTHFR C677T, and plasminogen activator inhibitor-1 4G/5G mutations. The group also measured levels of anticardiolipin antibodies immunoglobulin G and M, homocysteine, protein C, protein S, antithrombin III, and plasminogen activator inhibitor-1. The study demonstrated that factor-V Leiden mutation was more common in Perthes patients than in the controls and that the odds ratio for the development of Perthes disease in the presence of the factor-V Leiden mutation was 3.39. Also, a high level of anticardiolipin antibodies was found in a higher and statistically significant percentage of the Perthes patients as compared to the controls.

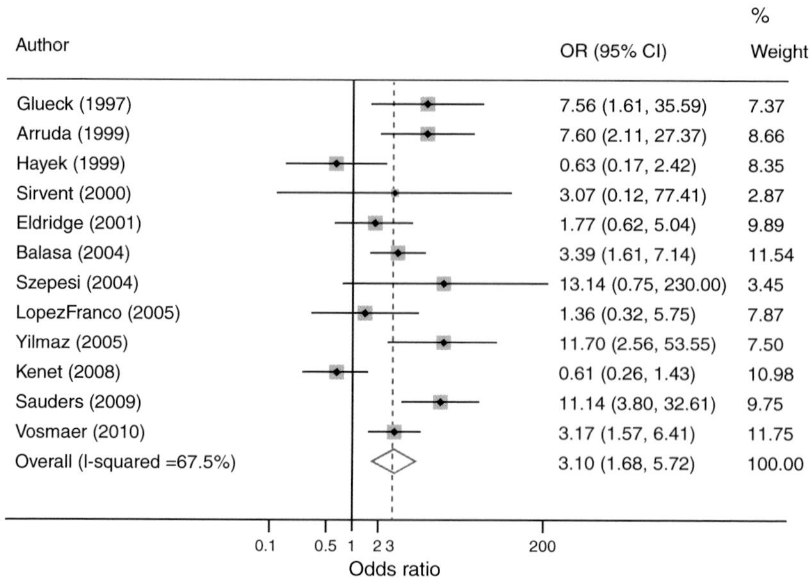

Fig. 13.3. Forest plot of factor-V Leiden gene effects on Perthes. *Source*: Woratanarat P, Thaveeratitharm C, Woratanarat T, Angsanuntsukh C, Attia J, Thakkinstian A (2014). Meta-analysis of hypercoagulability genetic polymorphisms in Perthes disease. *J Orthop Res*, 1–7. Reproduced with permission.

The odds ratio of patients with Perthes disease having one or more abnormalities in factor V, anticardiolipin antibody IgG, or anticardiolipin antibody IgM as opposed to normal values for all three variables was 3.29. The other variables tested did not demonstrate a significant difference between the two groups. It should be recognized that this study group included Gruppo and Glueck who had published previous papers confirming the association of factor-V Leiden mutations with Perthes disease.[32–36]

In an attempt to increase the power of these studies, a large meta-analysis has recently been performed to review the association between genetic determinants of hypercoagulability and Perthes disease.[87] This group chose to look at factor-V Leiden, prothrombin II, and MTHFR as they have been shown to not be confounded by age, vaccination, or infection.[51] Their findings were consistent with those of Balasa *et al.* above. This work supported the association between factor-V Leiden and Perthes disease revealing a population attributable risk of 3.1%. There was a non-significant association of prothrombin II polymorphism with Perthes with a population attributable risk of 1.48. MTHFR demonstrated an effect size close to 1. This meta-analysis attempted to include all relevant genetic association studies assessing gene effects on Perthes disease.

Certainly, these studies do not mean to imply that all cases of Perthes disease are directly related to inheritable or environmental conditions related to hypercoagulability. However, they do seem to indicate at least some association between the disorders.

13.4.2 *Medications*

The medications most commonly associated with AVN of the femoral head are the corticosteroids. The pathophysiology of AVN associated with glucocorticoid use differs from that of ischemic AVN; however, there are some similarities. It is thought that the glucocorticoids induce AVN through a combination of direct effects on osteocytes, as well as indirect mechanisms.[85,86] These medications have been shown to induce apoptosis of osteocytes. However, if that were the only mechanism by which they created susceptibility to AVN, one would expect a more equitable distribution of AVN throughout the skeleton. It is believed that the indirect effects of these medications include hyperlipidemia, hypercoagulation, and hypofibrinolysis.[45] With the known tenuous vascular supply of the femoral epiphysis, along with its likely susceptibility to hypercoagulability, it seems to follow that the femoral head would be particularly susceptible to AVN following administration of these medications.

Chemotherapeutic agents also have a high association with AVN. However, their effects do tend to be more dispersed throughout the bones of the body. This is likely due to their cytotoxicity, and therefore, the more direct effect at the osteophyte level.

13.4.3 *Sickle cell disease*

In this disease, a homozygous individual with two alleles both carrying a mutation in the beta-globin chain of hemoglobin, produces red blood cells that are of the characteristic sickle shape, particularly in low oxygen tension.[1] The sickled red blood cells lose elasticity and gains adhesiveness. The tenuous arterial supply of the femoral head likely produces lower oxygen tensions than in other areas of the skeleton, thus increasing the sickling of the red blood cells. It is hypothesized that the increased adhesiveness of the sickled red blood cells makes it more difficult for them to traverse through the microvasculature and cause microvascular occlusions.[53] This may contribute to a further decrease in the already tenuous arterial supply of the femoral head, and could also cause in an increase in intraosseous pressure through congestion of venous outflow. The end result of either mechanism would lead to decreased vascularity in the femoral epiphysis, mimicking that which would be observed in a coagulopathy. However, the pathophysiology of AVN from sickle cell disease is much more similar to that produced by traumatic AVN than that of Perthes disease. The slowly progressive fragmentation and re-ossification demonstrated throughout the stages of Perthes disease do not tend to occur with AVN related to sickle cell disease.

13.5 Surgical Considerations Related to the Vascularity of the Hip

13.5.1 *Surgical dislocation of the hip*

Surgical dislocation of the hip is a useful procedure to assess and treat proximal femoral deformities resulting from a number of pathologic conditions, but particularly slipped capital femoral epiphysis and Perthes disease. The deformities are known to cause hip dysfunction with regard to range of motion and pain, and are likely to diminish the life span of the joint with a hastening of the onset of osteoarthritis. Reshaping the deformed proximal femur with osteoplasty and/or osteotomy can be performed safely;[64, 78, 79] however, there is a relatively high risk of inducing AVN through disruption of the blood supply. Shore *et al.* utilized high-resolution contrast-enhanced MRI to visualize the path of the medial femoral circumflex artery and the lateral epiphyseal artery branches supplying the femoral head in 22 Perthes hips and a matched control group of 20 hips with developmental hip dysplasia.[79] They demonstrated that the lateral epiphyseal arteries were wedged deep into the trochanteric notch, and that this was often exaggerated by proximal femoral deformities resulting from Perthes disease including coxa magna, a shortened femoral neck, and trochanteric overgrowth. These findings were similar to those of Chung that described the deep branch of the medial femoral circumflex artery crossing the hip joint capsule at the trochanteric notch between the femoral neck and greater trochanter.[18] To review, Chung also found that in children four to eight years of age this space was very narrow and could result in an area susceptible to vascular occlusion.[18]

The location of the lateral epiphyseal arteries places them in close proximity to the location of a proposed trochanteric osteotomy required for surgical dislocation. This holds particularly true for patients with healed

Perthes disease due to the anatomic considerations discussed above. Shore *et al.* were able to demonstrate even more specifically the insertion of the lateral epiphyseal arteries into the femoral neck utilizing high-resolution, contrast-enhanced MRI.[79] They found that in the Perthes hips, the lateral epiphyseal artery branches inserted on the posterior-superior aspect of the femoral neck in an arc from the 11 o'clock position (superior-anterior) to the 2 o'clock position (superior-posterior). The greatest concentration of vessels was seen between the 11 and 1 o'clock positions. The vessel configuration in the dysplasia group was quite similar, with the majority of the lateral epiphyseal arteries inserting into the postero-superior aspect of the femoral neck in a narrow arc from 12 to 1 o'clock. Also of note, all patients with healed Perthes disease had visualized lateral epiphyseal arteries inserting into the femoral head indicating at least some degree of reconstitution of this vasculature after healing of Perthes disease.

Knowledge of this anatomy is crucial in planning surgical dislocation of the femoral head from the acetabulum if one hopes to avoid the devastating consequences of AVN. The vessels supplying the femoral head are few in number following Perthes disease and in close proximity to the base of the overgrown greater trochanter, near the site of trochanteric osteotomy.[79]

13.5.2 *Core decompression*

Core decompression, or drilling into the avascular areas noted in AVN, has long been the first line treatment of AVN of the femoral head. However, the literature is quite varied with regard to the success of the treatment, with a general consensus reaching only around 50%. Not only is the success rate among studies highly variable, but the mechanism by which core decompression produces positive results is not well understood. There are numerous techniques described for this procedure, including simply drilling into the avascular area, versus performing vascularized bone grafting or even infusing bone marrow aspirate cells into the drilled-out core of bone. No specific technique has been reliably and repeatedly shown to produce consistently superior results.

Despite its use in AVN, core decompression or drilling of the femoral head has not been widely utilized in the treatment of Perthes disease.[8] The mainstay of treatment in Perthes disease is to maintain the femoral head entirely in the acetabulum. This treatment is termed "containment." Unlike adult AVN, and AVN following trauma in children, Perthes-related osteonecrosis has a remodeling phase as part of its natural history.[37]

In younger children with increased growth and subsequent remodeling potential, the prognosis of Perthes disease with regard to long-term clinical outcomes can be quite positive. It is believed that the effect of full containment of the femoral head in the acetabular socket allows for remodeling of the femoral head into a concentrically fitting spherical shape. The pressure of the acetabulum against the femoral head contained within the socket is believed to be the driving force behind this phenomenon. This is the same basic treatment approach utilized in the treatment of the dysplastic hip, the difference being that the roles are reversed. In the case of dysplasia, the completely contained femoral head is believed to exert pressure on the developing acetabulum so that it conforms to its spherical shape.

An area of concern regarding drilling of avascular areas in Perthes hips is that multiple insults to the physis could cause damage to the growth plate and subsequent growth disturbance. In a study utilizing a piglet model, Gong *et al.* assessed the macroscopic histologic effects of drilling on immature femoral heads following surgically induced ischemia.[37] Three weeks following induction of ischemia in the piglet femoral heads, utilizing the contralateral ischemic but undrilled side as a control; lateral, medial, central, and lateral drill holes were made in the femoral heads utilizing Kirschner wires. Femoral heads were then harvested and examined at 3, 6, 9, and 12 weeks. The results were consistent with many of the findings discussed previously. They found significantly increased revascularization of the capital femoral epiphyses that had been drilled (Fig. 13.4). However, the percent of osteoblast surface, capital femoral epiphyseal quotient (a measure of the deformity of the femoral head), and proximal femoral growth plate height showed no significant difference.[8]

A previous report has shown that less than 7% of drill injury to the growth plate did not seem to cause growth disturbance.[42] Gong's study above also did not demonstrate adverse effects on the physis from the Kirschner wire drilling.[37] However, it also produced similar findings of multiple previous reports that revascularization across the physis from the metaphysis into the epiphysis did not seem to have a protective effect on the femoral head (Fig. 13.5).

13.5.3 *Abduction of the hip to improve containment*

The treatment of both developmental dysplasia of the hip and Perthes disease often involves significant abduction of the pathologic hip joints. In hip dysplasia, infants are often placed in Pavlik harnesses and older children

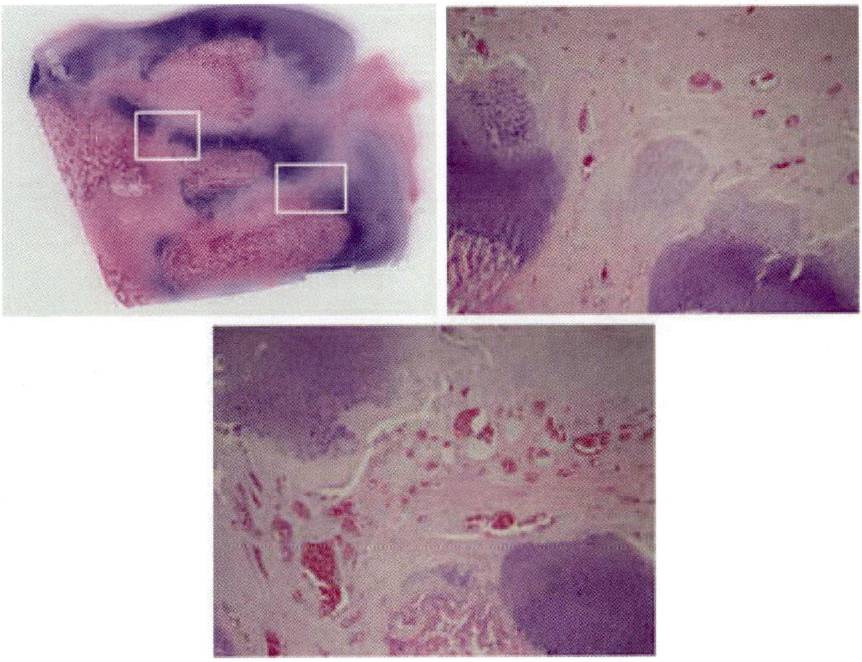

Fig. 13.4. Photomicrograph of the femoral head of immature piglet at three weeks following multiple drilling. [Top left] Polycut section view (H&E, x1). [Top right, bottom] The centro-medial and centro-lateral junctions of the proximal femoral growth plate are disrupted by drilling. From cervical metaphysis to the secondary ossification center though transphyseal hole, abundant fibrovascular invasion is observed (H&E, x4). *Source*: Gong SY, Kim HW, Park HW, Lee SY, Lee KS(2011). Effects of multiple drilling on the ischemic capital femoral epiphysis of immature piglets. *Yonsei Med J*, 809–817. Reproduced with permission.

in spica casts so that the hips can be maintained in an abducted position to allow direction of the femoral heads consistently into the acetabulum. The concept of containment is paramount in the treatment of Perthes disease. In some patients, this may involve placement of Petrie casts also meant to maintain the hips in an abducted position in order to maintain full coverage of the femoral head by the acetabulum.

However, there has been work done demonstrating that hips placed into a significant degree of abduction may in fact have decreased blood flow to the femoral capital epiphysis due to arterial hypoperfusion.[15,44,89] It has been previously postulated that the cause of the femoral head ischemia with abduction treatment was stretching of the medial circumflex artery

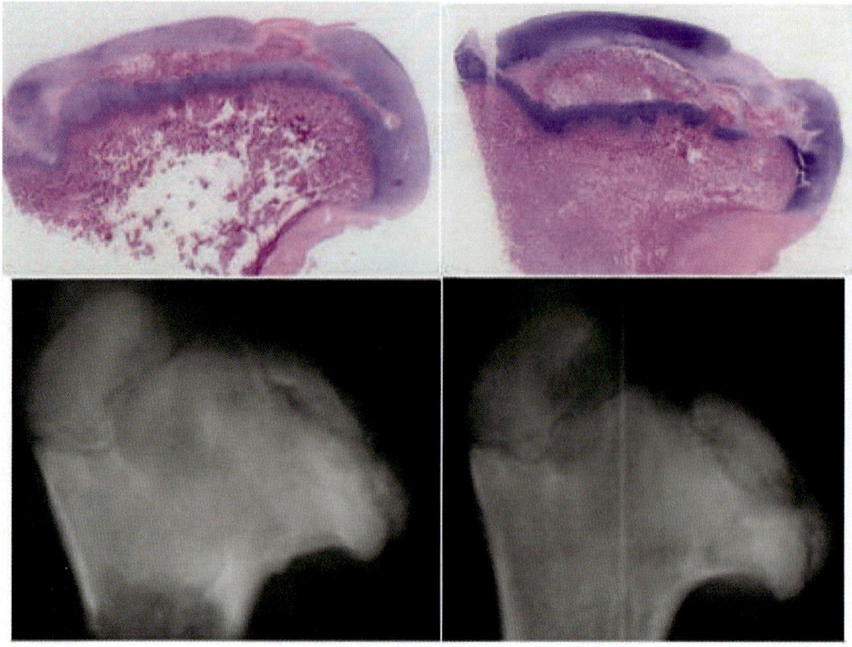

Fig. 13.5. Photomicrographs (H&E, x1) and AP radiographs of the femoral head of immature piglets at 12 weeks following drilling. Although multiple drilling provided increased revascularization on the ischemic capital femoral epiphysis, there was no significant difference in head collapse or proximal femoral growth plate height between untreated control group [left] and multiple drilling group [right]. *Source*: Gong SY, Kim HW, Park HW, Lee SY, Lee KS(2011). Effects of multiple drilling on the ischemic capital femoral epiphysis of immature piglets. *Yonsei Med J*, 809–817. Reproduced with permission.

or possibly obstruction of the profunda femoris artery which gives rise to the medial circumflex artery.[71,88] Jaramillo *et al.* demonstrated with gadolinium-enhanced MRI in a piglet model that greater than 70 degrees of abduction resulted in segmental ischemia in 100% of the femoral head epiphyses and 85% of the proximal femoral physes.[43] If the abduction angle was kept below 50 degrees, there was no evidence of ischemia.

In a perfusion study utilizing ultrasound,[61] observed the Doppler flow characteristics of the posterosuperior branch of the femoral head cartilage feeding vessels of 20 neonates held in varying degrees of abduction. These vessels can be thought of as the lateral epiphyseal vessels discussed in previous studies above. They first demonstrated that the posterosuperior branch

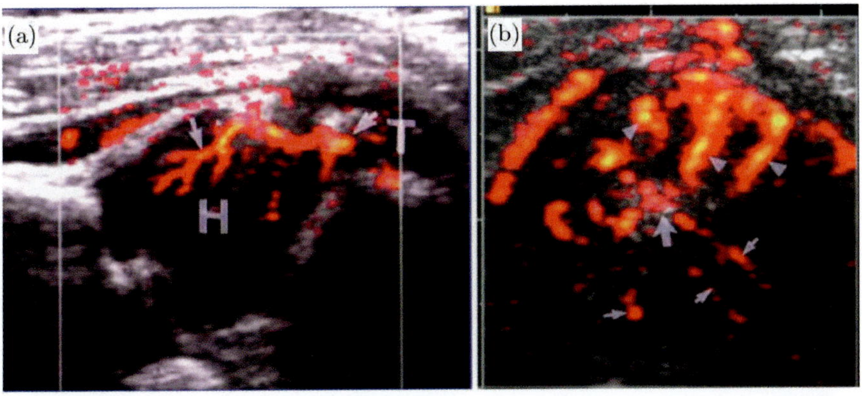

Fig. 13.6. Neutral position, epiphyseal perfusion. (a) Coronal view of the left femoral head demonstrates the dominance of the PS branch of the MCA in perfusion of the femoral head cartilage (arrows). (b) Transverse image shows the dominant contribution of the PS branch of MCA (arrowheads) versus the smaller and less contributing branches of the PI branch with lesser dimensions and velocities (smaller arrows). The ossific nucleus can be seen (large arrow). *Source*: Yousefzadeh DK, Doerger K, Sullivan C (2008). The blood supply of early, late, and nonossifying cartilage: Preliminary gray-scale and Doppler assessment and their implications. *Pediatr Radiol*, 146–158. Reproduced with permission.

of the medial circumflex artery was the most dominant feeding artery perfusing the femoral head epiphysis (Fig. 13.6). The artery was shown to enter the lateral aspect of the epiphysis just distal to the lower end of the acetabular labrum. Peak systolic arterial velocities declined significantly at 45 and 60 degrees of abduction. The diastolic flow was completely either absent or reversed at these angles of abduction, and no venous return was detectable. At 45 degrees, it was demonstrated that perfusion was absent in the domain of the posterosuperior branch of the medial circumflex artery. However, perfusion from the posteroinferior branch was unaffected as was flow to the femoral neck and greater trochanter (Fig. 13.7).

The authors of this study presented a few interesting ideas. First, they demonstrated that the zone of perfusion alterations were limited to the area supplied by the posterosuperior branch of the medial circumflex artery. If damage to the profunda femora or medial circumflex arteries was to blame for the ischemia, poor perfusion should be expected in a more complete area of the femoral head, not just those supplied by the posterosuperior branches. Second, they postulated that at fewer degrees of prolonged abduction, the vessels providing venous outflow, which they also demonstrated to accompany the posterosuperior arteries, would be more likely to be compressed

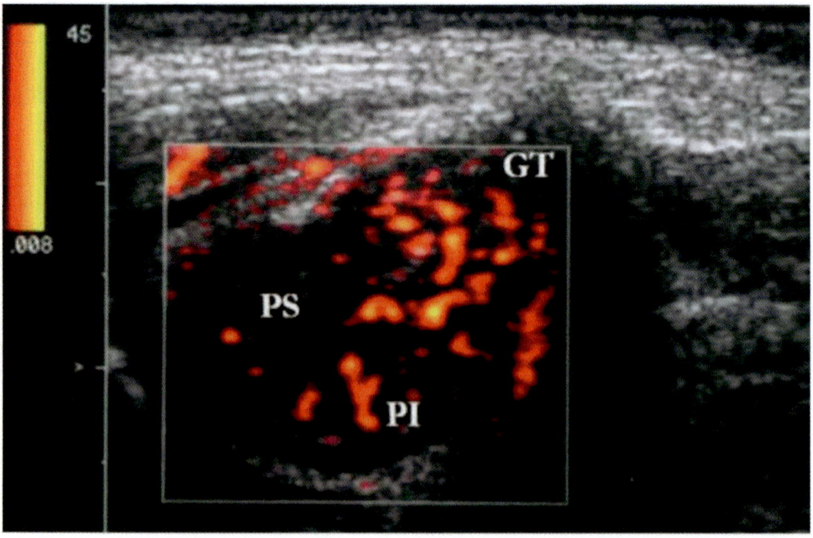

Fig. 13.7. Loss of blood flow in the PS branch of the MCA at 45-degree abduction. Power Doppler image of the entire chondroepiphysis in 45-degree abduction shows cessation of the femoral head perfusion in the domain of the PS branch of the MCA. However, the domain of the posteroinferior (PI) branch of the MCA, the flow within the femoral neck, and the greater trochanter remain intact. *Source*: Yousefzadeh DK, Jaramillo D, Johnson N, Doerger K, Sullivan C (2010). Biphasic threat to femoral head perfusion in abduction: Arterial hypoperfusion and venous congestion. *Pediatr Radiol*, 1517–1525. Reproduced with permission.

and occluded than the arteries themselves. This could indicate that venous hypertension could limit arterial flow into the femoral head and thus cause AVN, an idea that has been presented previously by multiple authors. Yousefzadeh *et al.* also proposed that the inferior aspect of the acetabular labrum was the structure compressing the posterosuperior vessels.[89] In hip disorders utilizing abduction treatment, they suggest that ultrasound-assisted measurement of the distance between the edge of the labrum and the point of entry of the posterosuperior branch may help predict safe angles of abduction to avoid hypoperfusion of the femoral head.

13.6 Pharmacologic Treatment of Perthes Disease

Possible pharmacologic alternatives for treatment of Perthes disease in its early stages have been presented. The bisphosphonate, ibandronate, was able to preserve the structure of the femoral head following ischemic necrosis by maintaining the trabecular number and separation. The retention of the bony trabeculae minimized the decrease in the epiphyseal quotient in a piglet model similar to Gong's study.[77] Ibandronate's protective effects are based upon its inhibition of osteoclastic bone resorption. In a similar paper, the group demonstrated the protective effects of receptor activator of NF-KB ligand (RANKL) inhibition on the epiphyseal quotient of ischemic piglet femoral heads.[67] RANKL has been previously shown to play a critical role in osteoclast formation, activation, and survival. By supplying a pharmacologic decoy receptor for RANKL, the group was able to reduce pathologic bone resorption that occurs during femoral head ischemia and protect the shape of the femoral head. Ultimately, preserving the normal shape of the femoral head, by preventing collapse, is the main goal in treatment of any osteonecrosis of the femoral head. By maintaining a normal spherically shaped femoral head, it is believed that the function and life of the hip joint can be preserved. Ibandronate and RANKL inhibition have yet to gain clinical use due to the possible systemic effects throughout the remainder of the skeleton. However, they may provide a promising new treatment alternative that can be developed in the future.

A significant amount of work has gone into the understanding of the vascularity of the hip joint. Furthermore, large amounts of data are available on pathologic conditions of the hip related to decreased perfusion of the proximal femoral epiphysis. Despite this significant amount of information and data, successfully treating these conditions with positive long-term results has proven extremely difficult. Many treatment options are available, but most are unproven and unreliable. Further study into the vascular supply of the femoral head, and the pathology that can inhibit it, is required if better and more reliable treatment options are to be created.

References

1. Aguilar C, Vichinsky E, Neumayr L (2005). Bone and joint disease in sickle cell disease. *Hematol Oncol Clin North Am*, 19(5), 929–941.
2. Aksoy MC, Aksoy DY Haznedaroglu IC, Sayinalp N, Kirazli S, Alpaslan M (2005). Enhanced tissue factor pathway inhibitor response as a defense mechanism against ongoing local microvascular events of Legg-Calve-Perthes disease. *Pediatr Hematol Oncol*, 22(5), 391–399.
3. Aksoy MC, Aksoy DY Haznedaroglu IC, Sayinalp N, Kirazli S, Alpaslan M (2005). Increments in the global fibrinolytic capacity in response to local endothelial impairment in Legg-Calve-Perthes disease (abstract). *EPOS Meeting*. Palma de Mallorca, Spain.

4. Alpaslan AM, Aksoy MC, Yazici M (2007). Interruption of the blood supply of femoral head: An experimental study on the pathogenesis of Legg-Calve-Perthes disease. *Arch Orthop Trauma Surg*, 127(6), 485–491.
5. Arruda VR, Belangero WD, Ozelo MC, Oliveira GB, Pagnano RG, Volpon JB, Annichino-Bizzacchi JM (1999). Inherited risks for thrombophilia among children with Legg-Calve-Perthes disease. *J Pediatr Orthop*, 19(1), 84–87.
6. Atsumi T, Yamano K, Muraki M, Yoshihara S, Kajihara T (2000). The blood supply of the lateral epiphyseal arteries in Perthes' disease. *J Bone Joint Surg Br*, 82(3), 392–398.
7. Axhausen G (1923). Kohler's disease and Perthes' disease. *Zentralbl Chir*, 48, 553.
8. Baksi DP (1995). Palliative operations for painful old Perthes' disease. *Int Orthop*, 19(1), 46–50.
9. Balasa VV, Gruppo RA, Glueck CJ, Wang P, Roy DR, Wall EJ, Mehlman CT, Crawford AH (2004). Legg-Calve-Perthes disease and thrombophilia. *J Bone Joint Surg Am*, 86(12), 2642–2647.
10. Barnewolt CE, Jaramillo D, Taylor GA, *et al.* (2003). Correlation of contrast-enhanced power Doppler sonography and conventional angiography of abduction-induced hip ischemia in piglets. *AJR*, 180(6), 1731–1735.
11. Basseett FH, Wilson JW, Allen BL, Azuma H (1969). Normal vascular anatomy of the head of the femur in puppies with emphasis on the inferior retinacular vessels. *J Bone Joint Surg Am*, 51(6), 1139–1153.
12. Beck M, Leunig M, Ellis T, Sledge B, Ganz R (2003). The acetabular blood supply: Implications for periacetabular osteotomies. *Surg Radiol Anat*, 25(50–6), 361–367.
13. Boutault JR, Baunin C, Berard E, Vial J, Labarre D, Domenech C, Sales de Gauzy J, Sans N(2012). Diffusion MRI of the neck of the femur in Legg-Calve-Perthes disease: Apreliminary study. *Diagn Interv Imaging*, 94(1),78–83.
14. Boyer D, Mickelson M, Ponset T (1981). Slipped capital femoral epiphysis: Long-term follow up and study of one hundred and twenty-one patients. *J Bone Joint Surg Am*, 63, 85.
15. Brougham DI, Broughton NS, Cole WG, *et al.* (1990). Avascular necrosis following closed reduction of congenital dislocation of the hip: Review of influencing factors and long-term follow-up. *J Bone Joint Surg Br*, 72, 557–562.
16. Carney BT, Weinstein SL, Noble J (1991). Long-term follow-up of slipped capital femoral epiphysis. *J Bone Joint Surg Am*,73(5), 667–674.
17. Cheng JC, Tang N (1999). Decompression and stable internal fixation of femoral neck fractures in children can affect the outcome. *J Pediatr Orthop*, 19(3), 338–343.
18. Chung SM (1976). The arterial supply of the head and neck of the human femur. *J Bone Joint Surg Am*, 58(7), 961–970.
19. Conway JJ (1993). A scintographic classification of Legg-Calve-Perthes disease. *Semin Nucl Med*, 23(4), 274–295.

20. Crock HV (1980). An atlas of the arterial supply of the head and neck of the femur in man. *Clin Orthop Relat Res*, 152, 17–27.
21. Daniel AB, Shah H, Kamath A, *et al.* (2012). Environmental tobacco and wood smoke increase the risk of Legg-Calve-Perthes disease. *Clin Orthop Relat Res*, 470(9), 2369–2375.
22. Dendane MA, Amrani A, El Alami ZF, El Medhi T, Gourina H (2010). Displaced femoral neck fractures in children: Are complications predictable? *Orthop & Trauma: Surg & Res*, 96, 161–165.
23. Doria AD, Cunha FG, Modena M, Maciel R, Molnar LJ, Luzo C, Moineddin R, Guarniero R (2008). Legg-Calve-Perthes disease: Multipositional power Doppler sonography of the proximal femoral vascularity. *Pediatr Radiol*, 38(4), 392–402.
24. Eldridge J, Dilley A, Austin H, El-Jamil M, Wolstein L, Doris J, Hooper WC, Meehan PL, Evatt B (2001). The role of protein C, protein S, and resistance to activated protein C in Legg- Perthes disease. *Pediatrics*, 107(6), 1329–1334.
25. Feigenberg Z, Pauker M, Levy M, *et al.* (1977). Fractures of the femoral neck in childhood: Results of conservative treatment. *J Trauma*, 17, 937–942.
26. Flynn JM, Wong KL, Yeh GL, *et al.* (2002). Displaced fractures of the hip in children. Management by early operation and immobilization in a hip spica cast. *J Bone Joint Surg Br*, 84(1), 108–112.
27. Gallisti S, Reitinger T, Linhart W, Muntean W (1999). The role of inherited thrombotic disorders in the etiology of Legg-Calve-Perthes disease. *J Pediatr Orthop*, 19(1), 82–83.
28. Ganey T, Ogden J (1998). Pre- and post-natal development of the hip. In Callaghan JJ, Rosenberg AG, Rubash HE (Eds)s.,*The Adult Hip*. Philadelphia: Lippincott-Raven, 39–55.
29. Ganz R, Gill TJ, Gautier E, Ganz K, Krugel N, Berlemann U (2001). Surgical dislocation of the adult hip a technique with full access to the femoral head and acetabulum without the risk of avascular necrosis. *J Bone Joint Surg Br*, 83(8), 1119–1124.
30. Garcia Mata S, Ardanaz Aicua E, Hidalgo Ovejero A, *et al.* (2000). Legg-Calve-Perthes disease and passive smoking. *J Pediatr Orthop*, 20(3), 326–330.
31. Gautier E, Ganz K, Krugel N, Gill T, Ganz R (2000). Anatomy of the medial femoral circumflex artery and its surgical implications. *J Bone Joint Surg Br*, 82, 679–683.
32. Glueck CJ, Brandt G, Gruppo R, Crawford A, Roy D, Tracy T, Stroop D, Wang P, Becker A (1997). Resistance to activated protein C and Legg-Perthes disease. *Clin Orthop*, 338, 139–152.
33. Glueck CJ, Crawford A, Roy D, *et al.* (1996). Association of antithrombotic factor deficiencies and hypofibrinolysis with Legg-Perthes disease. *J Bone Joint Surg Am*, 78(1), 3–13.
34. Glueck CJ, Freiberg RA, Crawford A, Gruppo R, Roy D, Tracy T, Sieve-Smith L, Wang P (1998). Secondhand smoke, hypofibrinolysis, and Legg-Perthes disease. *Clin Orthop*, 352, 159–167.

35. Glueck CJ, Frieberg R, Gruppo RM Crawford A, Roy D, Brandt G, McMahon RE, Bouquot J, Tracy T, Stroop D, Wang P, Becker A (1997). Thrombophilia and hypofibrinolysis: Reversible pathogenic etiologies of osteonecrosis. In Urbaniak JR, Jones JP Jr (Eds), *Osteonecrosis: Etiology, Diagnosis and Treatment.* Rosemont, IL: American Academy of Orthopaedic Surgeons, 105–110.
36. Glueck CJ, Glueck HI, Greenfield D, *et al.* (1994). Protein C and S deficiency, thrombophilia, and hypofibrinolysis: Pathophysiologic causes of Legg-Calve-Perthes disease. *Pediatr Res*, 35(4), 383–388.
37. Gong SY, Kim HW, Park HW, Lee SY, Lee KS (2011). Effects of multiple drilling on the ischemic capital femoral epiphysis of immature piglets. *Yonsei Med J*, 52(5), 809–817.
38. Griffith MJ (1975). Acute slipping of the capital femoral epiphysis. *J Bone Joint Surg Br*, 47, 1113.
39. Gruppo R, Glueck CJ, Wall E, Roy D, Wang P (1998). Legg-Perthes disease in three siblings, two heterozygous and one homozygous for the factor V Leiden mutation. *J Pediatr Orthop*, 132(5), 885–888.
40. Hresko MT, McDougall PA, Gorlin JB, Vamvakas EC, Kasser JR, Neufeld EJ (2002). Prospective re-evaluation of the association between thrombotic diathesis and Legg-Perthes disease. *J Bone Joint Surg Am*, 84(9), 1613–1618.
41. Hulth A, Norberg I, Olsson SE (1962). Coxa plana in dogs. *J Bone Joint Surg Am*, 44(5), 918–930.
42. Janarv PM, Wistrom B, Hirsch G (1998). The influence of transphyseal drilling and tendon grafting on bone growth: An experimental study in the rabbit. *J Pediatr Orthop*, 18(2), 149–154.
43. Jaramillo D, Connolly SA, Vajapeyam S, Robertson RL, Dunning PS, Mulkern RV, *et al.* (2003). Normal and ischemic epiphysis of the femur: Diffusion MR imaging study in piglets. *Radiology*, 227(3), 825–832.
44. Jaramillo D, Villegas-Medina OL, Doty DK, *et al.* (1995). Gadolinium-enhanced MR imaging demonstrates abduction-caused hip ischemia and its reversal in piglets. *Pediatr Radiol*, 25(8), 578–587.
45. Jones LC, Hungerford DS (2007). The pathogenesis of osteonecrosis. *Instr Course Lect*, 56, 179–196.
46. Joseph B, Pydisetty RK (1996). Chondrolysis and the stiff hip in Perthes' disease: An immunological study. *J Pediatr Orthop*, 16(1), 15–19.
47. Kaeley WD, Mayne EE, McDonald W, Murray P, Cosgrove AP (2000). The role of coagulation abnormalities in the development of Perthes' disease. *J Bone Joint Surg Br*, 82(5), 744–746.
48. Kallio P, Ryoppy S (1985). Transient synovitis and Perthes: Is there an etiologic connection? *J Bone Joint Surg Br*, 68, 608.
49. Kawelblum M, Lehman WB, Grant AD, Strongwater A (1993). Avascular necrosis of the femoral head as sequel of fracture of the greater trochanter. A case report and review of the literature. *Clin Orthop*, 294, 193–195.
50. Kay SP, Hall JE (1971). Fracture of the femoral neck in children and its complications. *Clin Orthop*, 80, 53–71.

51. Kenet G, Ezra E, Wientroub S, *et al.* (2008). Perthes' disease and the search for genetic associations: Collagen mutations, Gaucher's disease and thrombophilia. *J Bone Joint Surg Br*, 90, 1507–1511.
52. Kim HK, Stephenson N, Garces A, Aya-ay J, Bian H (2009). Effects of disruption of epiphyseal vasculature on the proximal femoral growth plate. *J Bone Joint Surg Am*, 91(5), 1149–1158.
53. Kim HK, Su PH, Qiu YS (2001). Histopathologic changes in growth-plate cartilage following ischemic necrosis of the capital femoral epiphysis: An experimental investigation in immature pigs. *J Bone Joint Surg Am*, 83(5), 688–697.
54. Kim HK, Su PH (2002). Development of flattening and apparent fragmentation following ischemic necrosis of the capital femoral epiphysis. *J Bone Joint Surg Am*, 84, 1329–1334.
55. Kim HKW, Larson AN, Fletcher ND, Winick N, Kim YJ (2011). Childhood femoral head osteonecrosis. *Clin Rev Bone Miner Metab*, 9(1), 2–12.
56. Kleinman RG, Bleck EE (1981). Increased blood viscosity in patients with Legg-Calve-Perthes disease: A preliminary report. *J Pediatr Orthop*, 1(2), 131–136.
57. Koeleman BP, van Rumpt D, Hamulyak K, *et al.* (1995). Factor V Leiden: An additional risk factor for thrombosis in protein S deficient families? *Throm Haemost*, 74, 580–583.
58. Lauritzen J (1974). The arterial supply to the femoral head in children. *Acta Orthop Scand*, 45, 724–736.
59. Lee MC, Eberson CP (2006). Growth and development of the child's hip. *Orthopclin N Amer*, 37(2), 119–133.
60. Li X, Qi J, Xia L, Li H, Hu J, Yu C, *et al.* (2008). Diffusion MRI in ischemic epiphysis of the femoral head: An experimental study. *J Mag Reson Imaging*, 28, 471–477.
61. Lim-Dunham JE, Ben-Ami TE, Yousefzadeh DK (1995). Septic arthritis of the elbow in children: the role of sonography. *Pediatr Radiol*, 25(7), 556–559.
62. Linhart W, Stampfel O, Ritter G (1984). Post-traumatic femur head necrosis following trochanter fracture. *Z Orthop Ihre Grenzgeb*, 122(6), 766–769.
63. Maeda S, Kita A, Funayama K, Kokubun S (2001). Vascular supply to slipped capital femoral epiphysis. *J Pediatr Orthop*, 21(5), 664–667.
64. Mardones RM, Gonzalez C, Chen Q, Zobitz M, Kaufman KR, Trousdale RT (2006). Surgical treatment of femoroacetabular impingement: Evaluation of the effect of the size of the resection. *J Bone Joint Surg Am*, 88, Supplement 1, Part 1, 84–91.
65. Menezes NM, Connolly SA, Shapiro F, Olear EA, Jimenez RM, Zurakowski D, *et al.* (2007). Early ischemia in growing piglet skeleton: MR diffusion and perfusion imaging. *Radiology*, 242(1), 129–136.
66. Moon ES, Mehlman CT. (2006). Risk factors for avascular necrosis after femoral neck fractures in children: 25 Cincinnati cases and meta-analysis of 360 cases. *J Orthop Trauma*, 20(5), 323–329.

67. Morgan-Bagley SA, Kostenuik P, Kim HKW (2006). RANKL inhibition decreases femoral head deformity following ischemic osteonecrosis of the capital femoral epiphysis, Proceedings of the 52nd Annual Meeting of the Orthopaedic Research Society.
68. Mukamel M, Litmanovitch M, Yosipovitch Z, *et al.* (1985). Legg Calve Perthes' disease following transient synovitis: How often? *Clin Pediatr*, 24, 629.
69. Nishiyami K, Sakamaki T, Ishii Y (1989). Follow-up study of slipped capital femoral epiphysis. *J Pediatr Orthop*, 9, 653–659.
70. O'Rourke MR, Weinstein SL (2003). Osteonecrosis following isolated avulsion fracture of the greater trochanter in children: A report of two cases. *J Bone Joint Surg Am*, 85(10), 2000–2005.
71. Ogden JA (1982). Normal and abnormal circulation. In Tachjden MO,(Ed),*Congenitul Dislocation of the Hip*. New York: Churchill Livingstone, 59–92.
72. Parke WM (1992). Chapter 1: The anatomy of the hip. In Balderston RA, Rothman RH, Booth RE, *et al.*, eds., *The Hip*. Philadelphia: Lea & Febige, 17–23.
73. Pforringer W, Rosemeyer B (1980). Fractures of the hip in children and adolescents. *Acta Orthop Scand*, 51(1), 91–108.
74. Phemister DB (1921). Operation of epiphysitis of the head of the femur (Perthes' disease). *Arch Surg*, 2, 221.
75. Phemister DB (1921). Perthes' disease. *Surg Gynecol Obstet*, 33, 87.
76. Ponseti IV, Maynard JA, Weinstein SL, *et al.* (1983). Legg-Calve-Perthes disease: Histochemical and ultrastructural observations of the epiphyseal cartilage and the physis. *J Bone Joint Surger Am*, 65(6), 797.
77. Randall TS, Sanders M, Athavale S, Bian H, Bauss F, Kim HKW (2005). Delivery and distribution of systemically administered ibandronate in the infarcted femoral head, Proceedings of the 51st Annual Meeting of the Orthopaedic Research Society.
78. Rebello G, Spencer S, Millis MB, Kim YJ (2009). Surgical dislocation in the management of pediatric and adolescent hip deformity. *Clin Orthop Relat Res*, 467(3), 724–731.
79. Shore BJ, Millis MB, Kim YJ (2012). Vascular safe zones for surgical dislocation in children with healed Legg-Calve-Perthes disease. *J Bone Joint Surg Am*, 94(8), 721–727.
80. Sirvent N, Fisher F, el Hayek T, Appert A, Giudicelli H, Griffet J (2000). Absence of congenital prethrombotic disorders in children with Legg-Perthes disease. *J Pediatr Orthop Br*, 9(1), 24–27.
81. Song KS, Kim YS, Sohn SW, *et al.* (2001). Arthrotomy and open reduction of the displaced fracture of the femoral neck in children. *J Pediatr Orthop Br*, 10(3), 205–210.
82. Strayer, LM (1971). Embryology of the human hip joint. *Clin Orthop*, 74, 221–240.